Optical Coherence Tomography Imaging: Advances in Ophthalmology

Optical Coherence Tomography Imaging: Advances in Ophthalmology

Editors

Jay Chhablani
Sumit Randhir Singh

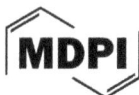

Editors
Jay Chhablani
UPMC Eye Center
University of Pittsburgh
Pittsburgh, PA, USA

Sumit Randhir Singh
Sharp Sight Eye Hospital
Bihar, India

Editorial Office
MDPI
St. Alban-Anlage 66
4052 Basel, Switzerland

This is a reprint of articles from the Special Issue published online in the open access journal *Journal of Clinical Medicine* (ISSN 2077-0383) (available at: https://www.mdpi.com/journal/jcm/special_issues/O_C_T_Ophthalmology).

For citation purposes, cite each article independently as indicated on the article page online and as indicated below:

Lastname, A.A.; Lastname, B.B. Article Title. *Journal Name* **Year**, *Volume Number*, Page Range.

ISBN 978-3-0365-9250-3 (Hbk)
ISBN 978-3-0365-9251-0 (PDF)
doi.org/10.3390/books978-3-0365-9251-0

© 2023 by the authors. Articles in this book are Open Access and distributed under the Creative Commons Attribution (CC BY) license. The book as a whole is distributed by MDPI under the terms and conditions of the Creative Commons Attribution-NonCommercial-NoDerivs (CC BY-NC-ND) license.

Contents

About the Editors ix

Sumit Randhir Singh and Jay Chhablani
Optical Coherence Tomography Imaging: Advances in Ophthalmology
Reprinted from: *J. Clin. Med.* **2022**, *11*, 2858, doi:10.3390/jcm11102858 1

Jens Julian Storp, Nils Hendrik Storp, Moritz Fabian Danzer, Nicole Eter and Julia Biermann
Evaluation of Retinal Nerve Fiber Layer and Macular Ganglion Cell Layer Thickness in Relation to Optic Disc Size
Reprinted from: *J. Clin. Med.* **2023**, *12*, 2471, doi:10.3390/jcm12072471 3

Sonny Caplash, Thamolwan Surakiatchanukul, Supriya Arora, Dmitri S. Maltsev, Sumit Randhir Singh, Niroj Kumar Sahoo, et al.
Multimodal Imaging Based Predictors for the Development of Choroidal Neovascularization in Patients with Central Serous Chorioretinopathy
Reprinted from: *J. Clin. Med.* **2023**, *12*, 2069, doi:10.3390/jcm12052069 17

Firuzeh Rajabian, Alessandro Arrigo, Lorenzo Bianco, Alessio Antropoli, Maria Pia Manitto, Elisabetta Martina, et al.
Optical Coherence Tomography Angiography in *CRB1*-Associated Retinal Dystrophies
Reprinted from: *J. Clin. Med.* **2023**, *12*, 1095, doi:10.3390/jcm12031095 27

Junji Kanno, Takuhei Shoji, Hirokazu Ishii, Hisashi Ibuki, Yuji Yoshikawa, Takanori Sasaki and Kei Shinoda
Deep Learning with a Dataset Created Using Kanno Saitama Macro, a Self-Made Automatic Foveal Avascular Zone Extraction Program
Reprinted from: *J. Clin. Med.* **2023**, *12*, 183, doi:10.3390/jcm12010183 35

Dmitrii S. Maltsev, Alexei N. Kulikov, Yaroslava V. Volkova, Maria A. Burnasheva and Alexander S. Vasiliev
Retinal Macrophage-Like Cells as a Biomarker of Inflammation in Retinal Vein Occlusions
Reprinted from: *J. Clin. Med.* **2022**, *11*, 7470, doi:10.3390/jcm11247470 51

Filippo Confalonieri, Huy Bao Ngo, Helga Halldorsdottir Petersen, Nils Andreas Eide and Goran Petrovski
Iris Racemose Hemangioma Assessment with Swept Source Optical Coherence Tomography Angiography: A Feasibility Study and Stand-Alone Comparison
Reprinted from: *J. Clin. Med.* **2022**, *11*, 6575, doi:10.3390/jcm11216575 61

Marc Kukan, Matthew Driban, Kiran K. Vupparaboina, Swen Schwarz, Alice M. Kitay, Mohammed A. Rasheed, et al.
Structural Features of Patients with Drusen-like Deposits and Systemic Lupus Erythematosus
Reprinted from: *J. Clin. Med.* **2022**, *11*, 6012, doi:10.3390/jcm11206012 69

Caroline Bormann, Catharina Busch, Matus Rehak, Manuela Schmidt, Christian Scharenberg, Focke Ziemssen and Jan Darius Unterlauft
Two Year Functional and Structural Changes—A Comparison between Trabeculectomy and XEN Microstent Implantation Using Spectral Domain Optical Coherence Tomography
Reprinted from: *J. Clin. Med.* **2022**, *11*, 5840, doi:10.3390/jcm11195840 81

Timothy Y. Y. Lai, Ziqi Tang, Adrian C. W. Lai, Simon K. H. Szeto, Ricky Y. K. Lai and Carol Y. Cheung
Association of Fundus Autofluorescence Abnormalities and Pachydrusen in Central Serous Chorioretinopathy and Polypoidal Choroidal Vasculopathy
Reprinted from: *J. Clin. Med.* **2022**, *11*, 5340, doi:10.3390/jcm11185340 93

Julian A. Zimmermann, Nicole Eter and Julia Biermann
Acute Idiopathic Blind Spot Enlargement Syndrome—New Perspectives in the OCT Era
Reprinted from: *J. Clin. Med.* **2022**, *11*, 5278, doi:10.3390/jcm11185278 101

Muneeswar G. Nittala, Federico Corvi, Jyotsna Maram, Swetha B. Velaga, Jonathan Haines, Margaret A. Pericak-Vance, et al.
Risk Factors for Progression of Age-Related Macular Degeneration: Population-Based Amish Eye Study
Reprinted from: *J. Clin. Med.* **2022**, *11*, 5110, doi:10.3390/jcm11175110 113

Khaldoon O. Al-Nosairy, Elisabeth V. Quanz, Julia Biermann and Michael B. Hoffmann
Optical Coherence Tomography as a Biomarker for Differential Diagnostics in Nystagmus: Ganglion Cell Layer Thickness Ratio
Reprinted from: *J. Clin. Med.* **2022**, *11*, 4941, doi:10.3390/jcm11174941 123

Pasquale Loiudice, Giuseppe Covello, Michele Figus, Chiara Posarelli, Maria Sole Sartini and Giamberto Casini
Choroidal Vascularity Index in Central and Branch Retinal Vein Occlusion
Reprinted from: *J. Clin. Med.* **2022**, *11*, 4756, doi:10.3390/jcm11164756 133

Makoto Inoue, Takashi Koto and Akito Hirakata
Large Amplitude Iris Fluttering Detected by Consecutive Anterior Segment Optical Coherence Tomography Images in Eyes with Intrascleral Fixation of an Intraocular Lens
Reprinted from: *J. Clin. Med.* **2022**, *11*, 4596, doi:10.3390/jcm11154596 141

Patryk Sidorczuk, Iwona Obuchowska, Joanna Konopinska and Diana A. Dmuchowska
Correlation between Choroidal Vascularity Index and Outer Retina in Patients with Diabetic Retinopathy
Reprinted from: *J. Clin. Med.* **2022**, *11*, 3882, doi:10.3390/jcm11133882 153

Rita Serra, Giuseppe D'Amico Ricci, Stefano Dore, Florence Coscas and Antonio Pinna
Evaluation of Radial Peripapillary Capillary Density in G6PD Deficiency: An OCT Angiography Pilot Study
Reprinted from: *J. Clin. Med.* **2022**, *11*, 3282, doi:10.3390/jcm11123282 167

Kuo-Chen Su, Hong-Ming Cheng, Yu Chu, Fang-Chun Lu, Lung-Hui Tsai and Ching-Ying Cheng
Correlating Ocular Physiology and Visual Function with Mild Cognitive Loss in Senior Citizens in Taiwan
Reprinted from: *J. Clin. Med.* **2022**, *11*, 2624, doi:10.3390/jcm11092624 175

Rita Serra, Antonio Pinna, Francine Behar-Cohen and Florence Coscas
OCT Angiography Fractal Analysis of Choroidal Neovessels Secondary to Central Serous Chorioretinopathy, in a Caucasian Cohort
Reprinted from: *J. Clin. Med.* **2022**, *11*, 1443, doi:10.3390/jcm11051443 187

Do-Young Park, Hoon Noh, Changwon Kee and Jong-Chul Han
Topographic Relationships among Deep Optic Nerve Head Parameters in Patients with Primary Open-Angle Glaucoma
Reprinted from: *J. Clin. Med.* **2022**, *11*, 1320, doi:10.3390/jcm11051320 197

Carla Danese and Paolo Lanzetta
Optical Coherence Tomography Findings in Rhegmatogenous Retinal Detachment:
A Systematic Review
Reprinted from: *J. Clin. Med.* **2022**, *11*, 5819, doi:10.3390/jcm11195819 . . . . **209**

Joshua Ong, Arman Zarnegar, Giulia Corradetti, Sumit Randhir Singh and Jay Chhablani
Advances in Optical Coherence Tomography Imaging Technology and Techniques for
Choroidal and Retinal Disorders
Reprinted from: *J. Clin. Med.* **2022**, *11*, 5139, doi:10.3390/jcm11175139 . . . . **223**

About the Editors

Jay Chhablani

Jay Chhablani is a Professor of Ophthalmology and a Vitreo-Retinal Surgeon at the Department of Ophthalmology at the University of Pittsburgh, Pittsburgh, USA. He is the Director of Clinical Research at the UPMC Vision Institute. He established the "Choroid Analysis and Research (CAR) Lab" at the University of Pittsburgh, which focuses on computational as well as biological research on the choroid. His areas of interest are macular disorders, automated retinal image analysis, and advanced imaging techniques. He has been consistently funded by the National Institute of Health (NIH) and various foundations. He has published more than 550 articles in peer-reviewed journals with a focus on the choroid. He is the editor of books "Choroidal Disorders", "Central Serous Chorioretinopathy", and "Choroidal Neovascularization". He is on the reviewing boards of several high-impact journals including Science Translational Medicine and Lancet. He is also on the editorial board of several other journals, including the American Journal of Ophthalmology. He serves on the grant-reviewing board of various funding agencies. He is a member of many esteemed societies such as the Macula Society and the Gonin Club. He is a member of various scientific committees in various national and international societies, including the American Academy of Ophthalmology. He has delivered more than 200 invited lectures and has been invited for visiting professorship by many universities around the world. He has won several national and international awards and delivered multiple named lectures.

Sumit Randhir Singh

Dr Sumit Randhir Singh completed his basic medical degree and Master of Surgery (MS) in Ophthalmology at Jawaharlal Institute of Postgraduate Medical Education & Research (JIPMER), Puducherry, Indi,. and was awarded a gold medal as the best outgoing student in his post-graduation examination. He also won the best paper award in clinical sciences from the JIPMER Scientific Society (JSS awards, 2015-16). He subsequently completed a two-year fellowship in vitreo-retina and uveitis at LVPEI, Hyderabad, India (2016-2018). Later, he served as faculty at LVPEI, GMRV campus, Visakhapatnam, India (2018-19), before moving to pursue a one-year research fellowship at Jacobs Retina Center, Shiley Eye Institute, University of California, San Diego, USA, till November 2020. He is currently working as a consultant at Sharp Sight Eye Hospital, Patna, Bihar, India.

His main areas of clinical interest include diseases of the macula and newer imaging modalities such as OCT angiography, wide field OCT, FFA, and imaging biomarkers for various retinal and choroidal diseases. He has to his credit more than 100 indexed publications in various national and international journals. He has co-authored three book chapters and multiple non-peer-reviewed publications with presentations at national and international meetings, and was awarded Best Paper Presentation in vitreo-retina at the AIOS Mid-Term Conference, 2023. He is a reviewer for various international journals such as the Asia–Pacific Journal of Ophthalmology and Scientific Reports.

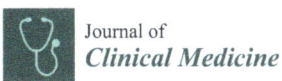

Editorial

Optical Coherence Tomography Imaging: Advances in Ophthalmology

Sumit Randhir Singh [1] and Jay Chhablani [2,*]

[1] Nilima Sinha Medical College & Hospital, Rampur 852122, India; sumit.jipmer@gmail.com
[2] UPMC Eye Center, University of Pittsburgh, Pittsburgh, PA 15213, USA
* Correspondence: jay.chhablani@gmail.com; Tel.: +1-412-377-1943; Fax: +1-412-647-5119

Citation: Singh, S.R.; Chhablani, J. Optical Coherence Tomography Imaging: Advances in Ophthalmology. *J. Clin. Med.* 2022, *11*, 2858. https://doi.org/10.3390/jcm11102858

Received: 6 May 2022
Accepted: 12 May 2022
Published: 18 May 2022

Publisher's Note: MDPI stays neutral with regard to jurisdictional claims in published maps and institutional affiliations.

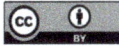

Copyright: © 2022 by the authors. Licensee MDPI, Basel, Switzerland. This article is an open access article distributed under the terms and conditions of the Creative Commons Attribution (CC BY) license (https://creativecommons.org/licenses/by/4.0/).

Since its advent in 1991, optical coherence tomography (OCT) has become the most commonly used imaging modality in vitreo-retina practice [1]. OCT, a non-invasive imaging modality, has a fast acquisition time, usually within seconds, and provides in vivo, high resolution, three-dimensional (3-D) imaging of the retina and choroid, akin to the histologic section [2]. These inherent advantages have enabled OCT installation in eye clinics throughout the world, thereby providing invaluable insights about the chorioretinal architecture in diverse ocular diseases.

Based on the principle of low coherence interferometry, OCT uses an infrared light wavelength ranging from 840 nm to 1050 nm [3]. Several technical modifications from the earlier time domain OCT (TD-OCT) to recent upgrades, including spectral domain (SD-OCT) and swept source OCT (SS-OCT), have significantly improved the image resolution, reaching up to 3–5 µm [3,4]. Deeper ocular penetration with higher wavelength SS-OCT allows clinicians to visualize additional details of the choroid, i.e., the choriocapillaris, Haller's layer, Sattler's layer, choroidoscleral interface and even the scleral tissue in special scenarios [5]. Features like eye tracking and scanning the same area during follow up help the clinicians to accurately detect the subtle change at the site of pathology.

En-face OCT scans, also referred as C-scans, based on the coronal plane are generated post 3-D scan acquisition and are different compared to the routinely performed cross-sectional scans [6]. Another significant milestone deserving special mention is OCT angiography, which uses motion contrast to identify the blood flow in capillaries and has found wide usage to perform qualitative analyses on microaneurysms, macular edema, macular ischemia, retinal neovascularization and choroidal neovascular membranes, and quantitative analyses on the capillary density and measurement of chorioretinal lesion size [7]. Moreover, volumetric analysis with segmentation to specific depths provides significant advantages compared to dye-based angiography.

Initial OCT protocols were limited to the macular area covering an area of 6 × 6 mm. Subsequent improvements, especially wide-field OCT, provided additional insights on the peripheral retina, with clinical utility in eyes with peripheral retinal ischemia, retinal degeneration and peripheral choroidal lesions [8]. This was made possible with a much higher A-scan acquisition rate (>100,000/s) compared to earlier generation TD-OCT (approximately 400/s), thereby reducing scan acquisition time and increasing the field of view [8]. Now, multiple 12 × 12 mm or even 18- or 20-mm scans can be captured and montaged using additional software to create a much wider field of view reaching up to the equator and beyond. Another breakthrough is the integration of OCT imaging with surgical microscopes, which can be helpful in intraoperative anatomical assessment, especially in macular surgeries, for instance, on the macular hole and epiretinal membrane [9]. Surgeons can therefore assess the anatomical details intraoperatively and predict the surgical success rates. Though hand-held OCT and home-based OCT are other additions to the armamentarium, image resolution is typically lower than standard OCT machines [10]. Apart from retina and uveitis clinics, OCT is commonly used in glaucoma clinics to quantitively analyze retinal nerve fiber layer thickness and cornea clinics to assess the corneal thickness and anterior chamber depth.

Despite the innumerable benefits, high purchase and maintenance cost of OCT systems prevent widespread adoption in poor resource settings and low-income countries. Ongoing technical improvements can hopefully bring OCT size and cost down to more affordable levels. Moreover, the commercial instruments are bulky, not portable and tabletop mounted, which becomes challenging with pediatric patients, mentally disabled patients with the inability to fixate and elderly bedridden patients [10].

To conclude, OCT imaging, in a span of three decades, has undergone several modifications and now is a standard of care in ophthalmology clinics throughout the world. In this special edition, we focus on these recent advances in OCT technology.

Author Contributions: Conceptualization, S.R.S. and J.C.; writing—original draft preparation, S.R.S.; writing—review and editing, S.R.S. and J.C. All authors have read and agreed to the published version of the manuscript.

Funding: This research received no external funding.

Conflicts of Interest: The authors declare no conflict of interest.

References

1. Huang, D.; Swanson, E.A.; Lin, C.P.; Schuman, J.S.; Stinson, W.G.; Chang, W.; Hee, M.R.; Flotte, T.; Gregory, K.; Puliafito, C.A.; et al. Optical Coherence Tomography. *Science* **1991**, *254*, 1178–1181. [CrossRef] [PubMed]
2. Balaratnasingam, C.; Messinger, J.D.; Sloan, K.R.; Yannuzzi, L.A.; Freund, K.B.; Curcio, C.A. Histologic and Optical Coherence Tomographic Correlates in Drusenoid Pigment Epithelium Detachment in Age-Related Macular Degeneration. *Ophthalmology* **2017**, *124*, 644–656. [CrossRef]
3. Potsaid, B.M.; Baumann, B.; Huang, D.; Barry, S.; Cable, A.E.; Schuman, J.S.; Duker, J.S.; Fujimoto, J.G. Ultrahigh speed 1050nm swept source / Fourier domain OCT retinal and anterior segment imaging at 100,000 to 400,000 axial scans per second. *Opt. Express* **2010**, *18*, 20029–20048. [CrossRef]
4. Lavinsky, F.; Lavinsky, D. Novel perspectives on swept-source optical coherence tomography. *Int. J. Retin. Vitr.* **2016**, *2*, 1–11. [CrossRef] [PubMed]
5. Singh, S.R.; Vupparaboina, K.K.; Goud, A.; Dansingani, K.K.; Chhablani, J. Choroidal imaging biomarkers. *Surv. Ophthalmol.* **2019**, *64*, 312–333. [CrossRef] [PubMed]
6. Rosen, R.B.; Hathaway, M.; Rogers, J.; Pedro, J.; Garcia, P.; Laissue, P.; Dobre, G.M.; Podoleanu, A.G. Multidimensional en-face OCT imaging of the retina. *Opt. Express* **2009**, *17*, 4112–4133. [CrossRef] [PubMed]
7. De Carlo, T.E.; Romano, A.; Waheed, N.K.; Duker, J.S. A review of optical coherence tomography angiography (OCTA). *Int. J. Retin. Vitr.* **2015**, *1*, 1–15. [CrossRef] [PubMed]
8. Kolb, J.P.; Klein, T.; Kufner, C.; Wieser, W.; Neubauer, A.S.; Huber, R. Ultra-widefield retinal MHz-OCT imaging with up to 100 degrees viewing angle. *Biomed. Opt. Express* **2015**, *6*, 1534–1552. [CrossRef] [PubMed]
9. Ehlers, J.P.; Tao, Y.K.; Srivastava, S.K. The value of intraoperative optical coherence tomography imaging in vitreoretinal surgery. *Curr. Opin. Ophthalmol.* **2014**, *25*, 221–227. [CrossRef] [PubMed]
10. Chopra, R.; Wagner, S.K.; Keane, P.A. Optical coherence tomography in the 2020s—outside the eye clinic. *Eye* **2020**, *35*, 236–243. [CrossRef] [PubMed]

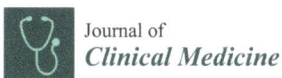

Article

Evaluation of Retinal Nerve Fiber Layer and Macular Ganglion Cell Layer Thickness in Relation to Optic Disc Size

Jens Julian Storp [1,*,†], Nils Hendrik Storp [1,†], Moritz Fabian Danzer [2], Nicole Eter [1] and Julia Biermann [1]

1. Department of Ophthalmology, University of Muenster Medical Center, 48149 Muenster, Germany
2. Institute of Biostatistics and Clinical Research, University of Muenster, 48149 Muenster, Germany
* Correspondence: jens.storp@ukmuenster.de; Tel.: +49-251-83-56001
† These authors contributed equally to this work.

Abstract: To investigate whether optic nerve ganglion cell amount is dependent on optic disc size, this trial analyzes the correlation between Bruch's membrane opening area (BMOA) and retinal nerve fiber layer (RNFL) thickness as well as macular ganglion cell layer thickness (mGCLT). Additionally, differences in RNFL and mGCLT regarding various optic disc cohorts are evaluated. This retrospective, monocentric study included 501 healthy eyes of 287 patients from the University Hospital Münster, Germany, who received macular and optic disc optical coherence tomography (OCT) scans. Rank correlation coefficients for clustered data were calculated to investigate the relationship between BMOA and thickness values of respective retinal layers. Furthermore, these values were compared between different optic disc groups based on BMOA. Statistical analysis did not reveal a significant correlation between BMOA and RNFL thickness, nor between BMOA and mGCLT. However, groupwise analysis showed global RNFL to be significantly decreased in small and large discs in comparison to medium discs. This was not observed for global mGCLT. This study extends existing normative data for mGCLT taking optic disc size into account. While the ganglion cell amount represented by the RNFL and mGCLT seemed independent of BMOA, mGCLT was superior to global RNFL in displaying optic nerve integrity in very small and very large optic discs.

Keywords: OCT; BMO; optic disc size; macrodisc; microdisc; macular ganglion cell layer; retinal nerve fiber layer; RNFL; thickness

Citation: Storp, J.J.; Storp, N.H.; Danzer, M.F.; Eter, N.; Biermann, J. Evaluation of Retinal Nerve Fiber Layer and Macular Ganglion Cell Layer Thickness in Relation to Optic Disc Size. *J. Clin. Med.* **2023**, *12*, 2471. https://doi.org/10.3390/jcm12072471

Academic Editors: Sumit Randhir Singh and Jay Chhablani

Received: 18 February 2023
Revised: 21 March 2023
Accepted: 22 March 2023
Published: 24 March 2023

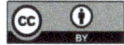

Copyright: © 2023 by the authors. Licensee MDPI, Basel, Switzerland. This article is an open access article distributed under the terms and conditions of the Creative Commons Attribution (CC BY) license (https://creativecommons.org/licenses/by/4.0/).

1. Introduction

Optical coherence tomography (OCT) allows for the non-invasive, quantitative assessment of individual retinal layers, such as the retinal nerve fiber layer (RNFL) around the optic disc and macular ganglion cell layer thickness (mGCLT). OCT measurement results can be compared to a normative reference database and can, therefore, allow for the differentiation between pathological and physiological findings [1–3]. In clinical routine, RNFL values are consulted most often to complement fundoscopic findings of conspicuous optic disc morphologies. However, investigation of the mGCLT has proven to provide important information in addition to RNFL measurements [4]. mGCLT has been shown to be of high diagnostic value in optic neuropathies and optic disc abnormalities [5–8].

A quantitative dependence of retinal ganglion cells on optic disc area has been demonstrated for RNFL and for histological axon content [9] and may, therefore, also be postulated for mGCLT. This raises the question of whether mGCLT and RNFL correlate with optic disc size in OCT, and whether optic disc morphology should be considered when interpreting results of retinal layer thickness measurements.

This field of research remains controversial. While several studies report a positive correlation between RNFL thickness and optic disc area [10,11], others contrarily describe no significant association between RNFL thickness and optic disc area [12,13].

In clinical practice, optic discs will be described as small, medium or large, as this division can help in identifying certain risk factors associated with optic nerve head morphology, such as an increased risk of anterior ischemic optic neuropathy in small optic discs [14], or to differentiate pseudopapilledema from optic disc swelling in microdiscs. In turn, it can be challenging to discriminate macrodiscs from glaucomatous optic neuropathies due to an enlarged cupping. Traditionally, this attribution of optic discs to one group has been based on fundoscopic assessment or on measurement results of confocal scanning laser tomography (CSLT). In recent years, studies using OCT for the characterization of optic disc morphology have demonstrated that approaches based on Bruch´s membrane opening area (BMOA) can be used instead [7,15–17]; however, categorization and thresholds for micro- and macrodiscs are still not universally defined.

Since OCT is one of the most frequently used imaging modalities in ophthalmological practice, investigating the effect of optic disc size, more precisely BMOA, on retinal structures such as RNFL and mGCLT is of great interest. The primary aim of this work is to analyze RNFL and mGCLT in relation to optic disc size defined by BMOA in a healthy cohort. Secondly, RNFL and mGCLT findings will be compared between different study groups based on optic disc size. The diagnostic value of the findings reported will be evaluated. Furthermore, the results presented in this trial can act as a reference database for mGCLT and peripapillary RNFL thickness in normal and extreme optic disc size.

2. Materials and Methods

This monocentric, retrospective study included 501 eyes from 287 Caucasian patients, who were examined at the Department of Ophthalmology, Münster University Hospital, Germany between 1 January 2016 and 1 October 2022.

This study was approved by the ethics committee of the Medical Association of Westfalen-Lippe and the University of Münster (No.: 2022-493-f-S) and adhered to the tenets of the Declaration of Helsinki.

We conducted a search in the electronic patient file system FIDUS (Arztservice Wente GmbH, Darmstadt, Germany) filtering for patients who received both a macular and optic disc OCT (Spectralis®, Heidelberg Engineering GmbH, Heidelberg, Germany) in at least one eye. Patients were only eligible to be included in the study if both macula and optic disc OCT scans were conducted on the same day or at least in a time span of no more than 1 month. Only healthy eyes were included in the study, resulting from a holistic ophthalmological examination. Patients were not eligible to be included if any of the following exclusion criteria applied: higher myopic refraction errors (spherical equivalent of <-6.0 diopters), any retinal or optic nerve diseases or congenital anomalies. Furthermore, patients with central nervous system disorders or neurotoxic drug intake were excluded, except for patients taking quensyl with no signs of retinopathy on ERG. Artifacts and low quality in macular or optic disc scans were additional exclusion criteria.

OCT images were all taken in the same location under the same conditions by expert operators. Scans of the macula and optic disc were reviewed by an expert examiner (N.H.S.). Further, boundaries of the BMO were verified and adjusted if the automatic annotation software failed to properly place BMO boundary markers.

Data were recorded in the spreadsheet software Microsoft Office Excel (Microsoft, Redmond, WA, USA; Version 16.71). Descriptive data are presented as mean ± standard deviation (SD).

Global RNFL represents the mean value of all RNFL sectors and is provided automatically by the Heidelberg system. In accordance with this parameter, global mGCLT was defined as the mean value of all mGCLT sectors and was calculated separately.

The BMOA to RNFL correlation was firstly evaluated for global RNFL and subsequently for individual sectors of RNFL (Figure 1).

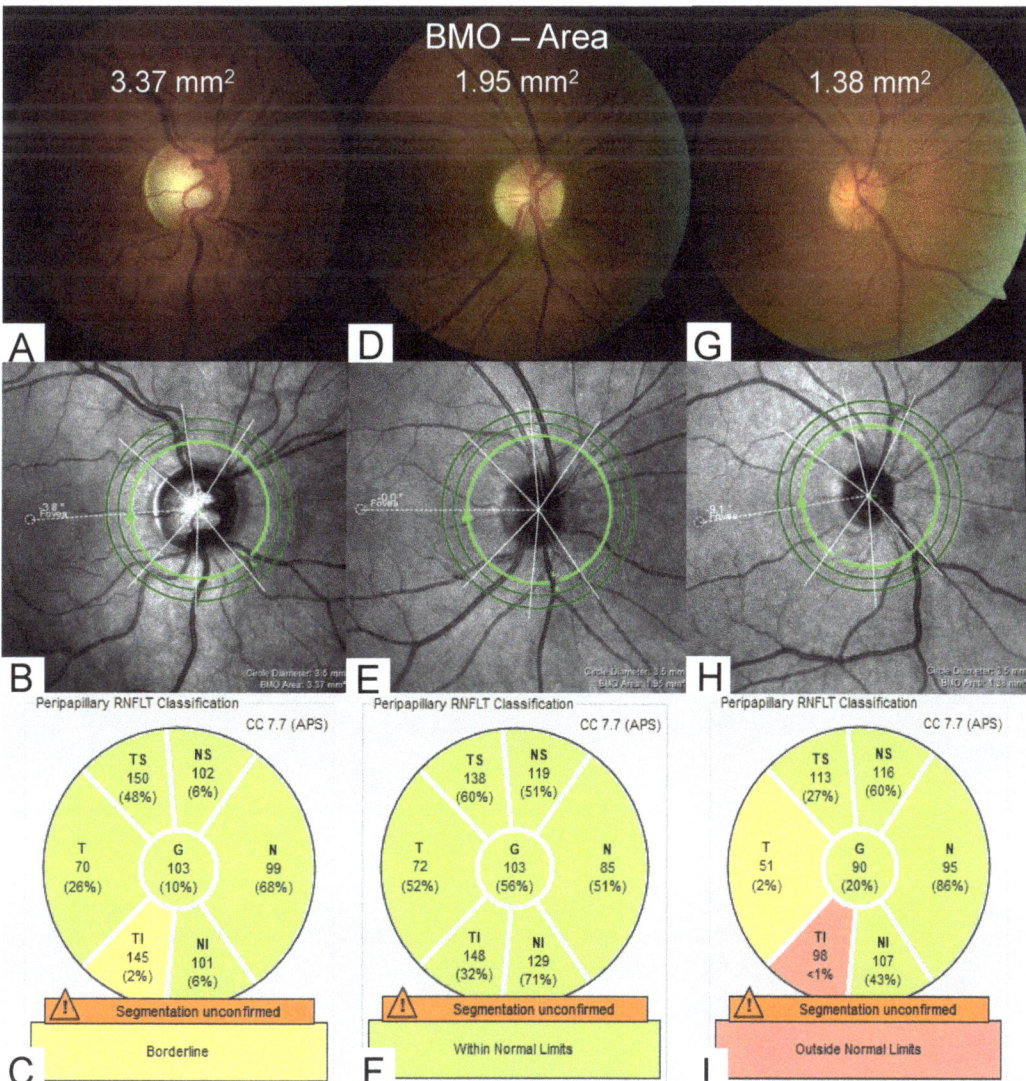

Figure 1. Examples for large, medium and small optic discs based on BMOA in fundoscopic view and optical coherence tomography scans. Upper row: fundus photographs of optic discs. Middle row: infrared images of the corresponding optic discs and illustration of the 3.5 mm, 4.1 mm and 4.7 mm diameter scan circles around the center of the optic nerve. Lower row: RNFL measurements of the corresponding optic discs (3.5 mm diameter) and valuation based on the database of Heidelberg Engineering GmbH. (**A–C**): large disc with a BMOA = 3.37 mm^2, (**D–F**) medium disc with a BMOA = 1.95 mm^2, (**G–I**): small disc with a BMOA = 1.38 mm^2. (**C,F,I**): values for RNFL measurements. G = global RNFL; NS = nasal superior RNFL; N = nasal RFNL; NI = nasal inferior RNFL; TI = temporal inferior RNFL; T = temporal RNFL; TS = temporal superior RNFL.

Likewise, the correlation between mGCLT and BMOA was firstly tested for global mGCLT and secondly for the individual mGCLT sectors. The latter are based on the Early Treatment Diabetic Retinopathy Study (ETDRS) grid (Figure 2).

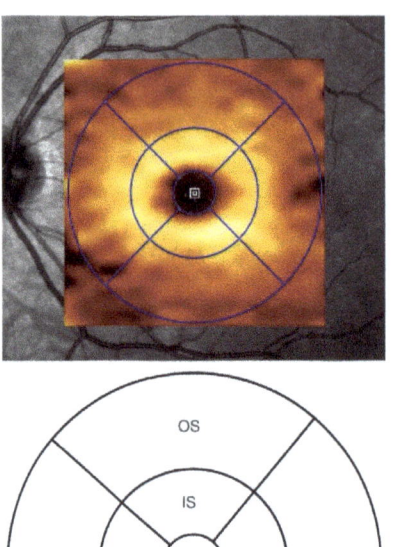

Figure 2. Location map for mGCLT data according to the Early Treatment Diabetic Retinopathy Study (ETDRS) grid. ETDRS sectors are labeled according to their location in relation to the fovea. C = Central area; IN = inner nasal; ON = outer nasal; II = inner inferior; OI = outer inferior; IT = inner temporal; OT = outer temporal; IS = inner superior; OS = outer superior.

In a next step, eyes were assigned to respective optic disc groups according to their BMOA.

Due to the lack of accepted cut-off values in BMO measurements by OCT, the allocation to the three cohorts was done as an approximation based on the HRT (Heidelberg Retina Tomograph) definition: Group 1 "small discs" (n = 80; BMOA: <1.63 mm^2), group 2 "medium discs" (n = 298; BMOA: 1.63–2.43 mm^2), group 3 "large discs" (n = 126; BMOA: >2.43 mm^2). Figure 1 displays examples for small, medium and large discs with their respective infrared images and RNFL values. In addition to this HRT-based division, groupwise comparison was also conducted via a quartile-based approach, comparing the 5% smallest and 5% largest optic discs to the remaining 90% (intermediate).

Statistical Analysis

For each retinal layer thickness variable, we computed correlations with BMOA to analyze the dependence between the variables. Since the normal distribution assumption could not be ensured, rank correlations were computed. However, the standard Spearman correlation coefficient does not take the clustering structure of our data into account. Hence, correspondingly adapted methods from Rosner et al. [18] with data from patients of which both eyes are available (n = 214) were applied. For each correlation coefficient, we also report 95% confidence intervals. No adjustments for multiple testing were made here, as our analyses are of an exploratory nature.

In order to discover non-monotonic effects, we executed pairwise comparisons of all variables between the three groups of eyes based on the HRT definition, and also between the three groups obtained by grouping the smallest 5% of BMOA, the largest 5% of BMOA and the remaining mean BMOA of the sample together. In order to account for the dependency structure, we applied a corresponding rank sum test as suggested by Rosner et al. [19] and implemented by Jiang et al. [20]. In keeping with the exploratory nature of our analysis, we report Bonferroni-adjusted p-values separately for each variable, i.e., the p-values are multiplied by 3 for the three comparisons made for each variable (small vs. medium discs, small vs. large discs, medium vs. large discs). Additionally, we report median values of the layer thickness variables for each group.

We report 95% confidence intervals that do not contain zero and p-values falling below 0.05 as significant findings. However, the purpose of this study is purely exploratory, and these findings should, therefore, be treated with care or confirmed in a separate study.

Statistical analysis was performed using R, version 4.1.2 [21]. The package clus-rank [20] was used to execute the rank sum tests from [19] and the package ggplot2 [22] was used to create plots.

3. Results

501 eyes from 287 patients were included in this trial. Study population characteristics are summarized in Table 1.

Table 1. General patient characteristics. Values are presented as absolute numbers (%) or as median (25% quartile; 75% quartile).

n (Eyes)	501 (100%)
n (patients)	287 (100%)
age (years)	35 (16; 56)
gender (M:F)	210 (42%):291 (58%)
n (eyes) according to optic disc size (HRT division):	
large (2.43–4.15 mm^2)	123 (25%)
medium (1.63–2.42 mm^2)	298 (59%)
small (0.91–1.62 mm^2)	80 (16%)
n (eyes) according to optic disc size (quantile division):	
largest (3.30–4.15 mm^2)	25 (5%)
intermediate (1.41–3.30 mm^2)	451 (90%)
smallest (0.91–1.40 mm^2)	25 (5%)
study eye (R:L)	249 (50%):252 (50%)
median visual acuity (logMAR)	0.10 (0.00; 0.20)
median spherical equivalent:	0.00 (−0.75; 0.63)
per group (HRT division)	
large	0.00 (−1.13; 0.63)
medium	0.00 (−0.75; 0.63)
small	0.00 (−0.38; 0.66)
per group (quantile division)	
large	−0.25 (−1.25; 0.13)
medium	0.00 (−0.63; 0.69)
small	0.00 (−1.50; 1.50)

n = number, M = male; F = female, R = right, L = left, logMAR = logarithm of minimum angle of resolution, HRT = Heidelberg Retina Tomograph.

Nominal values for RNFL and mGCLT are summarized in Figures 3 and 4.

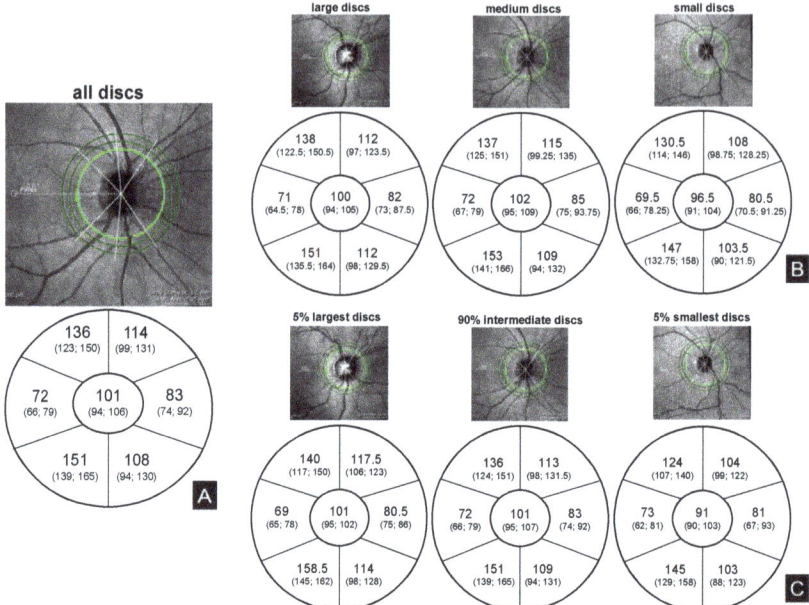

Figure 3. Illustration of median (25% quartile, 75% quartile) RNFL thickness values (μm). Note that, while right eye images are displayed as examples, the values shown were calculated on the basis of both right and left eye measurements. (**A**): median RNFL values for the entire patient population. (**B**): median RNFL values for the different cohorts based on HRT division. (**C**): median RNFL values for the different groups based on quartile division (5-90-5).

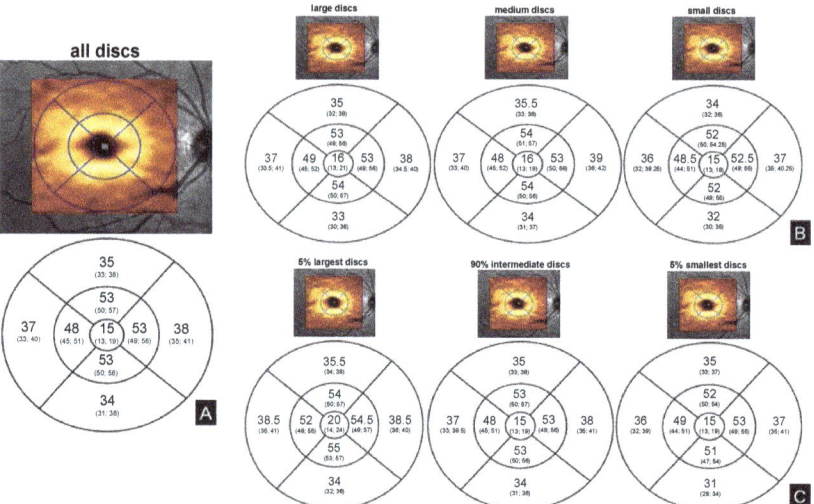

Figure 4. Illustration of median (25% quartile, 75% quartile) mGCLT values (μm). Note that, while right eye images are displayed as examples, the values shown were calculated on the basis of both right and left eye measurements. (**A**): median mGCLT values for the entire patient population according to the Early Treatment Diabetic Retinopathy Study (ETDRS) grid. (**B**): median mGCLT values for the different cohorts based on HRT division. (**C**): median mGCLT values for the different groups based on quartile division (5-90-5).

Statistical analysis did not show any significant correlation between global RNFL and BMOA, nor between global mGCLT and BMOA (Table 2 and Figure 5).

Table 2. Estimates and confidence intervals for correlation analysis between global RNFL and BMOA, as well as for correlation analysis between global mGCLT and BMOA.

	Estimate	Lower 95% CI	Upper 95% CI
RNFL global	0.04	−0.08	0.15
mGCLT global	0.04	−0.08	0.16

CI = confidence interval.

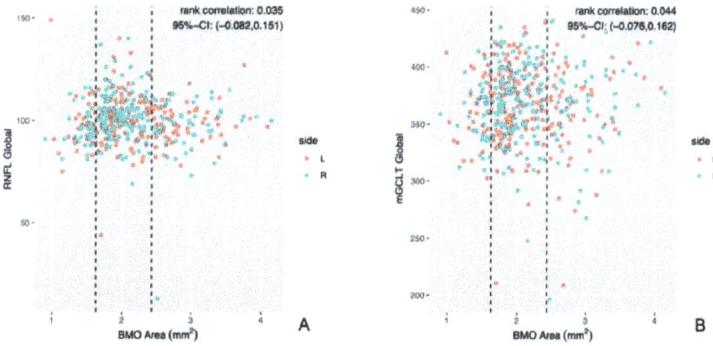

Figure 5. Scatter plots of global RNFL and global mGCLT in μm in relation to BMOA. (**A**): scatter plot of global RNFL and BMOA; dashed lines show bounds grouping by HRT definition. (**B**): scatter plot of global mGCLT and BMOA; dashed lines show bounds grouping by HRT definition. L = left eye; R = right eye.

3.1. Correlation Analysis

While a small effect could be seen for the central area of the mGCLT, no significant correlation could be demonstrated for the remaining individual sectors of the RNFL and mGCLT (Table 3 and Figure S1).

Table 3. Estimates and 95% confidence intervals of rank correlation coefficients of the individual RNFL and mGCLT sectors with BMOA.

RNFL	Estimate	Lower 95% CI Bound	Upper 95% CI Bound
NS	−0.04	−0.15	0.08
N	0.02	−0.09	0.14
NI	0.05	−0.07	0.16
TI	0.06	−0.06	0.17
T	−0.02	−0.14	0.10
TS	0.09	−0.02	0.21
mGCLT			
C	0.11	0.00	0.23
IN	0.02	−0.09	0.14
ON	−0.07	−0.18	0.05
II	0.06	−0.05	0.18
OI	0.00	−0.12	0.11
IT	0.09	−0.03	0.20
OT	0.05	−0.07	0.16
IS	0.03	−0.08	0.15
OS	0.01	−0.11	0.13

CI = confidence interval. RNFL sectors: NS = nasal superior; N = nasal; NI = nasal inferior; TI = temporal inferior; T = temporal; TS = temporal superior; mGCLT sectors: C = central area; IN = inner nasal; ON = outer nasal; II = inner inferior; OI = outer inferior; IT = inner temporal; OT = outer temporal; IS = inner superior; OS = outer superior.

3.2. Optic Disc Groups (HRT Division)

Statistical analysis of the secondary hypothesis looked at possible differences between BMO-based optic disc size groups. In the HRT division, global RNFL differed significantly between small and medium discs as well as between medium and large discs. In contrast, global mGCLT did not show significant differences among the various cohorts (Table 4).

Table 4. Differences in global RNFL and global mGCLT between optic disc cohorts based on HRT division. p-values ≤ 0.05 are highlighted in bold. Median thickness values are given in μm.

	Small vs. Medium	Medium vs. Large	Small vs. Large	Median Thickness Small	Median Thickness Medium	Median Thickness Large
RNFL Global	**<0.01**	**0.05**	0.42	96.50	102.00	100.00
mGCLT Global	0.08	1.00	0.94	40.11	41.22	40.89

Results of the HRT-based comparison of the individual RNFL and mGCLT sectors among the three cohorts are displayed in Table S1. Statistical analysis revealed significant differences between small and medium discs in various RNFL and mGCLT sectors as well as significant differences between medium and large optic discs in the nasal sector of the RNFL.

3.3. Optic Disc Groups (Quantile Division)

To analyze the largest and smallest optic discs based on BMOA, this study also allocated the data based on a quantile division (5-90-5), comparing the 5% smallest optic discs, the 5% largest optic discs and the residual 90% intermediate discs. Results of this quantile-based approach are summarized in Table 5. Results of the quantile-based comparison of the individual RNFL and mGCLT sectors among the three groups are displayed in Table S2.

Table 5. Differences in global RNFL and global mGCLT between optic disc cohorts in the 5 percent quantile division. Variable-wise Bonferoni-corrected p-values ≤ 0.05 are highlighted in bold. Median thickness values for the respective groups are given in μm.

	Smallest vs. Intermediate	Intermediate vs. Largest	Smallest vs. Largest	Median Thickness Smallest	Median Thickness Intermediate	Median Thickness Largest
RNFL Global	0.05	1.00	0.37	91.00	101.00	101.00
mGCLT Global	0.83	0.25	0.23	37.00	38.00	38.50

4. Discussion

The results of this retrospective study can be summarized as follows: Statistical analysis did not reveal a significant correlation between BMOA and RNFL thickness, nor between BMOA and mGCLT. Groupwise analysis showed global RNFL to be significantly decreased in micro- and macrodiscs when compared to medium sized discs. This was not observed for global mGCLT. This study extends existing normative data for mGCLT taking optic disc size into account.

This is the first study to examine the relationship between BMOA and RNFL, as well as between BMOA and mGCLT, using OCT in a large healthy study population.

In this monocentric analysis, neither RNFL nor mGCLT correlated significantly with optic disc size determined by BMOA.

However, noticeable differences were found among various optic disc groups, showing that while in the HRT division, global RNFL was reduced in small and large discs in comparison to medium discs, global mGCLT did not differ between these cohorts. In the quantile-based approach, this observation was reproducible for the smallest optic discs. These findings imply that mGCLT is affected less by optic disc size anomaly than RNFL thickness.

This observation is in line with data reported by Seo et al. [10]. The authors investigated the relation between optic disc size determined by CSLT and axial length on RNFL and ganglion cell–inner plexiform layer (GCIPL) in healthy individuals. While GCIPL and GCL are not entirely equivalent, both encompass similar retinal structures and can be considered equivalent with regard to their significance in clinical diagnostics [23]. While Seo et al. did not observe a significant correlation between GCIPL thickness and optic disc size, they report a positive correlation between optic disc size and RNFL thickness [10]. This is in line with reports by Savini et al., who describe a positive correlation between RNFL and optic disc size determined by OCT in their study of 54 healthy eyes [11]. Interestingly, we did not observe a noticeable correlation between RNFL or mGCLT and optic disc size in our study population. It should, however, be noted that optic disc size determination in the study by Savini et al. was based on the identification of the retinal pigment epithelium/choriocapillaris border and the addition of a 150 µm margin in papillary OCT scans, rather than BMO, which limits comparability. For the same reason, comparability to the CSLT based approach by Seo et al. is also limited. Nevertheless, the findings reported by Seo et al., and the findings reported in our study, consistently hint toward relatively constant values of the GCL/GCIPL irrespective of optic disc size variability [10].

While influencing factors on RNFL measurements are well described in the literature [24–31], there are little data on parameters that affect measurements of the mGCLT, such as axial length and spherical equivalent [10,32,33]. The findings of this study suggest that the size of the optic disc has little to no influence on mGCLT measurement results.

Optic disc size is a key aspect for correct optic disc assessment. Defining universally acknowledged thresholds to discriminate small from medium and large optic discs has posed a challenge due to the large variety of available methods [34–36]. Historically, optic disc size classification has been conducted during slit-lamp examination or on the basis of fundus photographs, both of which only allow for a certain degree of precision. For a long time, the assessment of the exact morphology and size of the optic disc was limited to findings in histological examinations [9]. The advances in retinal imaging of the past decades have enabled quantitative and reproducible measurements of optic disc parameters. CSLT devices have been applied extensively in order to investigate optic disc morphology. Nowadays, with the advancement of OCT, optic disc morphology can be computed three-dimensionally, allowing for precise illustration of optic nerve anatomy. Most importantly, OCT is capable of precisely identifying the termination of Bruch's membrane, the anatomical landmark determining optic disc size, making BMOA a suitable anatomical structure for the assessment of optic nerve head morphology and disc size [37]. When assessing BMOA, it is important to rule out possible imaging artifacts that might otherwise confound tomographic scanning results, such as signal voids in Bruch's membrane caused by overlying vessels.

Reports on the exact determination of optic disc size based on HRT and OCT are inconclusive. While some authors report no correlation between HRT and OCT optic disc measurements [38], Cazana et al. have recently demonstrated transferability of HRT measurements to an OCT-based BMOA assessment. They report a BMOA of ≥ 2.19 mm^2 to resemble the adequate threshold value for optic discs to be considered macrodiscs; however, they did not include microdiscs in their analysis [15]. Therefore, as definitive BMOA reference values for micro-, norm- and macrodiscs remain elusive, this study adhered to the traditional HRT division for optic discs size classification and added a 5% quantile approach in order to examine extreme optic nerve heads.

Our data on the average GCL thickness are in line with normative data reported by a number of spectral-domain OCT trials [32,39–41]. Similar to our study, Invernizzi et al. investigated retinal layer thickness in 200 Caucasian patients [32]. Studies that investigated patients of Asian descent [40–42] also report absolute values for mGCLT, which are comparable to the median values presented here. While some of these studies have analyzed correlations between systemic parameters, such as gender and age, and thickness of different retinal layers, they do not report on the correlation between retinal layer thickness and optic disc size.

This study used the Heidelberg Spectralis® Spectral-domain OCT (Heidelberg Engineering GmbH, Heidelberg, Germany), which comes with an integrated, color-coded reference database to help classify individual optic disc measurements. This reference database consists of 246 eyes of 246 patients, of whom 61 had a BMOA < 1.50 mm^2 and 8 had a BMOA > 2.50 mm^2. The authors of this manuscript are under the impression that micro- and macrodiscs can pose a challenge for the system when it comes to accurately rating RNFL values. Healthy individuals with very large or very small optic discs are frequently referred to our clinic due to abnormalities in the color-coded RNFL measurements (as demonstrated in Figure 1). Further work-up usually rules out any form of underlying disease which could cause such changes. We assume, therefore, that rather than being of actual pathological relevance, these RNFL abnormalities might occur due to a limited number of cases with optic disc anomalies being included in the reference database. This study included patients with normal visual function. Since our approach revealed mGCLT to be more stable in regards to changes in optic disc size, we suggest consulting mGCLT in micro- or macrodiscs in addition to RNFL measures if RNFL values appear implausible.

Limitations

As has been shown by several authors, axial length/spherical equivalent can exert a significant effect on RNFL, mGCLT and BMO measurements [10,28–30,32,43]. By excluding patients with a spherical equivalent < −6 diopters, we limited a possible influence on the results in this study. Cognitive function, vascular health, age, ethnicity, OCT signal strength and gender have further been identified as confounding parameters for both RNFL and mGCLT measurements [24–27,44–46]. Since these parameters differ among trials, comparison of results must be done with caution. For instance, as this trial only included patients of Caucasian descent, our findings may not be transferable to other study populations.

One major limitation of this study lies in its design. Due to its retrospective nature, we are unable to comment on prospective estimates related to optic disc size and OCT measurements. Further prospective studies are needed here.

This study included patients with normal visual function who passed a holistic ophthalmological examination to exclude eye diseases. However, in daily clinical practice, early or preperimetric changes in retinal ganglion cell number and integrity may happen to soma and axon at different timepoints; for example, optic nerve compression may alter RNFL thickness prior to mGCLT, and mitochondrial optic neuropathy might affect mGCLT prior to RNFL thinning. Thus, taking other diagnostic modalities and parameters into account is crucial for the correct interpretation of OCT values.

5. Conclusions

To summarize, we did not observe a noticeable correlation between RNFL or mGCLT and BMOA in this study. In contrast to RNFL, mGCLT appeared to be independent of optic disc size in this cohort of healthy patients, thus suggesting that mGCLT should be consulted when investigating large or small discs and inconclusive findings in OCT–RNFL analysis. The display of RNFL and mGCLT standard values for various disc size groups in this study can further help distinguish pathological from physiological findings in clinical practice.

Supplementary Materials: The following supporting information can be downloaded at: https://www.mdpi.com/article/10.3390/jcm12072471/s1, Figure S1: Scatter plots of RNFL sectors in relation to BMOA; Table S1: Differences in individual RNFL and mGCLT sectors between optic disc cohorts based on HRT division; Table S2: Differences in individual RNFL and mGCLT sectors between optic disc cohorts based on quantile division.

Author Contributions: Conceptualization, J.J.S., N.H.S. and J.B.; data curation, J.J.S. and N.H.S.; formal analysis, J.J.S. and N.H.S.; investigation, J.J.S. and N.H.S.; methodology, J.J.S., N.H.S. and J.B.; project administration, J.B.; resources, N.E. and J.B.; software, J.J.S. and M.F.D.; supervision, J.B.; validation, M.F.D.; writing—original draft, J.J.S., N.H.S. and J.B.; writing—review and editing, M.F.D., N.E. and J.B. All authors have read and agreed to the published version of the manuscript.

Funding: This research received no external funding.

Institutional Review Board Statement: The study was conducted in accordance with the Declaration of Helsinki and was approved by the ethics committee of the Medical Association of Westfalen-Lippe and the University of Münster (No.: 2022-493-f-S).

Informed Consent Statement: Patient consent was waived due to local regulations of the Ethics Committee of the University of Muenster, Germany, as this study meets the criteria of § 6 health data protection law NRW.

Data Availability Statement: Not applicable.

Conflicts of Interest: The authors declare no conflict of interest.

References

1. Wu, H.; De Boer, J.F.; Chen, T.C. Diagnostic capability of spectral-domain optical coherence tomography for glaucoma. *Am. J. Ophthalmol.* **2012**, *153*, 815–826. [CrossRef] [PubMed]
2. Ghasia, F.F.; El-Dairi, M.; Freedman, S.F.; Rajani, A.; Asrani, S. Reproducibility of spectral-domain optical coherence tomography measurements in adult and pediatric glaucoma. *J. Glaucoma* **2015**, *24*, 55–63. [CrossRef] [PubMed]
3. Lee, S.H.; Kim, S.H.; Kim, T.W.; Park, K.H.; Kim, D.M. Reproducibility of retinal nerve fiber thickness measurements using the test-retest function of spectral OCT/SLO in normal and glaucomatous eyes. *J. Glaucoma* **2010**, *19*, 637–642. [CrossRef]
4. Hood, D.C.; Raza, A.S.; de Moraes, C.G.; Liebmann, J.M.; Ritch, R. Glaucomatous damage of the macula. *Prog. Retin. Eye Res.* **2013**, *32*, 1–21. [CrossRef]
5. Na, J.H.; Sung, K.R.; Baek, S.; Kim, Y.J.; Durbin, M.K.; Lee, H.J.; Kim, H.K.; Sohn, Y.H. Detection of glaucoma progression by assessment of segmented macular thickness data obtained using spectral domain optical coherence tomography. *Investig. Ophthalmol. Vis. Sci.* **2012**, *53*, 3817–3826. [CrossRef]
6. Iverson, S.M.; Feuer, W.J.; Shi, W.; Greenfield, D.S. Advanced Imaging for Glaucoma Study Group. Frequency of abnormal retinal nerve fibre layer and ganglion cell layer SDOCT scans in healthy eyes and glaucoma suspects in a prospective longitudinal study. *Br. J. Ophthalmol.* **2014**, *98*, 920–925. [CrossRef] [PubMed]
7. Gardiner, S.K.; Boey, P.Y.; Yang, H.; Fortune, B.; Burgoyne, C.F.; Demirel, S. Structural Measurements for Monitoring Change in Glaucoma: Comparing Retinal Nerve Fiber Layer Thickness with Minimum Rim Width and Area. *Investig. Ophthalmol. Vis. Sci.* **2015**, *56*, 6886–6891. [CrossRef]
8. Schild, A.M.; Ristau, T.; Fricke, J.; Neugebauer, A.; Kirchhof, B.; Sadda, S.R.; Liakopoulos, S. SDOCT thickness measurements of various retinal layers in patients with autosomal dominant optic atrophy due to OPA1 mutations. *Biomed. Res. Int.* **2013**, *2013*, 121398. [CrossRef]
9. Jonas, J.B.; Schmidt, A.M.; Müller-Bergh, J.A.; Schlötzer-Schrehardt, U.M.; Naumann, G.O. Human optic nerve fiber count and optic disc size. *Investig. Ophthalmol. Vis. Sci.* **1992**, *33*, 2012–2018.
10. Seo, S.; Lee, C.E.; Jeong, J.H.; Park, K.H.; Kim, D.M.; Jeoung, J.W. Ganglion cell-inner plexiform layer and retinal nerve fiber layer thickness according to myopia and optic disc area: A quantitative and three-dimensional analysis. *BMC Ophthalmol.* **2017**, *17*, 22. [CrossRef]
11. Savini, G.; Zanini, M.; Carelli, V.; Sadun, A.A.; Ross-Cisneros, F.N.; Barboni, P. Correlation between retinal nerve fibre layer thickness and optic nerve head size: An optical coherence tomography study. *Br. J. Ophthalmol.* **2005**, *89*, 489–492. [CrossRef] [PubMed]
12. Resch, H.; Deak, G.; Vass, C. Influence of optic-disc size on parameters of retinal nerve fibre analysis as measured using GDx VCC and ECC in healthy subjects. *Br. J. Ophthalmol.* **2010**, *94*, 424–427. [CrossRef] [PubMed]
13. Huang, D.; Chopra, V.; Lu, A.T.; Tan, O.; Francis, B.; Varma, R. Advanced Imaging for Glaucoma Study-AIGS Group: Does optic nerve head size variation affect circumpapillary retinal nerve fiber layer thickness measurement by optical coherence tomography? *Investig. Ophthalmol. Vis. Sci.* **2012**, *53*, 4990–4997. [CrossRef]
14. Arnold, A.C. Pathogenesis of nonarteritic anterior ischemic optic neuropathy. *J. Neuroophthalmol.* **2003**, *23*, 157–163. [CrossRef] [PubMed]
15. Cazana, I.M.; Böhringer, D.; Reinhard, T.; Evers, C.; Engesser, D.; Anton, A.; Lübke, J. A comparison of optic disc area measured by confocal scanning laser tomography versus Bruch's membrane opening area measured using optical coherence tomography. *BMC Ophthalmol.* **2021**, *21*, 31. [CrossRef]

16. Enders, P.; Adler, W.; Schaub, F.; Hermann, M.M.; Dietlein, T.; Cursiefen, C.; Heindl, L.M. Novel Bruch's Membrane Opening Minimum Rim Area Equalizes Disc Size Dependency and Offers High Diagnostic Power for Glaucoma. *Investig. Ophthalmol. Vis. Sci.* **2016**, *57*, 6596–6603. [CrossRef]
17. Reis, A.S.; Sharpe, G.P.; Yang, H.; Nicolela, M.T.; Burgoyne, C.F.; Chauhan, B.C. Optic disc margin anatomy in patients with glaucoma and normal controls with spectral domain optical coherence tomography. *Ophthalmology* **2012**, *119*, 738–747. [CrossRef]
18. Rosner, B.; Glynn, R.J. Interval estimation for rank correlation coefficients based on the probit transformation with extension to measurement error correction of correlated ranked data. *Stat. Med.* **2007**, *26*, 633–646. [CrossRef]
19. Rosner, B.; Glynn, R.J.; Lee, M.L. Extension of the rank sum test for clustered data: Two-group comparisons with group membership defined at the subunit level. *Biometrics* **2006**, *62*, 1251–1259. [CrossRef]
20. Jiang, Y.; Lee, M.-L.T.; He, X.; Rosner, B.; Yan, J. Wilcoxon Rank-Based Tests for Clustered Data with R Package clusrank. *J. Stat. Softw.* **2020**, *96*, 1–26. [CrossRef]
21. R Core Team. *R: A Language and Environment for Statistical Computing*; R Foundation for Statistical Computing: Vienna, Austria, 2013. Available online: https://www.R-project.org/ (accessed on 5 October 2021).
22. Wickham, H. *ggplot2: Elegant Graphics for Data Analysis*; Springer: New York, NY, USA, 2016. Available online: https://ggplot2.tidyverse.org/ (accessed on 5 October 2022).
23. Mahmoudinezhad, G.; Mohammadzadeh, V.; Martinyan, J.; Edalati, K.; Zhou, B.; Yalzadeh, D.; Amini, N.; Caprioli, J.; Nouri-Mahdavi, K. Comparison of Ganglion Cell Layer and Ganglion Cell/Inner Plexiform Layer Measures for Detection of Early Glaucoma. *Ophthalmol. Glaucoma* **2023**, *6*, 58–67. [CrossRef]
24. Peng, P.H.; Lin, H.S. Retinal nerve fiber layer thickness measured by optical coherence tomography in non-glaucomatous Taiwanese. *J. Formos. Med. Assoc.* **2008**, *107*, 627–634. [CrossRef] [PubMed]
25. Jun, J.H.; Lee, S.Y. The effects of optic disc factors on retinal nerve fiber layer thickness measurement in children. *Korean J. Ophthalmol.* **2008**, *22*, 115–122. [CrossRef] [PubMed]
26. Kampougeris, G.; Spyropoulos, D.; Mitropoulou, A.; Zografou, A.; Kosmides, P. Peripapillary retinal nerve fibre layer thickness measurement with SD-OCT in normal and glaucomatous eyes: Distribution and correlation with age. *Int. J. Ophthalmol.* **2013**, *6*, 662–665. [CrossRef]
27. Yoo, Y.C.; Lee, C.M.; Park, J.H. Changes in peripapillary retinal nerve fiber layer distribution by axial length. *Optom. Vis. Sci.* **2012**, *89*, 4–11. [CrossRef]
28. Leung, C.K.; Mohamed, S.; Leung, K.S.; Cheung, C.Y.; Chan, S.L.; Cheng, D.K.; Lee, A.K.; Leung, G.Y.; Rao, S.K.; Lam, D.S. Retinal nerve fiber layer measurements in myopia: An optical coherence tomography study. *Investig. Ophthalmol. Vis. Sci.* **2006**, *47*, 5171–5176. [CrossRef] [PubMed]
29. Kang, S.H.; Hong, S.W.; Im, S.K.; Lee, S.H.; Ahn, M.D. Effect of myopia on the thickness of the retinal nerve fiber layer measured by Cirrus HD optical coherence tomography. *Investig. Ophthalmol. Vis. Sci.* **2010**, *51*, 4075–4083. [CrossRef]
30. Rauscher, F.M.; Sekhon, N.; Feuer, W.J.; Budenz, D.L. Myopia affects retinal nerve fiber layer measurements as determined by optical coherence tomography. *J. Glaucoma* **2009**, *18*, 501–505. [CrossRef]
31. Alasil, T.; Wang, K.; Keane, P.A.; Lee, H.; Baniasadi, N.; de Boer, J.F.; Chen, T.C. Analysis of normal retinal nerve fiber layer thickness by age, sex, and race using spectral domain optical coherence tomography. *J. Glaucoma* **2013**, *22*, 532–541. [CrossRef]
32. Invernizzi, A.; Pellegrini, M.; Acquistapace, A.; Benatti, E.; Erba, S.; Cozzi, M.; Cigada, M.; Viola, F.; Gillies, M.; Staurenghi, G. Normative Data for Retinal-Layer Thickness Maps Generated by Spectral-Domain OCT in a White Population. *Ophthalmol. Retin.* **2018**, *2*, 808.e1–815.e1. [CrossRef]
33. Koh, V.T.; Tham, Y.C.; Cheung, C.Y.; Wong, W.L.; Baskaran, M.; Saw, S.M.; Wong, T.Y.; Aung, T. Determinants of ganglion cell-inner plexiform layer thickness measured by high-definition optical coherence tomography. *Investig. Ophthalmol. Vis. Sci.* **2012**, *53*, 5853–5859. [CrossRef] [PubMed]
34. Littmann, H. Determination of the real size of an object on the fundus of the living eye. *Klinische Monatsblatter fur Augenheilkunde* **1982**, *180*, 286–289. [CrossRef] [PubMed]
35. Crowston, J.G.; Hopley, C.R.; Healey, P.R.; Lee, A.; Mitchell, P. Blue Mountains Eye Study. The effect of optic disc diameter on vertical cup to disc ratio percentiles in a population based cohort: The Blue Mountains Eye Study. *Br. J. Ophthalmol.* **2004**, *88*, 766–770. [CrossRef]
36. Jonas, J.B.; Gusek, G.C.; Naumann, G.O. Optic disc, cup and neuroretinal rim size, configuration and correlations in normal eyes. *Investig. Ophthalmol. Vis. Sci.* **1988**, *29*, 1151–1158.
37. Lee, E.J.; Lee, K.M.; Kim, H.; Kim, T.W. Glaucoma Diagnostic Ability of the New Circumpapillary Retinal Nerve Fiber Layer Thickness Analysis Based on Bruch's Membrane Opening. *Investig. Ophthalmol. Vis. Sci.* **2016**, *57*, 4194–4204. [CrossRef] [PubMed]
38. Scheuble, P.; Petrak, M.; Brinkmann, C.K. Glaucoma Diagnostic Testing: The Influence of Optic Disc Size. *Klinische Monatsblatter fur Augenheilkunde* **2022**, *239*, 1043–1051. [CrossRef]
39. Palazon-Cabanes, A.; Palazon-Cabanes, B.; Rubio-Velazquez, E.; Lopez-Bernal, M.D.; Garcia-Medina, J.J.; Villegas-Perez, M.P. Normative Database for All Retinal Layer Thicknesses Using SD-OCT Posterior Pole Algorithm and the Effects of Age, Gender and Axial Lenght. *J. Clin. Med.* **2020**, *9*, 3317. [CrossRef] [PubMed]
40. Ooto, S.; Hangai, M.; Tomidokoro, A.; Saito, H.; Araie, M.; Otani, T.; Kishi, S.; Matsushita, K.; Maeda, N.; Shirakashi, M.; et al. Effects of age, sex, and axial length on the three-dimensional profile of normal macular layer structures. *Investig. Ophthalmol. Vis. Sci.* **2011**, *52*, 8769–8779. [CrossRef]

41. Najeeb, S.; Ganne, P.; Damagatla, M.; Chaitanya, G.; Krishnappa, N.C. Mapping the thickness of retinal layers using Spectralis spectral domain optical coherence tomography in Indian eyes. *Indian J. Ophthalmol.* **2022**, *70*, 2990–2997. [CrossRef]
42. Choovuthayakorn, J.; Chokesuwattanaskul, S.; Phinyo, P.; Hansapinyo, L.; Pathanapitoon, K.; Chaikitmongkol, V.; Watanachai, N.; Kunavisarut, P.; Patikulsila, D. Reference Database of Inner Retinal Layer Thickness and Thickness Asymmetry in Healthy Thai Adults as Measured by the Spectralis Spectral-Domain Optical Coherence Tomography. *Ophthalmic Res.* **2022**, *65*, 668–677. [CrossRef]
43. Sung, M.S.; Heo, M.Y.; Heo, H.; Park, S.W. Bruch's membrane opening enlargement and its implication on the myopic optic nerve head. *Sci. Rep.* **2019**, *9*, 19564. [CrossRef] [PubMed]
44. Budenz, D.L.; Anderson, D.R.; Varma, R.; Schuman, J.; Cantor, L.; Savell, J.; Greenfield, D.S.; Patella, V.M.; Quigley, H.A.; Tielsch, J. Determinants of normal retinal nerve fiber layer thickness measured by Stratus OCT. *Ophthalmology* **2007**, *114*, 1046–1052. [CrossRef] [PubMed]
45. Ward, D.D.; Mauschitz, M.M.; Bönniger, M.M.; Merten, N.; Finger, R.P.; Breteler, M.M.B. Association of retinal layer measurements and adult cognitive function: A population-based study. *Neurology* **2020**, *95*, e1144–e1152. [CrossRef] [PubMed]
46. Xu, X.; Xiao, H.; Lai, K.; Guo, X.; Luo, J.; Liu, X. Determinants of macular ganglion cell-inner plexiform layer thickness in normal Chinese adults. *BMC Ophthalmol.* **2021**, *21*, 267. [CrossRef] [PubMed]

Disclaimer/Publisher's Note: The statements, opinions and data contained in all publications are solely those of the individual author(s) and contributor(s) and not of MDPI and/or the editor(s). MDPI and/or the editor(s) disclaim responsibility for any injury to people or property resulting from any ideas, methods, instructions or products referred to in the content.

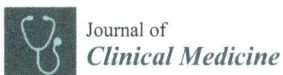

Article

Multimodal Imaging Based Predictors for the Development of Choroidal Neovascularization in Patients with Central Serous Chorioretinopathy

Sonny Caplash [1,*], Thamolwan Surakiatchanukul [2], Supriya Arora [3], Dmitrii S. Maltsev [4], Sumit Randhir Singh [5], Niroj Kumar Sahoo [6], Deepika Parameshwarappa [6], Alexei N. Kulikov [4], Claudio Iovino [7], Filippo Tatti [7], Ramkailash Gujar [8], Ramesh Venkatesh [9], Nikitha Gurram Reddy [9], Ram Snehith [9], Enrico Peiretti [7], Marco Lupidi [8] and Jay Chhablani [1]

[1] Department of Ophthalmology, University of Pittsburgh Medical Center, 203 Lothrop Street, Pittsburgh, PA 15213, USA
[2] Department of Ophthalmology, Jamaica Hospital Medical Center, 8900 Van Wyck Expy, New York Medical College, New York, NY 11418, USA
[3] Princess Margaret Hospital, 3MF7+P9G, Shirley St, Nassau P.O. Box N-3730, Bahamas
[4] Department of Ophthalmology, Military Medical Academy, 194044 St. Petersburg, Russia
[5] Scheie Eye Institute, 51 N 39th St, Philadelphia, PA 19104, USA
[6] LV Prasad Eye Institute, Kode Venkatadri Chowdary Campus, Penamaluru Rd, Tadigadapa, Vijayawada 521134, India
[7] Department of Surgical Sciences, Eye Clinic, University of Cagliari, Via Università, 40, 09124 Cagliari, Italy
[8] Department of Ophthalmology, University of Perugia, S. Maria della Misericordia Hospital, Piazza Università, 1, 06156 Perugia, Italy
[9] Department of Retina and Vitreous, Narayana Nethralaya Foundation, 1st Main, Binnamangala, Defence Colony, 100 Feet Road, Bengaluru 560099, India
* Correspondence: sonnycaplash@gmail.com

Abstract: This study evaluated predictors for choroidal neovascularization (CNV) associated with central serous chorioretinopathy (CSCR) based on multimodal imaging. A retrospective multicenter chart review was conducted on 134 eyes of 132 consecutive patients with CSCR. Eyes were classified as per the multimodal imaging-based classification of CSCR at baseline into simple/complex CSCR and primary episode/recurrent/resolved CSCR. Baseline characteristics of CNV and predictors were evaluated with ANOVA. In 134 eyes with CSCR, 32.8% had CNV (n = 44) with 72.7% having complex CSCR (n = 32), 22.7% having simple (n = 10) and 4.5% having atypical (n = 2). Primary CSCR with CNV were older (58 vs. 47, p = 0.00003), with worse visual acuity (0.56 vs. 0.75, p = 0.01) and of longer duration (median 7 vs. 1, p = 0.0002) than those without CNV. Similarly, recurrent CSCR with CNV were older (61 vs. 52, p = 0.004) than those without CNV. Patients with complex CSCR were 2.72 times more likely to have CNV than patients with simple CSCR. In conclusion, CNV associated with CSCR was more likely in complex CSCR and older age of presentation. Both primary and recurrent CSCR are implicated in CNV development. Patients with complex CSCR were 2.72 times more likely to have CNV than patients with simple CSCR. Multimodal imaging-based classification of CSCR supports detailed analysis of associated CNV.

Keywords: central serous chorioretinopathy (CSCR); central serous; choroidal neovascularization; multimodal imaging; central serous chorioretinopathy

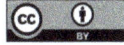

1. Introduction

First described by von Graefe in 1866, central serous chorioretinopathy (CSCR) is a disease characterized by a serous neurosensory retinal detachment due to choriocapillaris leakage [1–4]. The vast majority of cases of CSCR resolve spontaneously, usually within 3 to 6 months [5–7]. However, there is a minority of patients that progress to chronic

CSCR, which is often complicated by progressive retinal pigment epithelium (RPE) atrophy, bullous retinal detachment, and choroidal neovascularization (CNV). These sequelae (particularly CNV) offer a poor visual prognosis for patients. Conventionally, the incidence of CNV was estimated to be from 2–18% [7,8]. Investigations examining chronic CSCR patients found that roughly one-third will go on to develop CNV [9,10]. The advent of optical coherence tomography angiography (OCTA) has demonstrated an incidence closer to 30% [11]. This is likely due to the increased sensitivity and specificity of OCTA relative to fluorescein angiography and its overall convenience as a non-invasive imaging modality [11,12].

OCTA alone, however, may not be sufficient in detecting all cases of CNV in patients with CSCR [13]. Multimodal imaging often serves as the most comprehensive approach in detecting and characterizing neovascularization in patients with CSCR. The pathophysiologic mechanism for the development of CNV in patients with CSCR is postulated to involve decompensation of the RPE with subsequent disruption of Bruch's membrane; reminiscent of the proposed mechanism in age-related macular degeneration (ARMD) [4,11,14–16]. Previously, CNV associated with CSCR has been characterized broadly as a downstream sequela of the disease, with the assumption that all CNV associated with CSCR are similar in their presentation, prognosis, and effective treatment. Some studies have investigated long-term outcomes in patients with CSCR, finding that the majority of patients develop a Type I CNVM, with roughly 69 to 80% requiring either anti-VEGF or PDT [17–19].

Our group has recently published a revised classification that functions to standardize the terminology surrounding CSCR, allowing for more nuanced explorations into the diagnosis, management, and prognosis of the disease [16]. Our classification begins with classifying cases as simple, complex, and atypical based principally on RPE morphology. Simple and complex are differentiated by a size threshold of 2-disc diameters of clinically detectable retinal pigment epitheliopathy. Atypical cases served to include those cases of CSCR in which other retinal pathologies were also present as well as bullous CSCR. In order to further standardize the time course of CSCR, simple and complex cases were further reclassified, based on clinical course, as primary, recurrent, or resolved, and subsequently qualified as a persistent subtype [20].

Given the poor visual prognosis of patients with CSCR complicated by neovascularization, it is of particular clinical interest to stratify the risk of CNV development in patients with CSCR [4,5,7,14]. The purpose of this investigation is to establish the incidence of CNV development in relation to our recently described classification system and treatment outcome at one-year follow up for CNV associated with CSCR based on multimodal imaging

2. Materials and Methods

This was a retrospective, multicenter study on patients with a known diagnosis of CSCR. The study adhered to the tenets of the Declaration of Helsinki and ethical clearance was obtained by the Institutional Review Board. Informed consent was obtained from all patients.

Retrospective data were gathered from the Departments of Ophthalmology across multiple centers in the U.S., Italy, India, and Russia from 2015–2020. The charts of all patients with a diagnosis of CSCR were evaluated. Subsequent inclusion criteria were imposed, including (i) availability of demographic, clinical and reliable treatment details; (ii) availability of good quality multimodal imaging including fundus autofluorescence (FAF), spectral domain optical coherence tomography (SD OCT) (B scan), and OCTA or fundus fluorescein angiography (FFA) with indocyanine angiography (ICGA). Importantly, image quality on OCT and OCTA must have exceeded a signal strength of 7/10. With regard to angiographic imaging, patients must have had a full sequence of early, middle, and late phases without motion or lid artifacts. Exclusion criteria included were (i) any other retinal disease such as ARMD or any other cause of macular neovascularization, and (ii) poor quality imaging as discussed earlier.

Baseline data collected from patients included age, sex, best corrected visual acuity (BCVA), duration of complaints, reliable history of any previous such episodes, previous retinal treatment, or steroid use.

FAF, fundus photographs, FFA, and ICGA were obtained from Spectralis HRA + OCT (Heidelberg Engineering, Heidelberg, Germany) or F-10 scanning laser ophthalmoscope (NIDEK, Gamagori, Japan). OCTA examinations were performed with the RTVue-XR Avanti (Optovue, Fremont, CA, USA) or Spectralis HRA + OCT. For each eye, horizontal raster pattern scan through the center of the macula was obtained. OCTA examination including a 6 × 6 mm (2 orthogonal volumes with 400 × 400 A scans) pattern centered in the center of the fovea was performed with RTVue-XR Avanti.

Double blind classification was performed by two retinal experts [SA and DM] as per the new multimodal imaging-based classification system of CSCR. In cases of non-consensus, senior investigator (JC) was consulted. All images were made available by SC for all graders with images deidentified and randomly assigned by numeric generator to either expert. Eyes were classified as per the multimodal imaging-based classification of CSCR at baseline into (i) simple/complex CSCR, (ii) primary episode/recurrent/resolved CSCR, (iii) persistent SRF (>6 months) or not, (iv) outer retinal atrophy (ORA) presence or absence, (v) foveal involvement presence or absence, (vi) CNV presence or absence. Representative cases of simple and complex CSCR are illustrated in Figures 1 and 2, respectively.

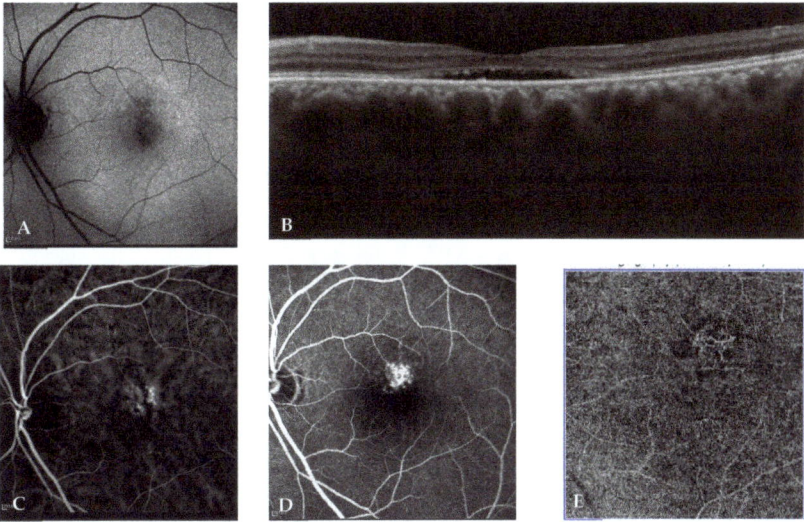

Figure 1. Eye of a 52-year-old male with a visual acuity of 20/20 and metamorphopsia for 4 months (**A**) shows <1–2 DD of RPE abnormality (simple CSCR) (**B**) OCT (B scan) passing through the fovea shows subretinal fluid along with flat irregular pigment epithelium detachment suspicious of CNV (**C**), (**D**,**E**) show ICG-A, FA and OCTA, respectively, all of which confirm the choroidal neovascular complex.

All patients selected by the above criteria were classified as previously published by our group [20]. Parameters evaluated at baseline, 3 months, 6 months, and 12 months included BCVA, subfoveal choroidal thickness (SFCT), and central macular thickness (CMT). Presence of CNV and treatment instituted for each of the above time intervals was also noted. Statistical analysis, including baseline characteristics of CNV and predictors, were evaluated with one-way analysis of variance (ANOVA), chi-square test, and odds ratio calculation via Microsoft Excel.

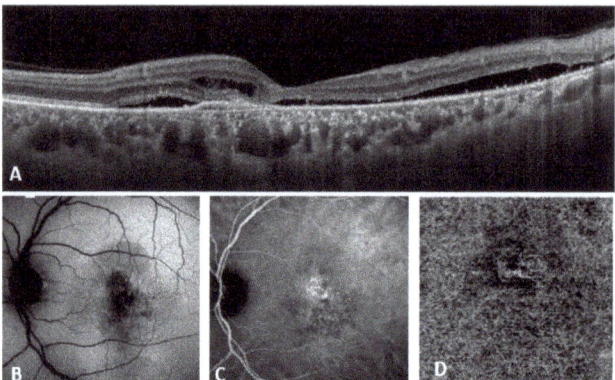

Figure 2. Eye of a 47-year-old male with a visual acuity of 20/320 and duration of complaints for 2 years. (**A**) OCT (B scan) passing through the fovea shows intraretinal and subretinal fluid along with flat irregular pigment epithelium detachment, suspicious for likely CNV. (**B**) Demonstrates > 2 DD area of RPE abnormality (Complex CSCR). (**C,D**) show corresponding ICG-A and OCTA, respectively, that confirm the choroidal neovascular complex in the outer retina and choriocapillaris slab.

3. Results

Included in this analysis were 134 eyes from 132 patients with six eyes having non-consensus requiring consultation of senior investigator JC. The median age of patients was 48 years (range: 23–67). There was a strong male gender predisposition with 84.6% being male. Seven eyes had previous histories of treatment at presentation: five eyes with focal laser, one eye with photodynamic therapy (PDT), and one patient on Eplerenone.

Of the 134 eyes with CSCR, CNV was present in 32.8% (n = 44), and demographic data for this group is summarized in Table 1. Of all patients with CNV, 15% were detected primarily by OCT-A, though ICG-A and FA showed suspicious lesions. Of the 44 patients with CNV, 32 had complex CSCR (72.7%), 10 had simple CSCR (22.7%), and 2 had atypical CSCR (4.5%). Demographic breakdown and visual acuity per each CSCR subtype in patients with CNV is summarized in Table 2. Among the 90 patients without CNV, 50 had simple CSCR (55.6%) and 40 had complex CSCR (44.4%). There was no statistically significant difference in the prevalence of simple CSCR between patients with CNV and those without (p = 0.08). Patients with complex CSCR were 2.72 times more likely to have CNV than patients with simple CSCR (95% CI 1.199 to 6.166; p = 0.016). Table 3 summarizes the incidence of CNV among CSCR subtypes.

Table 1. Choroidal Neovascularization in Central Serous Chorioretinopathy: Initial Presentation (N = 44).

Feature	Cases (%)
Age, years Mean (median, range, 95% CI)	59 (58, 40–82, 37–81)
Age distribution <45 45–60 60–75 >75	 4 (9) 22 (50) 16 (36) 2 (5)
Gender Male Female	 37 (84) 7 (16)
Visual acuity (decimal) Mean (median, range)	0.54 (0.50, 0.06–1.20)

Table 2. Demographics of CNV and Non-CNV in Central Serous Chorioretinopathy: Multimodal Imaging-Based Classification: Simple, Complex vs. Atypical.

	Simple		Complex		Atypical	
	Non CNV (N = 50)	CNV (N = 10)	Non CNV (N = 40)	CNV (N = 32)	Non CNV (N = 0)	CNV (N = 2)
Mean Age, years (N)	47	59	49	59		53
Median (range)	47 (23–67)	56 (45–77)	49 (32–67)	59 (40–82)		53 (48–58)
Age distribution (%)						
<45	21 (42)	0	12 (30)	4 (13)		
45–60	22 (44)	6 (60)	20 (50)	14 (44)		2 (100)
60–75	7 (14)	3 (30)	8 (20)	13 (41)		
>75	0	1 (10)	0	1 (2)		
Gender (%)						
Male	35 (70)	8 (80)	38	27 (84)		2 (100)
Female	15 (30)	2 (20)	2	5 (16)		
Mean Visual acuity (decimal)	0.73	0.72	0.67	0.49		0.5
Median (range)	0.80 (0.03–1.20)	0.67 (0.30–1.20)	0.70 (0.06–1.20)	0.50 (0.06–1.00)		0.50 (0.33–0.66)

Table 3. Incidence of CNV among CSCR sub-types (% of total patients).

	Primary	Recurrent	Resolved	Total
Simple	6 (12%)	4 (50%)	0	10 (17%)
Complex	13 (36%)	15 (48%)	4 (100%)	32 (43%)
Atypical	1 (100%)	1 (100%)	0	2 (100%)
Total	20 (22%)	20 (50%)	4 (100%)	44 (33%)

Patients with simple CSCR with CNV had better baseline BCVA than those with complex CSCR (0.72 vs. 0.49, $p = 0.03$) without differences in age (mean 59 vs. 59 years, $p = 0.76$), SFCT 393 vs. 390 μm, ($p = 0.997$), and reported duration of symptoms (median 6 vs. 18 weeks, $p = 0.38$).

Based on presentation, there was an equal incidence of CNV in both primary and recurrent cases ($n = 20$, 45.5% each) with the remainder of CNV found in resolved cases (9.1%, $n = 4$). Data is summarized in Table 4. There was no age-related, statistically significant difference between primary, recurrent, and resolved cohorts, with the mean age being 58 ± 10.8, 61 ± 9.8, and 62 ± 10.8, respectively ($p = 0.27$). BCVA was also not statistically significantly different among primary, recurrent, and resolved cases of CSCR with mean BCVA Snellen equivalent(logMAR) of 20/73 (0.56, standard deviation [SD] 0.29), 20/63 (0.50, SD 0.31) and 20/89 (0.65, SD 0.33), respectively ($p = 0.66$). Demographic and visual acuity data are summarized in Table 3. SFCT did not differ among these cohort as well with their mean values as $414 \pm SD$, $383 \pm SD$, and $329 \pm SD$ μ, respectively ($p = 0.55$). Differences in overall duration among the three cohorts were not statistically significant with median values of 7 and 30 months, respectively ($p = 0.42$). A summary of duration in months across various sub-groups is listed in Table 5.

In comparing patients with primary CSCR with CNV to those without CNV, the mean age was 58 years (SD 10 years) as compared to 47 years (SD 10 years) with a p-value of 0.00003. The mean BCVA logMAR (Snellen fraction) was 0.75 (20/112) as compared to 0.56 (20/73) with a p-value of 0.01. The average duration was 7 months as compared to 1 month ($p − 0.0002$).

Table 4. Demographics of CNV and Non-CNV in Central Serous Chorioretinopathy: Onset Status Multimodal Imaging-Based Classification: Primary and Recurrent vs. Resolved.

	Primary		Recurrent		Resolved	
	Non CNV (N = 69)	CNV (N = 20)	Non CNV (N = 20)	CNV (N = 20)	Non CNV (N = 1)	CNV (N = 4)
Mean Age, years	47	58	52	61	69	52
Median (range)	47 (23–67)	57 (44–77)	50 (39–65)	59 (42–82)	69	50 (40–67)
Age distribution (%)						
<45	33 (48)	1 (5)	2 (10)	1 (5)		2 (50)
45–60	29 (42)	11 (55)	12 (60)	10 (50)		1 (25)
60–75	8 (11)	7 (35)	6 (30)	8 (40)	1 (100)	1 (25)
>75	0	1 (5)	0	1 (5)		0 (0)
Gender (%)						
Male	55 (80)	15 (75)	20 (100)	17 (85)	1 (100)	4 (100)
Female	14 (20)	5 (25)		3 (15)		0 (0)
Mean Visual acuity (decimal)	0.75	0.56	0.61	0.5	0.0625	0.65
Median (range)	0.80 (0.03–1.20)	0.60 (0.10–1.00)	0.56 (0.10–1.20)	0.50 (0.06–1.20)	0.0625	0.68 (0.25–1.00)

Table 5. Median Duration in Months of Central Serous Chorioretinopathy per Classification and presence of CNV (N).

		Primary	Recurrent	Resolved
Simple	Non-CNV	1 (31)	1.5 (4)	
	CNV	7 (5)	4 (3)	
Complex	Non-CNV	4 (15)	60 (4)	
	CNV	12 (7)	7 (4)	30 (2)
Atypical	Non-CNV			144 (1)
	CNV	2 (1)	7 (1)	

When comparing patients with recurrent CSCR with CNV to those without, there was no statistically significant difference in mean logMAR BCVA (0.50 vs. 0.61, $p = 0.31$), duration (median 7 vs. 2 months, $p = 0.32$), and mean SFCT (383 ± 75 vs. 424 ± 85 μm, $p = 0.21$). An exception to this trend of similarity between the two groups is in the mean age of presentation, which was 60.7-years-old in patients with recurrent CSCR with CNV and 52-years-old in recurrent CSCR patients without CNV ($p = 0.003$).

Forty-three out of the forty-four patients with CNV had foveal involvement, compared to the eighty-five out of ninety patients without CNV, which was not statistically significant ($p = 0.38$). In comparing foveal involvement between patients with CNV and patients without CNV, there was no statistically significant difference. Regarding ORA, among all CSCR patients with CNV, 36 (78%) had ORA as opposed to 29 (32%) among CSCR patients without CNV ($p < 0.01$).

4. Discussion

Our investigation yields several key risk factors for the development of CNV in patients with CSCR. Patients with complex CSCR were at a significantly higher risk for CNV with an odds ratio of 2.72. In both primary and recurrent CSCR, there was a significant difference in age of presentation when comparing patients that developed CNV with those who did not. Specifically, in both primary and complex CSCR, older patients were more likely to develop CNV. Our data also intuitively demonstrate that primary CSCR patients with CNV are predisposed to longer courses when compared to patients without CNV. The relative higher incidence of CNV in patients with primary CSCR compared to prior published data implies that a lower threshold should exist for use of OCTA or FA to evaluate for CNV in CSCR patients with SRF on initial presentation. Counterintuitively, our data did not support statistically significant differences in duration of disease course between primary, recurrent and atypical CSCR. This finding supports the idea that recurrence functions as a secondary measure more so than a primary prognostic measure.

The positive correlation between age upon presentation and the incidence of CNV can serve as an important determinant of pre-test probability for the development of CNV when evaluating patients with CSCR on initial work-up. These findings are in line with other studies of CSCR which found older patients with higher incidence of CNV and worse visual acuity [7,21].

Multimodal imaging-based classification provides objective approach to associate disease severity with CNV formation and progression. More broadly, increased CNV in patients with complex CSCR when taken in conjunction with our findings of increased ORA in patients with CNV, reinforce the notion of complex CSCR as retinal pigment epitheliopathy. The co-occurrence of ORA with CNV has been validated by other groups as well [22]. The importance of the association between CNV and complex CSCR has several important implications beyond elucidation of underlying pathophysiology. In the affected eye, CNV has been shown previously to be associated with cystoid macular degeneration, a marker of progressive CSCR damage [15]. Given that CSCR has been frequently demonstrated to progress to bilateral disease, it is reasonable that in patients with unilateral neovascular CSCR, there is a risk of CNV secondary to CSCR in the fellow eye. Previously published work by our group has shown that the fellow eye in patients with unilateral CSCR complicated by CNV can have early signs of neovascularization as detected by OCTA [14].

CSCR often takes an uncomplicated, self-resolving course, however, in patients in which this does not occur, morbidity and visual prognosis can be poor. Our data point towards a model of CSCR management in which early classification can allow for appropriate risk stratification with regard to the development of CNV and consequently appropriate screening via multi-modal imaging. The rise of OCTA, taken together with ICGA, FFA, and OCT allow for a layered approach to the early diagnosis of CNV in both the affected eye and the fellow eye, with early treatment mitigating complications of long-standing CSCR such as cystoid macular degeneration.

While our study provides nuance to the progression and prognosis of patients with CNV, it is limited by a relatively small sample size and retrospective nature. Studies of CSCR are often limited by the relatively low incidence. Our study's retrospective nature precludes an ability to assess patients at a long-term follow-up. This can create bias in the data towards patients that may develop CNV later in their course. Additionally, while efforts were made to ensure randomization of patient images for classification, the retrospective nature of this study provides an inherent limitation to the completeness of randomization. It is also important to note that CSCR with CNV is often confounded by the presence of pachychoroid neovasculopathy; this element may confound interpretation of patient presentation.

The investigation and subsequent data presented tie our previously published classification system to objective, discrete outcomes in patients with CSCR, specifically, the development of CNV. Age upon presentation and complex CSCR phenotype serve as early prognostic indicators to the development of CNV and consequently poorer visual outcomes. The importance of these findings is their purported role in driving more targeted treatment for patients with CSCR. Further studies will be conducted to prospectively evaluate patients' treatment response and to further explore the relative distribution of different types of CNV across different CSCR classifications.

Author Contributions: For conceptualization, S.C., J.C. and T.S. For data curation, resources and methodology, S.A., D.S.M., S.R.S., N.K.S., D.P., A.N.K., C.I., F.T., R.G., R.V., N.G.R., R.S., E.P. and M.L. For data analysis, S.C., J.C. and T.S. For Writing—original draft S.C. For writing—review and editing S.C., J.C. and S.A. All authors have read and agreed to the published version of the manuscript.

Funding: This research received no external funding.

Institutional Review Board Statement: Not applicable.

Informed Consent Statement: Informed consent was obtained from all subjects involved in the study.

Data Availability Statement: Not applicable.

Conflicts of Interest: The authors declare no conflict of interest.

References

1. Zhao, M.; Celerier, I.; Bousquet, E.; Jeanny, J.C.; Jonet, L.; Savoldelli, M.; Offret, O.; Curan, A.; Farman, N.; Jaisser, F.; et al. Mineralocorticoid receptor is involved in rat and human ocular chorioretinopathy. *J. Clin. Investig.* **2012**, *122*, 2672–2679. [CrossRef]
2. Michael, J.C.; Pak, J.; Pulido, J.; de Venecia, G. Central serous chorioretinopathy associated with administration of sympathomimetic agents. *Am. J. Ophthalmol.* **2003**, *136*, 182–185. [CrossRef]
3. Reiner, A.; Fitzgerald, M.E.C.; Del Mar, N.; Li, C. Neural control of choroidal blood flow. *Prog. Retin. Eye Res.* **2018**, *64*, 96–130. [CrossRef]
4. Chhablani, J. *Central Serous Chorioretinopathy*; Academic Press: Cambridge, MA, USA, 2019; p. 662.
5. Liegl, R.; Ulbig, M.W. Central serous chorioretinopathy. *Ophthalmologica* **2014**, *232*, 65–76. [CrossRef]
6. Wang, M.; Munch, I.C.; Hasler, P.W.; Prunte, C.; Larsen, M. Central serous chorioretinopathy. *Acta Ophthalmol.* **2008**, *86*, 126–145. [CrossRef]
7. Spaide, R.F.; Campeas, L.; Haas, A.; Yannuzzi, L.A.; Fisher, Y.L.; Guyer, D.R.; Slakter, J.S.; Sorenson, J.A.; Orlock, D.A. Central serous chorioretinopathy in younger and older adults. *Ophthalmology* **1996**, *103*, 2070–2080. [CrossRef]
8. Loo, R.H.; Scott, I.U.; Flynn, H.W., Jr.; Gass, J.D.; Murray, T.G.; Lewis, M.L.; Rosenfeld, P.J.; Smiddy, W.E. Factors associated with reduced visual acuity during long-term follow-up of patients with idiopathic central serous chorioretinopathy. *Retina* **2002**, *22*, 19–24. [CrossRef] [PubMed]
9. Savastano, M.C.; Rispoli, M.; Lumbroso, B. The Incidence of Neovascularization in Central Serous Chorioretinopathy by Optical Coherence Tomography Angiography. *Retina* **2021**, *41*, 302–308. [CrossRef] [PubMed]
10. Sulzbacher, F.; Schutze, C.; Burgmuller, M.; Vecsei-Marlovits, P.V.; Weingessel, B. Clinical evaluation of neovascular and non-neovascular chronic central serous chorioretinopathy (CSC) diagnosed by swept source optical coherence tomography angiography (SS OCTA). *Graefes Arch. Clin. Exp. Ophthalmol.* **2019**, *257*, 1581–1590. [CrossRef]
11. Bonini Filho, M.A.; de Carlo, T.E.; Ferrara, D.; Adhi, M.; Baumal, C.R.; Witkin, A.J.; Reichel, E.; Duker, J.S.; Waheed, N.K. Association of Choroidal Neovascularization and Central Serous Chorioretinopathy With Optical Coherence Tomography Angiography. *JAMA Ophthalmol.* **2015**, *133*, 899–906. [CrossRef] [PubMed]
12. Bansal, R.; Dogra, M.; Mulkutkar, S.; Katoch, D.; Singh, R.; Gupta, V.; Dogra, M.R.; Gupta, A. Optical coherence tomography angiography versus fluorescein angiography in diagnosing choroidal neovascularization in chronic central serous chorioretinopathy. *Indian J. Ophthalmol.* **2019**, *67*, 1095–1100. [CrossRef] [PubMed]
13. Ng, D.S.; Ho, M.; Chen, L.J.; Yip, F.L.; Teh, W.M.; Zhou, L.; Mohamed, S.; Tsang, C.W.; Brelen, M.E.; Chen, H.; et al. Optical Coherence Tomography Angiography Compared with Multimodal Imaging for Diagnosing Neovascular Central Serous Chorioretinopathy. *Am. J. Ophthalmol.* **2021**, *232*, 70–82. [CrossRef]
14. Mandadi, S.K.R.; Singh, S.R.; Sahoo, N.K.; Mishra, S.B.; Sacconi, R.; Iovino, C.; Berger, L.; Munk, M.R.; Querques, G.; Peiretti, E.; et al. Optical coherence tomography angiography findings in fellow eyes of choroidal neovascularisation associated with central serous chorioretinopathy. *Br. J. Ophthalmol.* **2021**, *105*, 1280–1285. [CrossRef] [PubMed]
15. Sahoo, N.K.; Mishra, S.B.; Iovino, C.; Singh, S.R.; Munk, M.R.; Berger, L.; Peiretti, E.; Chhablani, J. Optical coherence tomography angiography findings in cystoid macular degeneration associated with central serous chorioretinopathy. *Br. J. Ophthalmol.* **2019**, *103*, 1615–1618. [CrossRef]
16. Chhablani, J.; Cohen, F.B.; Aymard, P.; Beydoun, T.; Bousquet, E.; Daruich-Matet, A.; Zweifel, S. Multimodal Imaging-Based Central Serous Chorioretinopathy Classification. *Ophthalmol. Retin.* **2020**, *4*, 1043–1046. [CrossRef] [PubMed]
17. Hagag, A.M.; Chandra, S.; Khalid, H.; Lamin, A.; Keane, P.A.; Lotery, A.J.; Sivaprasad, S. Multimodal Imaging in the Management of Choroidal Neovascularization Secondary to Central Serous Chorioretinopathy. *J. Clin. Med.* **2020**, *9*, 1934. [CrossRef]
18. Moussa, M.; Leila, M.; Khalid, H.; Lolah, M. Detection of Silent Type I Choroidal Neovascular Membrane in Chronic Central Serous Chorioretinopathy Using En Face Swept-Source Optical Coherence Tomography Angiography. *J. Ophthalmol.* **2017**, *2017*, 6913980. [CrossRef] [PubMed]
19. Kim, R.Y.; Ma, G.J.; Park, W.K.; Kim, M.; Park, Y.G.; Park, Y.H. Clinical course after the onset of choroidal neovascularization in eyes with central serous chorioretinopathy. *Medicine* **2021**, *100*, e26980. [CrossRef]
20. Arora, S.; Kulikov, A.N.; Maltsev, D.S. Implementation of the new multimodal imaging-based classification of central serous chorioretinopathy. *Eur. J. Ophthalmol.* **2021**, *32*, 1044–1049. [CrossRef]

21. Zhou, X.; Komuku, Y.; Araki, T.; Terasaki, H.; Miki, A.; Kuwayama, S.; Nishi, T.; Kinoshita, T.; Gomi, F. Risk factors and characteristics of central serous chorioretinopathy with later development of macular neovascularisation detected on OCT angiography: A retrospective multicentre observational study. *BMJ Open Ophthalmol.* **2022**, *7*, e000976. [CrossRef]
22. Borrelli, E.; Battista, M.; Sacconi, R.; Gelormini, F.; Querques, L.; Grosso, D.; Vella, G.; Bandello, F.; Querques, G. OCT Risk Factors for 3-Year Development of Macular Complications in Eyes With "Resolved" Chronic Central Serous Chorioretinopathy. *Am. J. Ophthalmol.* **2021**, *223*, 129–139. [CrossRef] [PubMed]

Disclaimer/Publisher's Note: The statements, opinions and data contained in all publications are solely those of the individual author(s) and contributor(s) and not of MDPI and/or the editor(s). MDPI and/or the editor(s) disclaim responsibility for any injury to people or property resulting from any ideas, methods, instructions or products referred to in the content.

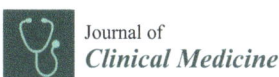

Article

Optical Coherence Tomography Angiography in *CRB1*-Associated Retinal Dystrophies

Firuzeh Rajabian [1], Alessandro Arrigo [1,*], Lorenzo Bianco [1], Alessio Antropoli [1], Maria Pia Manitto [1], Elisabetta Martina [1], Francesco Bandello [1], Jay Chhablani [2] and Maurizio Battaglia Parodi [1]

[1] Department of Ophthalmology, Vita-Salute San Raffaele University, IRCCS Ospedale San Raffaele, 20132 Milan, Italy
[2] Department of Ophthalmology, University of Pittsburgh School of Medicine, Pittsburgh, PA 15213, USA
* Correspondence: alessandro.arrigo@hotmail.com; Tel.: +39-0226432648

Abstract: Aim of the study: To report optical coherence tomography angiography (OCTA) findings in patients affected by *CRB1*-associated retinal dystrophies. Method: Patients affected by a genetically confirmed *CRB1*-associated retinal dystrophy were prospectively enrolled in an observational study, along with age- and sex-matched healthy volunteers as control subjects. All study and control subjects received a complete ophthalmic examination and multimodal retinal imaging, including OCTA. Result: A total of 12 eyes from 6 patients were included in the study. The mean BCVA of patients was 0.42 ± 0.25 logMAR. Two patients showed large central atrophy, with corresponding definite hypo-autofluorescence on fundus autofluorescence (FAF). Another four patients disclosed different degrees of RPE mottling, with uneven FAF. On OCTA, the macular deep capillary plexus and choriocapillaris had a lower vessel density in eyes affected by *CRB1*-associated retinopathy when compared to healthy controls. On the other hand, vessel density at the peripapillary radial capillary plexus, superficial capillary plexus, and deep capillary plexus was significantly altered with respect to control eyes. Statistical analyses disclosed a negative correlation between the deep capillary plexus and both LogMAR best corrected visual acuity and central retinal thickness. Conclusion: Our study reveals that *CRB1*-associated retinal dystrophies are characterized by vascular alterations both in the macular and peripapillary region, as assessed by OCTA.

Keywords: *CRB1*; crumbs homolog 1; retinal dystrophy; optical coherence tomography angiography; OCTA; multimodal imaging

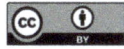

1. Introduction

CRB1-associated retinal dystrophy is a rare inherited disease (IRD) characterized by variable phenotypic manifestations, ranging from retinitis pigmentosa and Leber congenital amaurosis to isolated macular dystrophies [1–5]. While a recent study suggested that the more severe and early-onset forms of retinal degeneration are associated with null variants [6], a previous meta-analysis suggested that the different phenotype of patients with *CRB1* variants is possibly influenced by additional modifying factors rather than being determined by specific allelic combinations [7]. The degree of visual impairment is highly dependent on the specific phenotype—low vision in individuals with Leber congenital amaurosis and retinitis pigmentosa is reached in the second and fourth decade of life, respectively [8], while patients with macular dystrophy retain a relatively good visual function until adult age in at least one eye [6]. Optical coherence tomography (OCT) features of *CRB1*-associated retinal dystrophies have been extensively described and include abnormal retinal lamination, macular cystoid changes, and increased retinal nerve fiber layer thickness, and [6,9–11].

Optical coherence tomography angiography (OCTA) has been used in several IRDs to characterize the vascular anatomy in the macula and to identify vascular patterns associated with a faster progression. In particular, a reduction in vessel density at the level of the deep capillary plexus (DCP) has been described in several IRDs, including Stargardt disease [12], cone dystrophies [13], Best vitelliform macular dystrophy [14], X-linked retinoschisis [15], choroideremia [16], occult macular dystrophy [17], congenital stationary night-blindness [18], retinitis pigmentosa [19,20], and Bietti crystalline dystrophy [21]. This study aimed to describe the OCTA features in eyes affected by *CRB1*-associated retinal dystrophies, as no prior study has explored the vascular alterations in these disorders.

2. Methods

This cross-sectional case series included patients affected by an IRD related to a mono- or biallelic *CRB1* variant, detected by means of next-generation sequencing. A group of healthy age- and sex-matched control subjects was also enrolled. The study adhered to the tenets of the Declaration of Helsinki and was approved by the Institutional Review Board (MIRD2020) of IRCCS San Raffaele Hospital. Written informed consent was obtained from all the subjects included in the study.

The patients underwent an ophthalmological examination, complete with best corrected visual acuity (BCVA) measurement using standard ETDRS charts, slit-lamp examination, and multimodal retinal imaging. The standard imaging protocol included color photography, spectral-domain optical coherence tomography (OCT), and blue-light autofluorescence (FAF) (Spectralis HRA+OCT, Heidelberg Engineering, Heidelberg, Germany). Optical coherence tomography angiography (OCTA) (SS-DRI OCT Triton, Topcon, Tokyo, Japan) scans were of 4.5×4.5 mm volumes, acquired both in the macula and optic nerve head. Only high-quality images, assessed by Topcon image quality index ($\geq$70) [2], were considered.

In order to obtain macular and peripapillary vessel density (VD) measures, automatic segmentation of all vascular plexuses was first obtained from native OCTA acquisitions on ImageNet6 software; segmentations were manually corrected by an expert ophthalmologist (FR). Reconstructions of the superficial capillary plexus (SCP), deep capillary plexus (DCP), and choriocapillaris (CC), as well as the radial peripapillary capillary (RPC) plexus in optic nerve head scans, were then exported from the instrument in the .tiff format and imported into ImageJ software Version 1.53h (National Institutes of Health, Bethesda, MD, USA). All images were binarized using a mean threshold, to reduce the noise and highlight the blood vessels. Then, the white region was considered as the vascular area, and its number of pixels was quantified and expressed as a percentage over the total after exclusion of the foveal avascular zone (i.e., the VD parameter). Macular parameters will be referred to by means of the prefix "m", whereas the ones related to the optic nerve head with "n" (e.g., mSCP and nSCP for macular and peripapillary SCP, respectively) [22].

An unpaired two-tailed t-test (SPSS; Chicago, IL, USA) was used to compare the quantitative parameters among affected and control eyes. Correlations were assessed by means of the Pearson correlation coefficient. Statistical significance was set at $p \leq 0.05$.

3. Results

Overall, a total of 6 patients (12 eyes) affected by a genetically confirmed *CRB1*-associated retinal dystrophy were recruited, with ages ranging between 10 and 67 years (mean age 36.4 ± 25.7 years) and a mean BCVA of 0.4 ± 0.25 logMAR (Table 1). The control group consisted of six age- and sex-matched healthy volunteers.

Table 1. Clinical and imaging characteristics of patients affected by CRB1-associated retinal dystrophies.

	Gender	BCVA (logMAR)	CRT (μm)	SFCT (μm)	CRB1 Variants
Patient 1	M	0.4	173	465	c.772_779delinsG; c.498_506del
		0.4	163	340	
Patient 2	M	0	223	274	c.498_506del
		0.3	210	285	
Patient 3	M	0.2	220	239	c.1584C>A; c.498_506del
		0.3	158	251	
Patient 4	F	0.2	189	74	c.614T>C
		0.7	29	56	
Patient 5	M	0.7	151	290	c.2549G>T; c.4176_4177delAA
		0.7	131	238	
Patient 6	F	0.4	178	276	c.614T>C
		0.8	110	280	

Legend—For each patient, the first row refers to the right eye. Abbreviations—best corrected visual acuity (BCVA), central retinal thickness (CRT), subfoveal choroidal thickness (SFCT).

Anterior segment examination revealed no alteration in all patients. Two patients showed a large central atrophy, with corresponding definite hypo-autofluorescence on FAF. Another four patients disclosed different degrees of RPE mottling, with uneven FAF response. In all cases lesions turned out to be symmetrical between the two eyes of the same patient.

Central retinal thickness (CRT) was lower in CRB1 patients compared to control eyes (164 ± 56.7 vs. $256 + 45$ μm), while subfoveal choroidal thickness (SFCT) was similar (250 ± 95 vs. 251 ± 118 μm). Considering macular vascular plexa, OCTA detected an almost preserved VD at SCP ($p > 0.05$) while this was significantly reduced at DCP and CC ($p < 0.05$). At the level of the optic nerve head, VD at RCP, SCP, and DCP were significantly lower than control eyes ($p < 0.05$) (Table 2). Significant negative correlations were found between VD at macular DCP and both LogMAR BCVA ($r = -0.71$; $p < 0.001$) and CRT ($r = -0.62$; $p < 0.001$). The OCTA imaging in two cases of CRB1-associated retinal dystrophy is reported in Figures 1 and 2.

Table 2. Vessel density analysis at individual vascular plexa in CRB1-associated retinal dystrophy and control eyes.

	mSCP	mDCP	mCC	nRCP	nSCP	nDCP	nCC
CRB1	0.405 ± 0.013	0.360 ± 0.031	0.482 ± 0.014	0.398 ± 0.024	0.395 ± 0.037	0.305 ± 0.038	0.513 ± 0.042
Controls	0.413 ± 0.012	0.434 ± 0.005	0.500 ± 0.006	0.443 ± 0.007	0.426 ± 0.010	0.402 ± 0.019	0.542 ± 0.031
p-value	0.13352	4.46×10^{-9} *	0.000138 *	4.71×10^{-7} *	0.005277 *	1.70×10^{-8} *	0.060817

Legend—Data are presented as mean value and SD; * = p-value < 0.05; macular superficial capillary plexus (mSCP), macular deep capillary plexus (mDCP), macular choriocapillaris (mCC), nerve radial capillary plexus (nRCP), nerve superficial capillary plexus (nSCP), nerve deep capillary plexus (nDCP), nerve choriocapillaris (nCC).

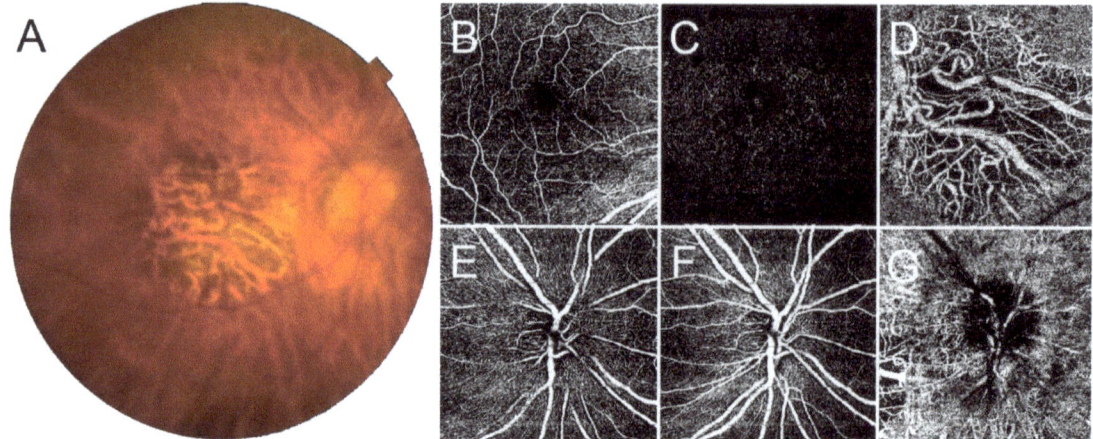

Figure 1. Optical coherence tomography angiography (OCTA) findings in *CRB1*-associated retinal dystrophy presenting with macular atrophy. Color fundus photography (**A**) shows complete atrophy of the macular region. Here, OCTA detects a partially spared superficial capillary plexus (**B**), markedly disrupted deep capillary plexus (**C**), and completely absent choriocapillaris (**D**) in the macula. At the level of the optic nerve head, it is possible to observe a loss of the radial peripapillary capillary plexus (**E**), together with a rarefied superficial and deep capillary plexus (**F**), while the choriocapillaris appears preserved (**G**).

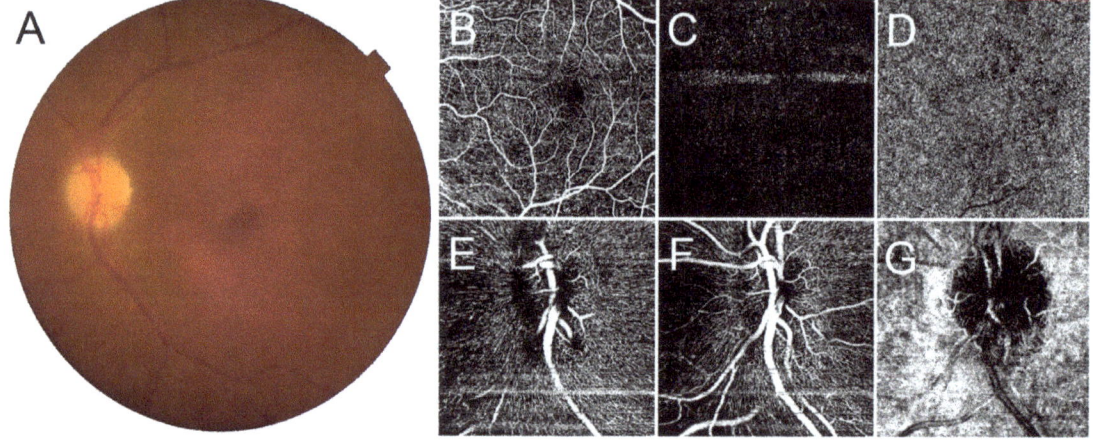

Figure 2. Optical coherence tomography angiography (OCTA) findings in *CRB1*-associated retinal dystrophy presenting with macular mottling. Color fundus photography (**A**) is characterized by macular pigmentary alterations in absence of clear atrophy. In the macula, OCTA detects a spared superficial capillary plexus (**B**), markedly disrupted deep capillary plexus (**C**), and choriocapillaris flow voids (**D**). At the level of the optic nerve head, the radial peripapillary capillary plexus appears rarefied (**E**), together with the involvement of the superficial and deep capillary plexus (**F**), while the choriocapillaris appears preserved (**G**).

4. Discussion

In the present study, we describe OCTA findings in six patients affected by genetically confirmed *CRB1*-associated retinal dystrophy. The OCTA examination indicates that this IRD is characterized by an extensive rarefaction of intraretinal vasculature and CC. In more detail, we detected a VD reduction at the level of DCP and CC in the macula, and at the level of RCP, SCP, and DCP in the peripapillary region. Our data are based on simple cross-sectional analyses, making it difficult to tell whether the vascular impairment is primary feature or, instead, a secondary phenomenon due to degenerative changes in the photoreceptor-RPE and inner retinal layers. However, it should be noted that *CRB1* variants been described in association with Coats-like exudative vasculopathy both in Leber congenital amaurosis and retinitis pigmentosa [23–25].

The CRB1 (Crumbs homologue 1) protein belongs to the CRB complex, which functions in the maintenance of apical–basal cell polarity and the formation of adherent junctions between cells [26]. As the *CRB1* gene in the human retina is expressed in Muller glial microvilli and photoreceptor cells but is absent in retinal pigment epithelium and choroid tissue [27,28], we believe that the vascular rarefaction detected within the macular region likely represents a secondary effect. However, significant rarefaction of intraretinal vasculature was also identified in the peripapillary region, and the interpretation of this latter finding may be related to a diffuse dysregulation of the retinal neurovascular unit, which is composed of neuronal cells, intraretinal vessels, and *CRB1*-expressing Muller cells [29]. Interestingly, the severity of the vessel density reduction was similar across the different phenotypical manifestations, which ranged from mere RPE mottling up to large atrophic changes, suggesting that this peripapillary vascular impairment is independent of the stage of the disease. Even though the comparison of the OCTA findings described in other IRDs is hard due to the different pathogenesis of each subform, we have to underline that DCP is always involved, often also showing a correlation with BCVA [12–21]. Thus, DCP may represent an important biomarker to better characterize the stage of the disease and the extent of functional damage.

We are aware that our case series has a number of limitations, including, first of all, the scant number of patients and the inclusion of both eyes in the analysis. Nevertheless, *CRB1*-associated retinal dystrophy is a rare condition. Moreover, the different phenotypic manifestations and the different stages could be characterized by variable vascular alterations. Multicenter studies with a longitudinal follow-up should be designed to collect a high number of patients affected by *CRB1*-associated retinal dystrophy to ascertain the natural history evolution, investigating the correlation between dystrophy severity and vascular damage. In addition, quantitative analysis of OCTA images in the setting of IRDs is hindered by the inherent difficulty of segmenting individual vascular plexuses, especially in the presence of extensive atrophy or severely altered retinal lamination [22]. Lastly, we cannot exclude that the phenotype and pattern of vascular impairment that we observed our cohort could have been modified by allelic variants in other genes related to IRDs.

In essence, our study highlights that *CRB1*-associated retinal dystrophy is characterized by vascular alterations on OCTA both in the macula and peripapillary region. Further investigations are warranted to confirm our results and the relationship between the severity of clinical phenotype and the extent of vascular damage. This knowledge could eventually provide new insights on the pathogenesis of this IRD, as well as useful criteria for patient selection in future gene therapy trials.

Author Contributions: Methodology, F.R. and A.A. (Alessandro Arrigo); Investigation, E.M.; Data curation, M.P.M.; Writing—review & editing, J.C.; Supervision, L.B., F.B. and M.B.P.; Project administration, A.A. (Alessio Antropoli). All authors have read and agreed to the published version of the manuscript.

Funding: This research received no external funding.

Institutional Review Board Statement: The study was conducted in accordance with the Declaration of Helsinki, and approved by the Institutional Review Board of IRCCS San Raffaele Hospital (MIRD2020).

Informed Consent Statement: Informed consent was obtained from all subjects involved in the study.

Data Availability Statement: The data presented in this study are available on request from the corresponding author. The data are not publicly available due to ethical restrictions.

Conflicts of Interest: The authors declare no conflict of interest.

References

1. Hollander, A.I.D.; Brink, J.B.T.; de Kok, Y.J.; van Soest, S.; Born, L.I.V.D.; van Driel, M.A.; van de Pol, D.J.; Payne, A.M.; Bhattacharya, S.S.; Kellner, U.; et al. Mutations in a human homologue of Drosophila crumbs cause retinitis pigmentosa (RP12). *Nat. Genet.* **1999**, *23*, 217–221. [CrossRef]
2. Khan, K.N.; Robson, A.; Mahroo, O.A.R.; Arno, G.; Inglehearn, C.F.; Armengol, M.; Waseem, N.; Holder, G.E.; Carss, K.J.; Raymond, L.F.; et al. A clinical and molecular characterisation of CRB1-associated maculopathy. *Eur. J. Hum. Genet.* **2018**, *26*, 687–694. [CrossRef]
3. Roshandel, D.; Thompson, J.A.; Jeffery, R.C.H.; Sampson, D.M.; Chelva, E.; McLaren, T.L.; Lamey, T.M.; De Roach, J.N.; Durkin, S.R.; Chen, F.K. Multimodal Retinal Imaging and Microperimetry Reveal a Novel Phenotype and Potential Trial End Points in *CRB1*-Associated Retinopathies. *Transl. Vis. Sci. Technol.* **2021**, *10*, 38. [CrossRef] [PubMed]
4. Henderson, R.H.H.; Mackay, D.; Li, Z.; Moradi, P.; Sergouniotis, P.; Russell-Eggitt, I.; Thompson, D.; Robson, A.; Holder, G.E.; Webster, A.R.; et al. Phenotypic variability in patients with retinal dystrophies due to mutations in CRB1. *Br. J. Ophthalmol.* **2010**, *95*, 811–817. [CrossRef] [PubMed]
5. Wang, Y.; Sun, W.; Xiao, X.; Li, S.; Jia, X.; Wang, P.; Zhang, Q. Clinical and Genetic Analysis of 63 Families Demonstrating Early and Advanced Characteristic Fundus as the Signature of CRB1 Mutations. *Am. J. Ophthalmol.* **2021**, *223*, 160–168. [CrossRef]
6. Varela, M.D.; Georgiou, M.; Alswaiti, Y.; Kabbani, J.; Fujinami, K.; Fujinami-Yokokawa, Y.; Khoda, S.; Mahroo, O.A.; Robson, A.G.; Webster, A.R.; et al. CRB1-Associated Retinal Dystrophies: Genetics, Clinical Characteristics, and Natural History. *Am. J. Ophthalmol.* **2022**, *246*, 107–121. [CrossRef]
7. Bujakowska, K.; Audo, I.; Mohand-Saïd, S.; Lancelot, M.-E.; Antonio, A.; Germain, A.; Léveillard, T.; Letexier, M.; Saraiva, J.-P.; Lonjou, C.; et al. *CRB1* mutations in inherited retinal dystrophies. *Hum. Mutat.* **2011**, *33*, 306–315. [CrossRef] [PubMed]
8. Talib, M.; Van Cauwenbergh, C.; De Zaeytijd, J.; Van Wynsberghe, D.; De Baere, E.; Boon, C.J.F.; Leroy, B.P. *CRB1*-associated retinal dystrophies in a Belgian cohort: Genetic characteristics and long-term clinical follow-up. *Br. J. Ophthalmol.* **2021**, *106*, 696–704. [CrossRef]
9. Jacobson, S.G.; Cideciyan, A.V.; Aleman, T.S.; Pianta, M.; Sumaroka, A.; Schwartz, S.B.; Smilko, E.E.; Milam, A.H.; Sheffield, V.; Stone, E.M. Crumbs homolog 1 (CRB1) mutations result in a thick human retina with abnormal lamination. *Hum. Mol. Genet.* **2003**, *12*, 1073–1078. [CrossRef]
10. Talib, M.; van Schooneveld, M.J.; van Genderen, M.M.; Wijnholds, J.; Florijn, R.J.; Brink, J.B.T.; Schalij-Delfos, N.E.; Dagnelie, G.; Cremers, F.P.; Wolterbeek, R.; et al. Genotypic and Phenotypic Characteristics of CRB1 -Associated Retinal Dystrophies. *Ophthalmology* **2017**, *124*, 884–895. [CrossRef]
11. Mathijssen, I.B.; Florijn, R.J.; Born, L.I.V.D.; Zekveld-Vroon, R.C.; Brink, J.B.T.; Plomp, A.S.; Baas, F.; Meijers-Heijboer, H.; Bergen, A.A.B.; van Schooneveld, M.J. Long-Term Follow-Up of Patients with Retinitis Pigmentosa Type 12 Caused by Crb1 Mutations: A Severe Phenotype with Considerable Interindividual Variability. *Retina* **2017**, *37*, 161–172. [CrossRef]
12. Arrigo, A.; Romano, F.; Aragona, E.; di Nunzio, C.; Sperti, A.; Parodi, M.B. OCTA-Based Identification of Different Vascular Patterns in Stargardt Disease. *Transl. Vis. Sci. Technol.* **2019**, *8*, 26. [CrossRef]
13. Toto, L.; Parodi, M.B.; D'Aloisio, R.; Mercuri, S.; Senatore, A.; Di Antonio, L.; Di Marzio, G.; Di Nicola, M.; Mastropasqua, R. Cone Dystrophies: An Optical Coherence Tomography Angiography Study. *J. Clin. Med.* **2020**, *9*, 1500. [CrossRef]
14. Battaglia Parodi, M.; Romano, F.; Cicinelli, M.V.; Rabiolo, A.; Arrigo, A.; Pierro, L.; Iacono, P.; Bandello, F. Retinal Vascular Impairment in Best Vitelliform Macular Dystrophy Assessed by Means of Optical Coherence Tomography Angiography. *Am. J. Ophthalmol.* **2018**, *187*, 61–70. [CrossRef]
15. Mastropasqua, R.; Toto, L.; Di Antonio, L.; Parodi, M.B.; Sorino, L.; Antonucci, I.; Stuppia, L.; Di Nicola, M.; Mariotti, C. Optical Coherence Tomography Angiography Findings in X-Linked Retinoschisis. *Ophthalmic Surg. Lasers Imaging Retin.* **2018**, *49*, e20–e31. [CrossRef]
16. Arrigo, A.; Romano, F.; Parodi, M.B.; Issa, P.C.; Birtel, J.; Bandello, F.; MacLaren, R.E. Reduced vessel density in deep capillary plexus correlates with retinal layer thickness in choroideremia. *Br. J. Ophthalmol.* **2021**, *105*, 687–693. [CrossRef]
17. Bianco, L.; Arrigo, A.; Antropoli, A.; Carrera, P.; Spiga, I.; Patricelli, M.G.; Bandello, F.; Parodi, M.B. Multimodal imaging evaluation of occult macular dystrophy associated with a novel RP1L1 variant. *Am. J. Ophthalmol. Case Rep.* **2022**, *26*, 101550. [CrossRef]
18. Parodi, M.B.; Arrigo, A.; Rajabian, F.; Mansour, A.; Mercuri, S.; Starace, V.; Bordato, A.; Manitto, M.P.; Martina, E.; Bandello, F. Multimodal imaging in Schubert-Bornschein congenital stationary night blindness. *Ophthalmic Genet.* **2022**, 1–6. [CrossRef]
19. Arrigo, A.; Bordato, A.; Romano, F.; Aragona, E.; Grazioli, A.; Bandello, F.; Parodi, M.B. Choroidal Patterns in Retinitis Pigmentosa: Correlation with Visual Acuity and Disease Progression. *Transl. Vis. Sci. Technol.* **2020**, *9*, 17. [CrossRef]
20. Arrigo, A.; Romano, F.; Albertini, G.; Aragona, E.; Bandello, F.; Parodi, M.B. Vascular Patterns in Retinitis Pigmentosa on Swept-Source Optical Coherence Tomography Angiography. *J. Clin. Med.* **2019**, *8*, 1425. [CrossRef]

21. Montemagni, M.; Arrigo, A.; Parodi, M.B.; Bianco, L.; Antropoli, A.; Malegori, A.; Bandello, F.; Tranfa, F.; Costagliola, C. Optical coherence tomography angiography in Bietti crystalline dystrophy. *Eur. J. Ophthalmol.* **2022**. [CrossRef] [PubMed]
22. Arrigo, A.; Aragona, E.; Parodi, M.B.; Bandello, F. Quantitative approaches in multimodal fundus imaging: State of the art and future perspectives. *Prog. Retin. Eye Res.* **2023**, *92*, 101111. [CrossRef] [PubMed]
23. Hollander, A.I.D.; Heckenlively, J.R.; Born, L.I.V.D.; de Kok, Y.J.; van der Velde-Visser, S.D.; Kellner, U.; Jurklies, B.; van Schooneveld, M.J.; Blankenagel, A.; Rohrschneider, K.; et al. Leber Congenital Amaurosis and Retinitis Pigmentosa with Coats-like Exudative Vasculopathy Are Associated with Mutations in the Crumbs Homologue 1 (CRB1) Gene. *Am. J. Hum. Genet.* **2001**, *69*, 198–203. [CrossRef] [PubMed]
24. Magliyah, M.; Alshamrani, A.A.; Schatz, P.; Taskintuna, I.; Alzahrani, Y.; Nowilaty, S.R. Clinical spectrum, genetic associations and management outcomes of Coats-like exudative retinal vasculopathy in autosomal recessive retinitis pigmentosa. *Ophthalmic Genet.* **2021**, *42*, 178–185. [CrossRef]
25. Hasan, S.M.; Azmeh, A.; Mostafa, O.; Megarbane, A. Coat's like vasculopathy in leber congenital amaurosis secondary to homozygous mutations in CRB1: A case report and discussion of the management options. *BMC Res. Notes* **2016**, *9*, 91. [CrossRef] [PubMed]
26. Alves, H.A.; Pellissier, L.P.; Wijnholds, J. The CRB1 and adherens junction complex proteins in retinal development and maintenance. *Prog. Retin. Eye Res.* **2014**, *40*, 35–52. [CrossRef]
27. Den Hollander, A.I.; Ghiani, M.; de Kok, Y.J.; Wijnholds, J.; Ballabio, A.; Cremers, F.P.; Broccoli, V. Isolation of Crb1, a mouse homologue of Drosophila crumbs, and analysis of its expression pattern in eye and brain. *Mech Dev.* **2002**, *110*, 203–207. [CrossRef]
28. Ray, T.A.; Cochran, K.; Kozlowski, C.; Wang, J.; Alexander, G.; Cady, M.A.; Spencer, W.J.; Ruzycki, P.A.; Clark, B.S.; Laeremans, A.; et al. Comprehensive identification of mRNA isoforms reveals the diversity of neural cell-surface molecules with roles in retinal development and disease. *Nat. Commun.* **2020**, *11*, 3328. [CrossRef]
29. Mairot, K.; Smirnov, V.; Bocquet, B.; Labesse, G.; Arndt, C.; Defoort-Dhellemmes, S.; Zanlonghi, X.; Hamroun, D.; Denis, D.; Picot, M.-C.; et al. *CRB1*-Related Retinal Dystrophies in a Cohort of 50 Patients: A Reappraisal in the Light of Specific Müller Cell and Photoreceptor *CRB1* Isoforms. *Int. J. Mol. Sci.* **2021**, *22*, 12642. [CrossRef]

Disclaimer/Publisher's Note: The statements, opinions and data contained in all publications are solely those of the individual author(s) and contributor(s) and not of MDPI and/or the editor(s). MDPI and/or the editor(s) disclaim responsibility for any injury to people or property resulting from any ideas, methods, instructions or products referred to in the content.

Article

Deep Learning with a Dataset Created Using Kanno Saitama Macro, a Self-Made Automatic Foveal Avascular Zone Extraction Program

Junji Kanno [1], Takuhei Shoji [1,2,*], Hirokazu Ishii [1], Hisashi Ibuki [1], Yuji Yoshikawa [1], Takanori Sasaki [1] and Kei Shinoda [1]

1. Department of Ophthalmology, Saitama Medical University School of Medicine, Iruma 350-0495, Japan
2. Koedo Eye Institute, Kawagoe 350-1123, Japan
* Correspondence: shoojii@gmail.com; Tel.: +81-49-276-1250

Abstract: The extraction of the foveal avascular zone (FAZ) from optical coherence tomography angiography (OCTA) images has been used in many studies in recent years due to its association with various ophthalmic diseases. In this study, we investigated the utility of a dataset for deep learning created using Kanno Saitama Macro (KSM), a program that automatically extracts the FAZ using swept-source OCTA. The test data included 40 eyes of 20 healthy volunteers. For training and validation, we used 257 eyes from 257 patients. The FAZ of the retinal surface image was extracted using KSM, and a dataset for FAZ extraction was created. Based on that dataset, we conducted a training test using a typical U-Net. Two examiners manually extracted the FAZ of the test data, and the results were used as gold standards to compare the Jaccard coefficients between examiners, and between each examiner and the U-Net. The Jaccard coefficient was 0.931 between examiner 1 and examiner 2, 0.951 between examiner 1 and the U-Net, and 0.933 between examiner 2 and the U-Net. The Jaccard coefficients were significantly better between examiner 1 and the U-Net than between examiner 1 and examiner 2 ($p < 0.001$). These data indicated that the dataset generated by KSM was as good as, if not better than, the agreement between examiners using the manual method. KSM may contribute to reducing the burden of annotation in deep learning.

Keywords: foveal avascular zone; automatic extraction; manually extract; U-Net; annotation

1. Introduction

With the advent of optical coherence tomography angiography (OCTA), studies on the foveal avascular zone (FAZ) have been actively conducted and yielded various findings in healthy eyes [1], retinal vascular diseases (e.g., diabetic retinopathy and retinal vein occlusion) [2,3], vitreous interface lesions (e.g., epiretinal membrane and macular hole) [4,5], hereditary degenerative diseases (e.g., retinitis pigmentosa) [6], glaucoma [7] and others [8]. In these studies, the methods used to extract FAZ features included manual methods with tools for manual selection, conventional automatic methods executed by algorithms, and deep learning [9,10], which has attracted increasing attention in recent years. Although the manual method is considered the gold standard for examination because it enables more detailed extraction, it imposes a heavy burden on the examiner performing the extraction and does not guarantee reproducibility. Conventional automated methods were developed to overcome the problems associated with manual methods. These included analyses using the device's built-in software. For example, several studies have reportedly used Python, which is a programming language and MATLAB® (MathWorks) numerical analysis software, as well as ImageJ (https://imagej.nih.gov/ij, accessed on 8 February 2021), an image processing software distributed free of charge by the National Institutes of Health [11–14]. The advantage of these automated methods is that good-quality extraction can be obtained with a simple procedure. Previously, we also reported on automated extraction (Kanno Saitama Macro,

KSM) using ImageJ Macro [15]. The advantage of KSM is that it can facilitate extraction that closely approximates the manual method with extremely high reproducibility with one click of a button. Furthermore, automatic extraction with a deep learning technique known as semantic segmentation is being actively promoted for medical imaging research in other specialties [16–21]. Although this method enables the simultaneous extraction of a large number of images, it requires a vast dataset and tremendous labor for the creation of the dataset (i.e., annotation). The dataset used in semantic segmentation consists of images pertaining to the question and the correct answer. In FAZ extraction, the question is the OCTA image (original image) and the correct answer is the image (label image) showing only the FAZ area. Extracting FAZ from en face images obtained with OCTA has conventionally been done manually, requiring 50 to 100 plots per image, which requires an enormous amount of time. Therefore, we investigated whether a useful data set could be created using automated methods. We used the dataset we created for training and testing using a typical U-Net. We then compared the results with the manual method to determine the usefulness of the dataset.

Although automatic extraction using artificial intelligence (AI) on healthy and diseased eyes has been introduced [9,10], to our knowledge, there are no previous reports in deep learning for FAZ extraction that aimed to automatically create FAZ datasets. Thus, we propose a method to reduce the burden of annotation using the ImageJ macro. The purpose of this study was to examine the utility of the dataset created by KSM for FAZ extraction.

2. Materials and Methods

2.1. Study Population

This study was conducted according to the Declaration of Helsinki after obtaining approval from the Saitama Medical University Hospital Ethics Committee (No. 19079.01). The study sample included 40 healthy volunteers, aged 20 years and above, who provided written informed consent for participation in the study between October and December 2017. Participants underwent comprehensive ophthalmic examinations including visual acuity measurement, visual field testing, slit-lamp examination, non-contact tonometry (TONOREFRII, Nidek, Gamagori, Japan), fundus photography (CX-1, Canon, Tokyo, Japan), axial length and central corneal thickness measurement (Optical Biometer OA-2000, Tomey Corporation, Nagoya, Japan), static visual field testing (Humphrey field analyzer, Carl Zeiss Meditec, Jena, Germany), retinal nerve fiber layer analysis using spectral-domain OCT (SD-OCT, Spectralis®HRA2, Heidelberg Engineering, Heidelberg, Germany), and swept-source OCTA (SS-OCTA) photography (PLEX® Elite 9000, Carl Zeiss Meditec, Jena, Germany).

Patients with a spherical equivalent of +3 D or more or −6 D or less; axial length of 26 mm or more; suspected glaucomatous change in the visual field test, fundus photograph or retinal nerve fiber layer analysis; ocular diseases, such as diabetic retinopathy, macular disease, severe myopia, pseudoexfoliation; and those with a history of ocular surgery, were excluded. The training and validation data were obtained from each fellow eye of patients with unilateral ocular diseases (idiopathic macular hole, vitreomacular traction syndrome, glaucoma, central serous chorioretinopathy, idiopathic epiretinal membrane, and rhegmatogenous retinal detachment) who visited our clinic and underwent SS-OCTA imaging between February 2018 and September 2019. A total of 227 of 257 eyes (from 257 patients) were used to create the training dataset and the remaining 30 eyes were used to create the validation dataset. Only images with an OCTA signal strength of 8/10 or higher were incorporated into the dataset.

2.2. Optical Coherence Tomography Angiography

An image, measuring 3 mm × 3 mm, that was centered on the macula was acquired using SS-OCTA, with a central wavelength of 1060 nm and scanning speed of 100,000 A scan/s. Each 3 mm × 3 mm OCTA image consists of 300 pixels × 300 pixels, and is output as a 1024 pixels × 1024 pixels image. The algorithm for creating vascular signals uses optical microangiography, which measures changes in both phase and amplitude [22]. The original image used in this study was an en face image of the superficial retinal layer (SRL), defined as extending from the inner limiting membrane to the inner plexiform layer, constructed using the OCTA device's built-in segmentation software.

2.3. KSM (Modified Version) and Annotation Simplification

KSM is a method that utilizes the dilation-erosion [23] morphological process, which is usually used in multiple consecutive processes, such as opening and closing, and is effective for noise reduction and edge detection [24]. In KSM, the interruptions in the vascular signal are connected with successive dilations, and the FAZ region is reproduced with successive erosions. Moreover, KSM can be customized using various processes implemented in ImageJ, since KSM is part of the ImageJ Macro. We added noise processing and changed the area expansion value to 4 pixels because the previously-reported macro did not include noise processing and had a slightly narrower extraction area. Changing these settings ensured improvements in the extraction of uneven areas and the extraction of high-brightness images (Figure 1).

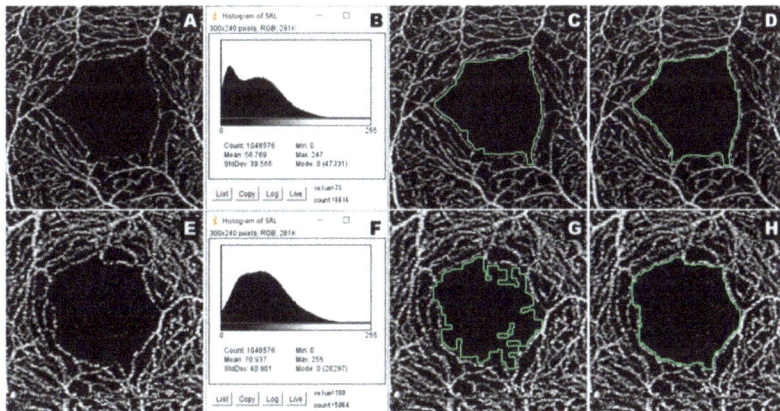

Figure 1. Effects of the change in KSM settings. A typical captured image (**A**) and its histogram (**B**). High-brightness images (**E**) and its histogram (**F**). Represent images extracted with the previously-reported settings (**C,G**), Represent images extracted after the settings were changed (**D,H**). PLEX® Elite 9000 can acquire images with high-brightness (**E**). The histogram (**F**) of an image with high-brightness is different from the histogram (**B**) of a typical captured image (**A**). The higher the brightness of the image, the stronger the influence of noise during region extraction, thus, resulting in poorer extraction (**G**). When noise processing is added, extraction can be improved, as (**H**) is better than (**G**). Moreover, noise processing can enhance the extraction quality for typical captured images, as (**D**) is better than (**C**). KSM: Kanno Saitama Macro.

The code of the setting change is presented below. (Please refer to Code S1: Modified KSM.)

(1) Noise processing

It was inserted in the first line of the previously-reported macro.
Run ("Bandpass Filter ... ", "filter_large = 1024 filter_small = 3.5 suppress = None tolerance = 5 process").

(2) Area expansion

The enlarged setting on the 9th line was changed to 4 pixels.
Run ("Enlarge ... ", "enlarge = 4 pixels").

Furthermore, since the previously-reported macro extracted images one-by-one, we created a macro to simplify the annotation process. In addition to the setting changes, the macro for continuous extraction was executed using the "stack" function that displays the

images in the folder in one window and the "region-of-interest (ROI) set" that specifies each slice.
(1) The interpolation processing setting was changed to "none" when enlarging/reducing the image.
(2) Extraction was performed with "analyze particles" instead of the wand tool and the size of the extraction area was specified.

In this study, continuous extraction was performed for every 5 images, and the ROI was saved after confirming the extraction. The procedure for dataset creation is as follows. (1) The FAZ was extracted. (2) The label image was created. (3) The label image was saved. The above-mentioned steps were repeated for the number of datasets. However, the repetition of these steps is monotonous and time-consuming even if the extraction is performed automatically. Therefore, each process was divided, and a macro of the process up to the saving step was created.

The annotation process is shown below. (Please refer to Code S2, Video S1: Annotation by Continuous Automatic Extraction).
(1) The folder containing the original image was loaded and displayed as a stack.
(2) The FAZ was extracted from all the original images using the continuous method for every 5 images using ROI sets that specified the slices and the ROI sets were saved.
(3) The entire window was selected and the "fill" command was used to suffuse all the original images with black (brightness value: 0). This image served as the background of the label image.
(4) The ROI set saved in step 2 was loaded. The ROI for each slice was specified and the images were filled with white (luminance value: 255) (completion of label image).
(5) The completed label images were saved one-by-one using the ROI sets specific to the slices.

The mechanism of label image creation is based on stack-based processing and extremely simple macros. Using this mechanism, dataset amplification can also be performed automatically using inversion and rotation. Creating training and validation datasets from 257 eyes, including the annotation process and FAZ extraction using KSM, required approximately 4 h—that is, approximately 1 min per eye.

Moreover, the dataset created in the above-mentioned process has a large image size of 1024 pixels × 1024 pixels, which was reduced to 512 pixels × 512 pixels to accommodate the deep learning networks. These were subsequently cropped to 256 pixels × 256 pixels.

2.4. Deep Learning Network

We used a typical U-Net for the semantic segmentation network [25]. The U-Net architecture is based on the fully convolutional neural network, which does not use fully-connected layers and allows images to be used as input and produces binary maps as output. As shown in Figure 2, the U-Net consists of a contracting (encoding) path and a symmetric expanding (decoding) path. In the contracting path, successive convolution layers are followed by pooling operations. In the expanding path, pooling operators are replaced by upsampling operators. The combination of the upsampled output and high-resolution features from the contracting path can supplement the information lost in the pooling process. The U-Net exhibits satisfactory performance in biomedical image segmentation because of its special structure [26]. This study used a 4-layered U-Net, binary cross entropy as the loss function, Adam [27] as the optimization algorithm, and binary accuracy as the evaluation function. Moreover, the environment was built using a graphics processing unit in Google Colaboratory Notebook. Python 3 was used as the programming language and Keras was used as the library.

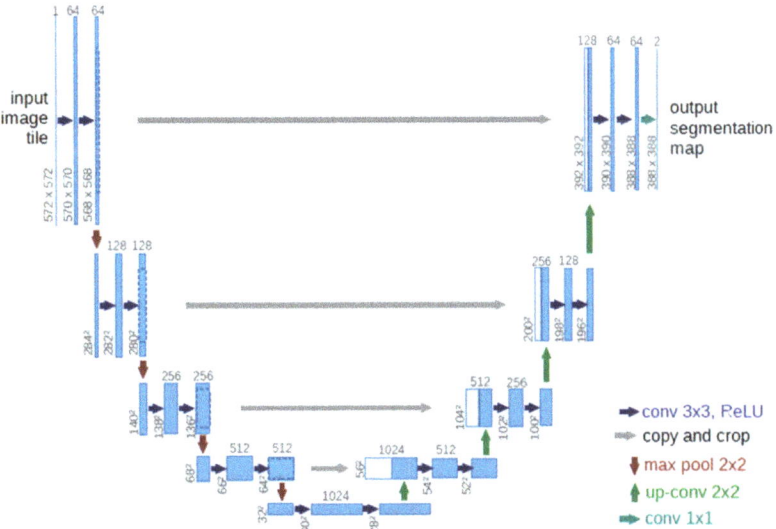

Figure 2. The U-Net architecture.

2.5. The FAZ Extraction Method

The 3 types and 4 methods of extraction used in this study are described below.

2.5.1. The Manual Method (Examiner 1 and Examiner 2)

The SRL image was imported into ImageJ. Subsequently, two examiners (H. Ibuki and H. Ishii) used the polygonal manual selection tool to trace the FAZ boundaries and save the ROI sets. An FAZ mask image was created using the above-mentioned method for the label image using the previously-obtained ROI sets.

2.5.2. The Conventional Automatic Method (ARI)

The Advanced Retina Imaging Zeiss Macular Algorithm (ARI; v 0.6.1) [15] is a prototype of Carl Zeiss's proprietary algorithm, which is available online and can be used to extract the FAZ in the SRL. Uploading an anonymized raw file to the ARI network portal causes an FAZ mask image, measuring 512 pixels × 512 pixels, to be downloaded in the Portable Network Graphics format.

2.5.3. Automatic Methods Using Deep Learning (U-Net)

The dataset created by KSM was used to train and test the U-Net. First, we performed several training sessions and adjusted the number of epochs to 20 and the batch size to 12. After setting the brightness of the output image to 0 for the background and 1 for the extraction area, training and testing were performed 5 times, and all the results were acquired. The extracted image obtained was captured in ImageJ, converted into an FAZ mask image, and compared with the mask image of the manual method. The images that possessed the best results in comparison with the manual method were used in this study.

2.6. Evaluation of the Extraction Accuracy

The FAZ mask image obtained by each method was imported into ImageJ and converted to the same size as the extracted image obtained by the U-Net. This was followed by the evaluation of the extraction accuracy using the following indices, with the manual method as the gold standard.

2.6.1. Coefficient of Variation and Correlation Coefficient of the Area

The area of the FAZ on the OCTA image was calculated using the correction formula of the magnification based on the axial length [28]. The area was quantified by inputting the measured values into a "set scale", followed by correction. The coefficient of variation (CV) and the correlation coefficient of the area obtained, were evaluated. CV was calculated from the mean and standard deviation of the area per subject between methods.

2.6.2. Measures of Similarity

The extraction accuracy is often evaluated using two measures of similarity [29,30]. However, since the evaluation differs due to the difference in the nature of the indices, both values were calculated. The similarity index evaluates the extraction target, extraction result, and the overlap between the two areas. Using the "image calculator," we calculated and quantified the intersection and union, and the false negative (FN) and false positive (FP), and evaluated the excess and deficiency of the extraction. The above-mentioned quantification was calculated from the number of pixels in each region.

Jaccard Similarity Coefficient

The Jaccard similarity coefficient (Jaccard index), [11,31] which is also called Intersection over Union, is calculated by dividing the intersection of two regions (extraction target: A, extraction result: B) by the union. The results are expressed as numerical values between 1.0 to 0.0, which are graded as follows: 0.4 or less, poor; 0.7, good; and 0.9 or more, excellent.

$$\text{Jaccard}(A, B) = \frac{A \cap B}{A \cup B}$$

Dice Similarity Coefficient

The Dice similarity coefficient [32,33] (DSC) is calculated by dividing the twice the value of intersection by the sum of the two regions. It is expressed as a numerical value between 1.0 to 0.0; the closer the value is to 1.0, the better the similarity. It is expressed as a higher value than the Jaccard coefficient due to the difference in the nature of the two indices.

$$\text{DSC}(A, B) = \frac{2(A \cap B)}{A \cup B}$$

2.7. Statistical Analysis

The participants' background variables were expressed as the median and interquartile range, and the FAZ area was expressed as the mean and standard deviation (SD). The CV, Jaccard coefficient, and DSC were represented as the mean and 95% confidence interval (CI). The FN and FP values were expressed as percentages (%).

We evaluated the extraction accuracy of the automatic method using the manual method as the gold standard, and also examined the accuracy between the manual methods. Nonparametric analysis was used for the obtained results since normality was rejected by the Shapiro-Wilk normality test. The area correlation coefficient was tested using Spearman's rank correlation coefficient, and each extraction method was compared using the Friedman and multiple comparison tests (Bonferroni). The FN and FP values were compared using the Wilcoxon signed rank sum test. A p-value of <0.05 was considered statistically significant. All statistical analyzes were performed using the R software (version 3.6.3; R Foundation for Statistical Computing, Vienna, Austria).

3. Results

In this study, we used the dataset created by KSM to extract the test data (40 eyes from 20 healthy subjects) with the typical U-Net and compared the extraction results with the manual method to verify its usefulness. The participants' background variables that were used in the test data were expressed as the median (interquartile range). The age of the target group was 30.00 (26.50 to 44.25) years. The corrected equivalent visual acuity was

−0.08 (−0.08 to −0.08) logarithm of the minimum angle of resolution. The axial length was 24.15 (23.56 to 24.85) mm. The spherical equivalent was −1.25 (−2.31 to 0.00) D. Three of the 20 participants (7.5%) had a history of smoking, 1 participant (2.5%) had hypertension, and 1 participant (2.5%) had dyslipidemia; none of them had diabetes or cardiovascular disease.

3.1. Coefficient of Variation and Correlation Coefficient of the Area

Table 1 shows the results of the FAZ area and the Friedman test for each extraction method. Figure 3A shows the results of multiple comparisons. The area of the FAZ was 0.271 mm^2 for examiner 1, which was significantly larger than that obtained by other methods ($p < 0.001$). The area of the FAZ for examiner 2 and the U-Net was 0.265 mm^2, which was not significantly different ($p = 1.00$). The area of the FAZ measured using ARI has the smallest value at 0.240 mm^2 ($p < 0.001$).

Table 1. The FAZ area obtained by each extraction method and results of the Friedman test.

Method	Area (Mean ± SD) (mm^2)
Examiner 1	0.271 ± 0.086
Examiner 2	0.265 ± 0.086
U-Net	0.265 ± 0.085
ARI	0.240 ± 0.081
p-value *	<0.001

* Friedman test. FAZ: foveal avascular zone, ARI: Advanced Retina Imaging.

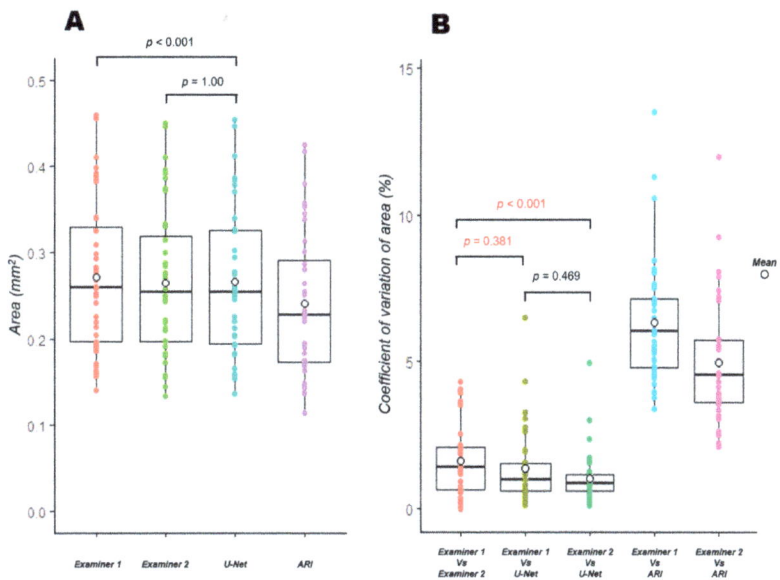

Figure 3. Multiple comparisons of the FAZ area and its coefficient of variation obtained by each extraction method. Results of the FAZ area (**A**) and the coefficient of variation of area (**B**) obtained by each extraction method. Comparing each combination of the four extraction methods, significant differences ($p < 0.001$) were found for all of those without a p-value listed. Moreover, the area obtained by U-Net is significantly different from examiner 1 ($p < 0.001$), but not from examiner 2 (**A**). ($p = 1.00$). The CV of the area between examiner 1 and the U-Net is not significantly different from that between the manual methods ($p = 0.381$), and the CV of the area between examiner 2 and the U-Net is significantly better than that between the manual methods (**B**). ($p < 0.001$). The Bonferroni correction was used to adjust the p-value. FAZ: foveal avascular zone.

Table 2 shows the results of the CV and Friedman tests for the extraction methods and the correlation between the FAZ areas obtained with each extraction method. The results of multiple comparisons are also shown in Figure 3B. The CV was 1.61% between the manual methods (examiner 1 and examiner 2) compared to 1.35% between examiner 1 and the U-Net ($p = 0.38$), and 1.01% between examiner 2 and the U-Net ($p < 0.001$), indicating that the CV between the manual methods and the U-Net was as good as or better than that between the manual methods, with the best value for the comparison between examiner 2 and the U-Net. The results of the manual method and ARI were both higher than 4% ($p < 0.001$). The correlation coefficient showed a strong association between all the extraction methods, but the values obtained with the manual method and ARI were slightly lower.

Table 2. The coefficient of variation and Friedman test results for each extraction method, and correlation of the FAZ area obtained by each extraction method.

Method	CV (Mean [95%CI]) (%)	rho	*p*-Value
Examiner 1 vs Examiner 2	1.61 (1.23–1.98)	0.995	<0.001 *
Examiner 1 vs U-Net	1.35 (0.95–1.75)	0.994	<0.001 *
Examiner 2 vs U-Net	1.01 (0.73–1.29)	0.995	<0.001 *
Examiner 1 vs ARI	6.35 (5.68–7.02)	0.987	<0.001 *
Examiner 2 vs ARI	4.99 (4.33–5.65)	0.987	<0.001 *
			<0.001 †

* Spearman's rank correlation. † Friedman test. FAZ: foveal avascular zone, ARI: Advanced Retina Imaging, CV: coefficient of variation, CI: confidence interval, vs: versus.

3.2. Two Types of Similarity, FN and FP (Excess or Deficiency of Extraction)

Table 3 shows the similarity results and the Friedman test. Figure 4 shows the results of multiple comparisons. The Jaccard index was 0.931 between the manual methods, 0.951 between examiner 1 and the U-Net ($p < 0.001$), and 0.933 between examiner 2 and the U-Net ($p = 1.00$). The Jaccard index between examiner 1 and ARI was 0.875 ($p < 0.001$) and 0.894 between examiner 2 and ARI ($p < 0.001$). The DSC was 0.964 between the manual methods, 0.975 between examiner 1 and the U-Net, and 0.965 between examiner 2 and the U-Net. The DSC between examiner 1 and ARI was 0.933, and 0.944 between examiner 2 and ARI. The Jaccard index and DSC for the combination of the manual and the U-Net methods was equal to or higher than that for the manual methods, similar to the CV results. The best value was for the combination of examiner 1 and the U-Net, unlike the CV. Table 4 shows the results of the FN and FP quantification. FN (insufficient extraction) was significantly more common for all combinations than FP (false extraction) ($p < 0.001$), except for the combination of examiner 2 and the U-Net.

Table 3. Two types of similarity and the results of each Friedman test.

	Jaccard (95%CI)	DSC (95%CI)
Examiner 1 vs Examiner 2	0.931 (0.923–0.940)	0.964 (0.959–0.969)
Examiner 1 vs U-Net	0.951 (0.943–0.959)	0.975 (0.971–0.979)
Examiner 2 vs U-Net	0.933 (0.924–0.942)	0.965 (0.960–0.970)
Examiner 1 vs ARI	0.875 (0.864–0.887)	0.933 (0.926–0.940)
Examiner 2 vs ARI	0.894 (0.881–0.906)	0.944 (0.936–0.951)
p value *	<0.001	<0.001

DSC: Dice similarity coefficient, ARI: Advanced Retina Imaging, CI: confidence interval, vs: versus. * Friedman test.

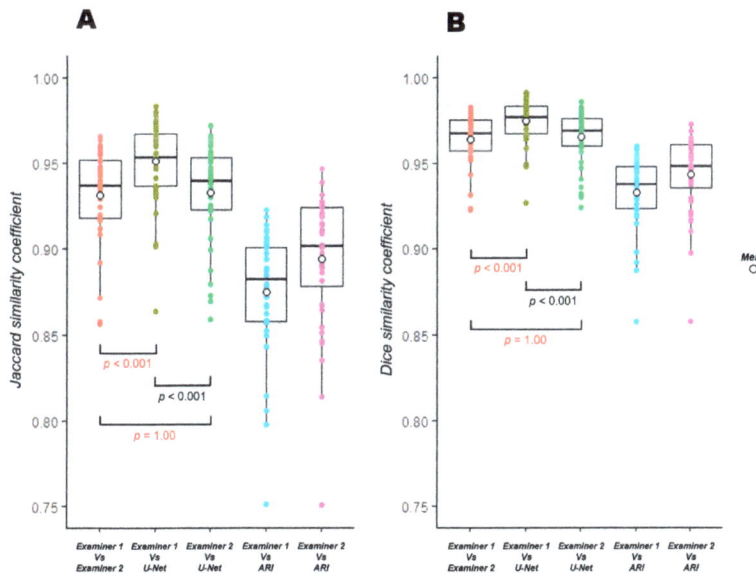

Figure 4. Multiple comparisons using the Jaccard index (**A**) and DSC (**B**). Results of the Jaccard index (**A**) and DSC (**B**). Comparing each 5 similarities coefficient of extraction methods, significant differences ($p < 0.001$) were found for all of those without a p-value listed. For similarities, the results between examiner 1 and the U-Net are significantly better than those between the manual methods (examiner 1 and 2) ($p < 0.001$), and the results between examiner 2 and the U-Net are not significantly different from those of the manual methods ($p = 1.00$). The Bonferroni correction was used to adjust the p-value.

Table 4. Significant differences between the false negatives (FN) and false positives (FP).

	Mean FN (%)	Mean FP (%)	p-Value *
Examiner 1 vs Examiner 2	4.87	2.21	<0.001
Examiner 1 vs U-Net	3.65	1.34	<0.001
Examiner 2 vs U-Net	3.3	3.66	0.128
Examiner 1 vs ARI	12.22	0.35	<0.001
Examiner 2 vs ARI	10.07	0.68	<0.001

* Wilcoxon signed rank sum test.

Figure 5 shows the extracted image for each method. It is apparent from the extraction results of each manual method that almost the same area was extracted by both examiners, but there was a difference in the recognition of the uneven parts (Figure 5, arrows). Figure 6 shows an image in which the extraction lines of the manual and automatic methods are superimposed. The comparison of the extraction lines of each manual method with respect to the extraction lines of the U-Net showed that examiner 1 extracted almost the same boundary as the U-Net, except for the uneven part. Conversely, the extraction of examiner 2 gave the impression of partial intersection.

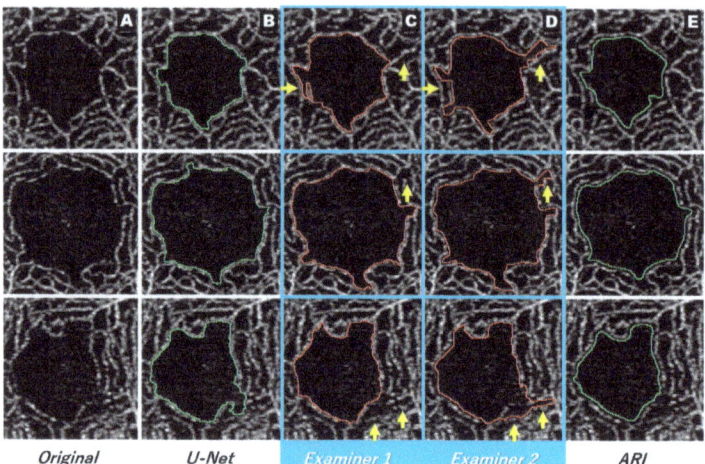

Figure 5. Extraction results for each method. Original image (column (**A**)), U-Net (column (**B**)). Examiners 1 and 2 (columns (**C**) and (**D**)), ARI (column (**E**)). There is a difference in the recognition of unevenness between the manual methods (Arrows in columns (**C**,**D**)). ARI: Advanced Retina Imaging.

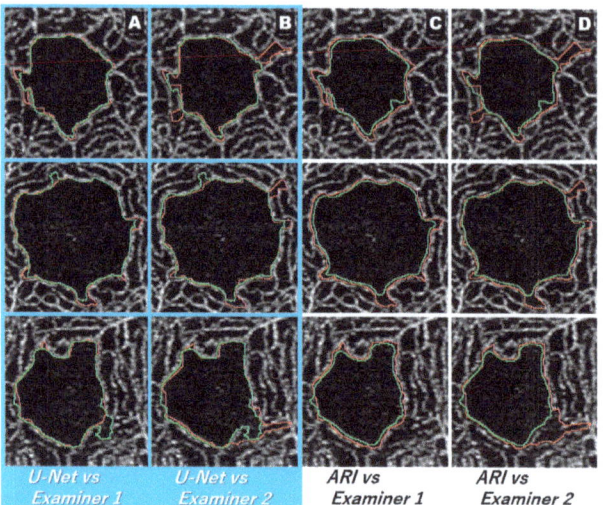

Figure 6. Superimposed images of the extraction lines of each automatic method and each manual method. Extraction lines for each automatic method (green line for U-Net and ARI). Extraction line for each manual method (red line). The extraction lines of examiners 1 and the U-Net demarcated almost the same area, except for the uneven area (column (**A**)). The extraction lines of examiners 2 and the U-Net appear to cross each other (column (**B**)). The extraction line for ARI looks smaller than any of the examiners (columns (**C**,**D**)). ARI: Advanced Retina Imaging.

4. Discussion

In this study, we used the dataset created by KSM to extract the test data (40 eyes from 20 healthy subjects) with the typical U-Net and compared the extraction results with the manual method to verify its usefulness. The U-Net results trained from this dataset were as good as or better than the manual results in terms of the CV of the area, correlation coefficient, and similarity evaluation. Diaz et al. [11] stated that the results of correlation coefficients between manual methods used as a gold standard will affect the performance evaluation of automatic methods. The correlation coefficient between the manual methods in this study was 0.995, which represented a strong association and seemed to be sufficiently accurate for use as the gold standard. The correlation coefficient between the manual method and ARI was also good at 0.987, but the correlation coefficient between the manual method and the U-Net was higher or equivalent to that of the than that of ARI and manual method (Table 2).

In some images, we have shown that the boundaries are different even between manual methods (Figures 5 and 6). Although relatively clear images were used in this study, such errors were also observed between the manual methods. Moreover, the evaluation of the CV revealed that the combination of the manual method and the U-Net elicited the same or better results compared to the combination of the manual methods. The CVs of the manual method and ARI were more than 4%, while the CVs of the manual method and the U-Net were less than 1.5%. These findings suggest that the CVs of the manual method and the U-Net were significantly better than those of the manual method and ARI (Table 2 and Figure 3B). Similar results were obtained for the evaluation of the degree of similarity. The combination of examiner 1 and the U-Net had the best value (Table 3 and Figure 4), which differed from the results of the CV. The reason for the difference in the combination with the best values may be attributed to the nature of CV evaluation. Evaluation based on the above-mentioned characteristics of manual extraction and the results of FP and FN (Table 4) showed that the extraction of the U-Net was similar to that of examiner 1 with respect to the shape, but the area obtained with U-Net was smaller than that of examiner 1 because the FN was significantly larger than the FP in the extraction achieved by the U-Net and examiner 1 (Table 1 and Figure 3A). The area measured by the U-Net was almost the same as that of examiner 2 (Table 1 and Figure 3A), probably because there was no significant difference between the FP and FN of U-Net and examiner 2. Hence, the CV of the FAZ area was lower for the combination of the U-Net and examiner 2 than that for the combination of the U-Net and examiner 1.

Currently, reports of automated FAZ extraction include both conventional automatic methods (built-in program) [11–15,34] and methods using deep learning [9,10]. Table 5 presents the details of previous studies that used the Jaccard index and DSC as indicators, as well as the maximum average for each similarity [9–12,14,34]. This study was the only one to obtain an excellent (0.9 or higher) value for the Jaccard coefficient from amongst the previous studies. The lowest value was reported by Diaz et al. [11] but the correlation coefficient between the manual methods was also low in that study, which seems to be the result of the influence of the accuracy of the gold standard (as mentioned in a previous study). Moreover, ARI, which showed the lowest value in this study, also seemed to show a good result compared to previous studies.

Table 5. Previous studies using the Jaccard index and DSC, and the maximum average of each similarity.

Study Using the Jaccard Similarity Coefficient

Author	Imaging Device	n	Slab	Method	Maximum Mean of Jaccard Similarity Coefficient	Area Correlation Coefficient *
Diaz et al. [11]	TOPCON DRI OCT Triton	144	SRL	Second observer	0.83	0.93
				System	0.82	0.90
Zhang et al. [34]	Optovue RTVue-XR	22	SRL	Automated Detection	0.85	
Lu et al. [12]	Optovue RTVue-XR	19	Inner Retinal	GGVF snake algorithm	0.87	
Current study	Zeiss PLEX Elite 9000	40	SRL	Second observer	0.931	0.995
				Typical U-Net (KSM Datasets)	0.951	0.994
				ARI	0.894	0.987

Study Using the Dice Similarity Coefficient

Author	Imaging Device	n	Slab	Method	Maximum Mean of Dice Similarity Coefficient	Area Correlation Coefficient
Lin et al. [14]	Zeiss Cirrus HD-OCT 5000	34	SRL	Second observer	0.931	
				Level-sets macro	0.924	
				Unadjusted KSM	0.910	
Guo et al. [9]	Zeiss Cirrus HD-OCT 5000	45	SRL	Improved U-Net (Manual Datasets)	0.976	0.997
Mirshahi et al. [10]	RTVue XR 100 Avanti	10	Inner Retinal	Mask R-CNN (Manual Datasets)	0.974	0.995
Current study	Zeiss PLEX Elite 9000	40	SRL	Second observer	0.964	0.995
				Typical U-Net (KSM Datasets)	0.975	0.994
				ARI	0.944	0.987

* Correlation coefficient is the highest Index value. DSC: Dice similarity coefficient, ARI: Advanced Retina Imaging, OCT: optical coherence tomography, KSM: Kanno Saitama Macro, SRL: superficial retinal layer, R-CNN: region based convolutional neural networks.

Previous studies that employed the DSC investigated conventional automated methods and deep learning. Lin et al. [14] used Level Sets, a plugin of ImageJ, to study the extraction accuracy for images with an image quality index of 6 to 10, obtained with the Cirrus HD-OCT 5000. The extraction accuracy of Level Sets was comparable to that of the manual method, and the results were stable with various image quality levels. KSM was also used for comparison in their study. The extraction accuracy of KSM was poor at low image quality and showed inadequate reproducibility, which seemed inappropriate for the Cirrus HD-OCT 5000. The authors speculated that this was due to the false extraction caused by high-luminance noise. We assumed that the images presented in the previous study seem to be strongly affected by noise. We opine that good results can be obtained by performing noise processing (Figure 1E,F) in such cases. We recommend adjusting the number of times "dilate" and "erode" are used in the event of poor extraction, since noise processing also affects the blood flow signal. The results of Lin et al. were the lowest among the previous studies that used DSC, but even in that study, the similarity between the manual methods was also low. In other words, the accuracy of the gold standard could have affected the results in the current study, as well as that undertaken by Diaz et al. [11]. Based on the results of these two studies, there is also a need for a way to evaluate the accuracy of the gold standard in the future.

Guo et al. [9] used an improved U-Net in their study. Interestingly, that study used a dataset that included a group that edited the OCTA image and changed the brightness/contrast (B/C) to flexibly handle the extraction of OCTA images with different levels of B/C. The appeal of deep learning is that it allows for the creation of models for various conditions using datasets that have been edited to meet this purpose. Moreover, Guo et al. [9] stated that the extraction accuracy would plummet significantly in the case of conventional automatic extraction if the B/C differs from the default settings. The extraction disorder becomes stronger as the setting tolerance is exceeded in the conventional automatic method. However, images whose signal strength is reduced to the point that extraction fails are usually excluded from the study because they adversely affect the reliability of the results. Rather, the major factor that causes poor extraction seems to be a localized decrease in signal strength.

Zhang et al. [34] reported a method to deal with localized signal intensity reduction in conventional image analysis. Such local signal intensity reduction can cause extraction failure if it interferes with the FAZ. Semantic segmentation may be able to deal with local signal strength degradation that interferes with FAZ by devising the dataset. Therefore, to perform ideal extraction for various OCTA images, it is necessary to create datasets according to various requirements. To reduce the burden of creating these datasets, there is also a need for an efficient way to reduce the burden of annotation. In this study, we used ImageJ macro to simplify the annotation process; ImageJ macro is a recommended tool for annotation because it can easily automate various processes.

In the comparison of similarity, the past studies using deep learning (Guo et al. [9] and Mirshahi et al. [10]) showed good results, but this is due to the performance of the deep learning network, probably because FAZ extraction of the dataset containing the test labels was also performed by the same person. In this study, we used a typical U-Net, the FAZ extraction of the data set was performed by KSM, and the test label was extracted by the manual method. In other words, the evaluation was performed using a test label that differed from the dataset. Therefore, the results obtained in this study are excellent, and the utility of the dataset created by KSM is high.

This study has some limitations. First, all images used in the dataset, including the test data, were images with OCTA signal strength of 8/10 or higher. As shown in the study by Guo et al. [9], there are images with different luminance and B/C variations in clinical practice, and this dataset is not sufficient to deal with images with various variations. Second, the cases used for the test data included only healthy subjects. In the future, studies including diseased eyes are warranted, as in the study by Diaz et al. [11]. Regardless, the results obtained in this study are still useful based on the accuracy of the extraction and the simplification of the annotation. The next step is to evaluate the feasibility of the current method for diseased eyes. Future studies should also examine whether KSM is useful for images with lower signal strength, and whether the dataset obtained by KSM from lower signal images is useful as a dataset for deep learning. Furthermore, we aim to follow the method of Guo et al. [9] to create a dataset that can handle images with various variations. The Training: Testing ratio in this study was 8.7:1.3; Guo et al. [9] reported a ratio of 8:2, and Mirshahi et al. [10] reported a ratio of 7.7:2.3, which is close to the present study. Third, this study aimed to test the usefulness of the KSM dataset, not the performance of the neural network, and we used a typical U-Net. Other practice may have yielded different results. We plan to conduct research using other programs in the future. Fourth, another limitation is the small sample size. Further studies with a larger number of cases are needed in the future. Finally, we compared the results of the measurement method proposed in this study with those of the manual method in the same way as previous reports. The manual method is not always correct. Automated methods have reproducibility and rapidity advantages. Establishment of a measurement method that requires less manual intervention is awaited. The current study demonstrates the validity of reducing the intervention of manual methods in establishing measurement methods using AI.

5. Conclusions

This study demonstrated that the deep learning dataset created by KSM provides comparable performance in the extraction of FAZ with conventional automatic methods. The results can contribute to reducing the burden of annotation in deep learning and promote AI research using OCTA images.

Supplementary Materials: The following supporting information can be downloaded at: https://www.mdpi.com/article/10.3390/jcm12010183/s1. Code S1: Modified KSM. Code S2: Annotation using continuous automatic extraction. Video S1: Annotation using continuous automatic extraction.

Author Contributions: J.K., T.S. (Takuhei Shoji) and K.S.: Designed and conducted the study; J.K., T.S. (Takuhei Shoji), H.I. (Hirokazu Ishii), H.I. (Hisashi Ibuki), Y.Y. and T.S. (Takanori Sasaki): Data collection; J.K., T.S. (Takuhei Shoji) and K.S.: Data analysis and interpretation; JK: Writing; T.S. (Takuhei Shoji) and K.S.: Critical revision; J.K., T.S. (Takuhei Shoji), H.I. (Hirokazu Ishii), H.I. (Hisashi Ibuki), Y.Y., T.S. (Takanori Sasaki) and K.S.: Manuscript approval. All authors have read and agreed to the published version of the manuscript.

Funding: This research received no external funding.

Institutional Review Board Statement: This study was conducted according to the tenets of the Declaration of Helsinki and was approved by the Ethics Committee of Saitama Medical University (No. 19079.01).

Informed Consent Statement: Informed consent was obtained from all subjects involved in the study.

Data Availability Statement: The datasets generated and/or analyzed during the current study are available from the corresponding author upon reasonable request.

Conflicts of Interest: The authors declare no conflict of interest.

References

1. Fujiwara, A.; Morizane, Y.; Hosokawa, M.; Kimura, S.; Shiode, Y.; Hirano, M.; Doi, S.; Toshima, S.; Takahashi, K.; Hosogi, M.; et al. Factors affecting foveal avascular zone in healthy eyes: An examination using swept-source optical coherence tomography angiography. *PLoS ONE* **2017**, *12*, e0188572. [CrossRef] [PubMed]
2. Ciloglu, E.; Unal, F.; Sukgen, E.A.; Koçluk, Y. Evaluation of Foveal Avascular Zone and Capillary Plexuses in Diabetic Patients by Optical Coherence Tomography Angiography. *Korean J. Ophthalmol.* **2019**, *33*, 359–365. [CrossRef] [PubMed]
3. Balaratnasingam, C.; Inoue, M.; Ahn, S.; McCann, J.; Dhrami-Gavazi, E.; Yannuzzi, L.A.; Freund, K.B. Visual Acuity Is Correlated with the Area of the Foveal Avascular Zone in Diabetic Retinopathy and Retinal Vein Occlusion. *Ophthalmology* **2016**, *123*, 2352–2367. [CrossRef]
4. Shiihara, H.; Terasaki, H.; Sonoda, S.; Kakiuchi, N.; Yamaji, H.; Yamaoka, S.; Uno, T.; Watanabe, M.; Sakamoto, T. Association of foveal avascular zone with the metamorphopsia in epiretinal membrane. *Sci. Rep.* **2020**, *10*, 170–192. [CrossRef]
5. Tsuboi, K.; Fukutomi, A.; Sasajima, H.; Ishida, Y.; Kusaba, K.; Kataoka, T.; Kamei, M. Visual Acuity Recovery After Macular Hole Closure Associated with Foveal Avascular Zone Change. *Transl. Vis. Sci. Technol.* **2020**, *9*, 20. [CrossRef] [PubMed]
6. Jauregui, R.; Park, K.S.; Duong, J.K.; Mahajan, V.; Tsang, S.H. Quantitative progression of retinitis pigmentosa by optical coherence tomography angiography. *Sci. Rep.* **2018**, *8*, 13130. [CrossRef]
7. Shoji, T.; Kanno, J.; Weinreb, R.N.; Yoshikawa, Y.; Mine, I.; Ishii, H.; Ibuki, H.; Shinoda, K. OCT angiography measured changes in the foveal avascular zone area after glaucoma surgery. *Br. J. Ophthalmol.* **2022**, *106*, 80–86. [CrossRef]
8. Araki, S.; Miki, A.; Goto, K.; Yamashita, T.; Yoneda, T.; Haruishi, K.; Ieki, Y.; Kiryu, J.; Maehara, G.; Yaoeda, K. Foveal avascular zone and macular vessel density after correction for magnification error in unilateral amblyopia using optical coherence tomography angiography. *BMC Ophthalmol.* **2019**, *19*, 171. [CrossRef]
9. Guo, M.; Zhao, M.; Cheong, A.M.Y.; Dai, H.; Lam, A.K.C.; Zhou, Y. Automatic quantification of superficial foveal avascular zone in optical coherence tomography angiography implemented with deep learning. *Vis. Comput. Ind. Biomed. Art* **2019**, *2*, 21. [CrossRef]
10. Mirshahi, R.; Anvari, P.; Riazi-Esfahani, H.; Sardarinia, M.; Naseripour, M.; Falavarjani, K.G. Foveal avascular zone segmentation in optical coherence tomography angiography images using a deep learning approach. *Sci. Rep.* **2021**, *11*, 1031. [CrossRef]
11. Díaz, M.; Novo, J.; Cutrín, P.; Gómez-Ulla, F.; Penedo, M.G.; Ortega, M. Automatic segmentation of the foveal avascular zone in ophthalmological OCT-A images. *PLoS ONE* **2019**, *14*, e0212364. [CrossRef] [PubMed]
12. Lu, Y.; Simonett, J.M.; Wang, J.; Zhang, M.; Hwang, T.; Hagag, A.; Huang, D.; Li, D.; Jia, Y. Evaluation of Automatically Quantified Foveal Avascular Zone Metrics for Diagnosis of Diabetic Retinopathy Using Optical Coherence Tomography Angiography. *Investig. Opthalmology Vis. Sci.* **2018**, *59*, 2212–2221. [CrossRef] [PubMed]
13. Tang, F.Y.; Ng, D.S.; Lam, A.; Luk, F.; Wong, R.; Chan, C.; Mohamed, S.; Fong, A.; Lok, J.; Tso, T.; et al. Determinants of Quantitative Optical Coherence Tomography Angiography Metrics in Patients with Diabetes. *Sci. Rep.* **2017**, *7*, 2575. [CrossRef] [PubMed]
14. Lin, A.; Fang, D.; Li, C.; Cheung, C.Y.; Chen, H. Improved Automated Foveal Avascular Zone Measurement in Cirrus Optical Coherence Tomography Angiography Using the Level Sets Macro. *Transl. Vis. Sci. Technol.* **2020**, *9*, 20. [CrossRef]
15. Ishii, H.; Shoji, T.; Yoshikawa, Y.; Kanno, J.; Ibuki, H.; Shinoda, K. Automated Measurement of the Foveal Avascular Zone in Swept-Source Optical Coherence Tomography Angiography Images. *Transl. Vis. Sci. Technol.* **2019**, *8*, 28. [CrossRef]
16. Jimenez, G.; Racoceanu, D. Deep Learning for Semantic Segmentation vs. Classification in Computational Pathology: Application to Mitosis Analysis in Breast Cancer Grading. *Front. Bioeng. Biotechnol.* **2019**, *7*, 145. [CrossRef]

17. Hollon, T.C.; Pandian, B.; Adapa, A.R.; Urias, E.; Save, A.V.; Khalsa, S.S.S.; Eichberg, D.G.; D'Amico, R.S.; Farooq, Z.U.; Lewis, S.; et al. Near real-time intraoperative brain tumor diagnosis using stimulated Raman histology and deep neural networks. *Nat. Med.* **2020**, *26*, 52–58. [CrossRef]
18. Bevilacqua, V.; Brunetti, A.; Cascarano, G.D.; Guerriero, A.; Pesce, F.; Moschetta, M.; Gesualdo, L. A comparison between two semantic deep learning frameworks for the autosomal dominant polycystic kidney disease segmentation based on magnetic resonance images. *BMC Med. Inform. Decis. Mak.* **2019**, *19*, 1244. [CrossRef]
19. Casalegno, F.; Newton, T.; Daher, R.; Abdelaziz, M.; Lodi-Rizzini, A.; Schürmann, F.; Krejci, I.; Markram, H. Caries Detection with Near-Infrared Transillumination Using Deep Learning. *J. Dent. Res.* **2019**, *98*, 1227–1233. [CrossRef]
20. Nemoto, T.; Futakami, N.; Yagi, M.; Kumabe, A.; Takeda, A.; Kunieda, E.; Shigematsu, N. Efficacy evaluation of 2D, 3D U-Net semantic segmentation and atlas-based segmentation of normal lungs excluding the trachea and main bronchi. *J. Radiat. Res.* **2020**, *61*, 257–264. [CrossRef]
21. Bakr, S.; Gevaert, O.; Echegaray, S.; Ayers, K.; Zhou, M.; Shafiq, M.; Zheng, H.; Benson, J.A.; Zhang, W.; Leung, A.N.C.; et al. A radiogenomic dataset of non-small cell lung cancer. *Sci. Data* **2018**, *5*, 180202. [CrossRef] [PubMed]
22. Bojikian, K.D.; Chen, C.-L.; Wen, J.C.; Zhang, Q.; Xin, C.; Gupta, D.; Mudumbai, R.C.; Johnstone, M.A.; Wang, R.K.; Chen, P.P. Optic Disc Perfusion in Primary Open Angle and Normal Tension Glaucoma Eyes Using Optical Coherence Tomography-Based Microangiography. *PLoS ONE* **2016**, *11*, e0154691. [CrossRef] [PubMed]
23. Tambe, S.B.; Kulhare, D.; Nirmal, M.D.; Prajapati, G. Image Processing (IP) Through Erosion and Dilation Methods. *Int. J. Emerg. Technol. Adv. Eng.* **2013**, *3*, 285–289.
24. Kumar, M.; Singh, S. Edge Detection and Denoising Medical Image Using Morphology. *Int. J. Emerg. Technol. Adv. Eng.* **2012**, *2*, 66–72.
25. Ronneberger, O.; Fischer, P.; Brox, T. U-Net: Convolutional networks for biomedical image segmentation. In *Medical Image Computing and Computer-Assisted Intervention 2015*; Navab, N., Hornegger, J., Wells, W.M., Frangi, A.F., Eds.; Springer International Publishing: Cham, Switzerland, 2015; pp. 234–241. [CrossRef]
26. Kou, C.; Li, W.; Liang, W.; Yu, Z.; Hao, J. Microaneurysms segmentation with a U-Net based on recurrent residual convolutional neural network. *J. Med. Imaging* **2019**, *6*, 025008. [CrossRef] [PubMed]
27. Kingma, D.P.; Ba, J. Adam: A method for stochastic optimization. *arXiv* **2014**, arXiv:1412.6980.
28. Moghimi, S.; Hosseini, H.; Riddle, J.; Lee, G.Y.; Bitrian, E.; Giaconi, J.; Caprioli, J.; Nouri-Mahdavi, K. Measurement of Optic Disc Size and Rim Area with Spectral-Domain OCT and Scanning Laser Ophthalmoscopy. *Investig. Opthalmology Vis. Sci.* **2012**, *53*, 4519–4530. [CrossRef]
29. Belgacem, R.; Malek, I.T.; Trabelsi, H.; Jabri, I. A supervised machine learning algorithm SKVMs used for both classification and screening of glaucoma disease. *New Front. Ophthalmol.* **2018**, *4*, 1–27. [CrossRef]
30. Bertels, J.; Eelbode, T.; Berman, M.; Vandermeulen, D.; Maes, F.; Bisschops, R.; Blaschko, M.B. Optimizing the Dice Score and Jaccard Index for Medical Image Segmentation: Theory and Practice. In *International Conference on Medical Image Computing and Computer-Assisted Intervention*; Springer: Cham, Switzerland, 2019; pp. 92–100. [CrossRef]
31. Jaccard, P. The Distribution of the Flora in the Alpine Zone. *New Phytol.* **1912**, *11*, 37–50. [CrossRef]
32. Dice, L.R. Measures of the Amount of Ecologic Association Between Species. *Ecology* **1945**, *26*, 297–302. [CrossRef]
33. Zou, K.H.; Warfield, S.; Bharatha, A.; Tempany, C.M.; Kaus, M.R.; Haker, S.J.; Wells, W.M., 3rd; Jolesz, F.A.; Kikinis, R. Statistical validation of image segmentation quality based on a spatial overlap index1: Scientific reports. *Acad. Radiol.* **2004**, *11*, 178–189. [CrossRef] [PubMed]
34. Zhang, M.; Hwang, T.S.; Dongye, C.; Wilson, D.J.; Huang, D.; Jia, Y. Automated Quantification of Nonperfusion in Three Retinal Plexuses Using Projection-Resolved Optical Coherence Tomography Angiography in Diabetic Retinopathy. *Investig. Opthalmol. Vis. Sci.* **2016**, *57*, 5101–5106. [CrossRef] [PubMed]

Disclaimer/Publisher's Note: The statements, opinions and data contained in all publications are solely those of the individual author(s) and contributor(s) and not of MDPI and/or the editor(s). MDPI and/or the editor(s) disclaim responsibility for any injury to people or property resulting from any ideas, methods, instructions or products referred to in the content.

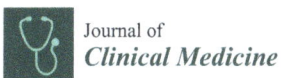

Article

Retinal Macrophage-Like Cells as a Biomarker of Inflammation in Retinal Vein Occlusions

Dmitrii S. Maltsev *, Alexei N. Kulikov, Yaroslava V. Volkova, Maria A. Burnasheva and Alexander S. Vasiliev

Department of Ophthalmology, Military Medical Academy, 21, Botkinskaya St, 194044 St. Petersburg, Russia
* Correspondence: glaz.med@yandex.ru

Abstract: Aim: To study the macrophage-like cells (MLC) of the inner retinal surface in eyes with retinal vein occlusions (RVO) and the association of MLC with clinical characteristics of RVO. Methods: In this retrospective cross-sectional study, the medical records and multimodal imaging data of treatment-naïve patients with unilateral RVO and no abnormalities of vitreoretinal interface electronic were reviewed and analyzed. To visualize MLC, structural projections of optical coherence tomography (OCT) angiography scans within a slab between two inner limiting membrane segmentation lines (with 0 and -9 μm offset) were evaluated. The density of MLC was calculated and compared between affected and fellow eyes of each patient with regards to OCT and clinical characteristics of RVO. Results: Thirty-six eyes (twenty-eight branch RVO and eight central RVO) of 36 patients (21 males and 15 females, mean age 48.9 ± 9.8 years) were included. The density of MLC in affected eye was statistically significantly higher than that of the fellow eye, 8.5 ± 5.5 and 4.0 ± 3.6 cells/mm^2, respectively ($p < 0.001$). The MLC density in the affected eye had a statistically significantly correlation with that of the fellow eye ($r = 0.76$, $p = 0.0001$), but with none of the OCT and clinical characteristics of the affected eye apart from the presence of subfoveal fluid. Eyes with subfoveal fluid had a statistically significantly higher mean number of MLC than that of eyes without subfoveal fluid, 12.6 ± 6.3 and 6.9 ± 4.0 cells/mm^2, respectively ($p = 0.009$). Conclusion: The number of MLC on the inner retinal surface increases in RVO eyes which may reflect the activation of inflammatory pathways.

Keywords: macrophage-like cells; retinal vein occlusion; optical coherence tomography; macular edema; subfoveal fluid; optical coherence tomography angiography

Citation: Maltsev, D.S.; Kulikov, A.N.; Volkova, Y.V.; Burnasheva, M.A.; Vasiliev, A.S. Retinal Macrophage-Like Cells as a Biomarker of Inflammation in Retinal Vein Occlusions. *J. Clin. Med.* **2022**, *11*, 7470. https://doi.org/10.3390/jcm11247470

Academic Editor: Fumi Gomi

Received: 2 November 2022
Accepted: 13 December 2022
Published: 16 December 2022

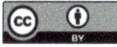

Copyright: © 2022 by the authors. Licensee MDPI, Basel, Switzerland. This article is an open access article distributed under the terms and conditions of the Creative Commons Attribution (CC BY) license (https://creativecommons.org/licenses/by/4.0/).

1. Introduction

Although retinal vein occlusion is a common retinal disorder affecting a significant proportion of the population, the pathophysiology of this condition is still not fully understood. Basic steps in the occlusion described by the Virchow's triad include venous congestion, alteration of endothelial sheet, and blood hypercoagulability [1]. However, clinically significant complications of the RVO, namely macular edema and neovascularization, are driven by the changes in specific molecular signaling pathways.

From studies which analyzed vitreous samples, it is known that RVO is followed by the increase of intraocular concentrations of vascular endothelial growth factor (VEGF) and several proinflammatory cytokines controlling the integrity of the inner blood-retinal barrier [2,3]. This leads to an increase of vascular permeability, exudation, macular edema, and to further neovascular complications. Any study of the relationship between angiogenic and proinflammatory cytokines in RVO is therefore of high practical value as it will help to optimize the therapeutic approach. In cases where VEGF plays a leading role, patients benefit from anti-VEGF treatment. Where inflammatory reactions play a greater role, corticosteroids may be a more favorable approach [4].

Several studies have considered clinical biomarkers indicating the role of inflammation in RVO pathophysiology, including the types of fluid associated with macular edema, choroidal thickness, intraretinal hyperreflective foci, and anterior chamber flare [4–6].

However, several recent studies have described a new biomarker with the potential to characterize intraocular inflammation: macrophage-like cells of the inner limiting membrane [7,8]. With clinical OCT, these cells were defined as being evenly distributed over the macula spindle or star-like motile cells located above the inner limiting membrane surface. MLC demonstrated substantial changes in diabetic retinopathy, which is driven by ischemia and inflammation [9]. Since ischemia and inflammation also play an important role in RVO, we may expect some changes of MLC in RVO.

The aim of this study was to investigate changes of the density of MLC in eyes with RVO and the association of the density of MLC with the clinical and OCT characteristics of RVO.

2. Materials and Methods

This was a retrospective cross-sectional study. The study followed the ethical standards stated in the Declaration of Helsinki and was approved by the Local Ethics Committee. All participants signed informed consent for the use of their clinical data for investigation. Only treatment-naïve unilateral RVO patients were included in this study. Exclusion criteria were the presence of any abnormalities of vitreoretinal interface in either eye, including any stage of posterior vitreous detachment detected using optical coherence tomography (OCT), diabetes mellitus, glaucoma, history or presence of active intraocular inflammation, retinal vascular occlusion in the fellow eye, or any concurrent ocular condition impeding OCT imaging.

For all patients, electronic medical records and multimodal imaging data were reviewed and analyzed. All patients received OCT and OCT angiography (OCTA) (RTVue-XR, Optovue, Fremont, CA, software version 2017.1.0.150), green scanning laser ophthalmoscopy (F-10, NIDEK, Gamagory, Japan), fluorescein angiography (F-10, Nidek or Visucam 524, Carl Zeiss Meditec AG, Jena, Germany), and color fundus photography (AFC-330, NIDEK or Visucam 524, Carl Zeiss Meditec AG). All imaging procedures were performed after medically induced mydriasis. OCTA scans with a 6 × 6 mm field of view centered on the center of the fovea were used to obtain structural and vascular parameters, including the density of MLC, central retinal thickness (CRT), vessel density in superficial capillary plexus (SCP), and deep capillary plexus (DCP). The presence of subfoveal fluid was defined on structural scans crossing the central subfield as a hyporeflective space between the photoreceptor outer segment layer and the retinal pigment epithelium (RPE). The subfoveal choroidal thickness (SCT) was measured with the caliper tool as the distance from the RPE to the choroidal-scleral junction beneath the center of the fovea. The mean of three measurements was taken for analysis. Ischemic RVO was established if the area of retinal nonperfusion based on FA was larger than five and ten optic disc areas for BRVO and CRVO, respectively.

To visualize MLC, structural projections of OCTA scans within a slab between two inner limiting membrane segmentation lines (with 0 and −9 μm offset) were evaluated for both the affected and fellow eyes (Figure 1). With these settings, MLC were defined as small moderately reflective spots, some portion of which demonstrated a star-like or spindle-shape appearance. Using a cell counter tool, the density of MLC was calculated in ImageJ (NIH, Bethesda, CA, USA) by two experienced masked graders as the number of MLC per mm^2. Correction of image magnification for myopic eyes was performed using Bennet's formula before calculating MLC. For BRVO eyes, the density of MLC was calculated separately for the affected and unaffected areas. Based on multimodal imaging data, the area of RVO was defined as an area of retinal capillary hypo- or nonperfusion and/or accumulation of intraretinal fluid and/or intraretinal hemorrhages with or without cotton wool-spots. The RVO area was manually delineated on en face OCTA projections in ImageJ, measured, and converted to a mask which was further used to calculate MLC outside the affected area. The number of MLC within the affected area was calculated as the difference between the total number of MLC and the MLC number outside the affected area (Figure 2). Finally, the MLC density was calculated for the affected and unaffected areas of BRVO eyes.

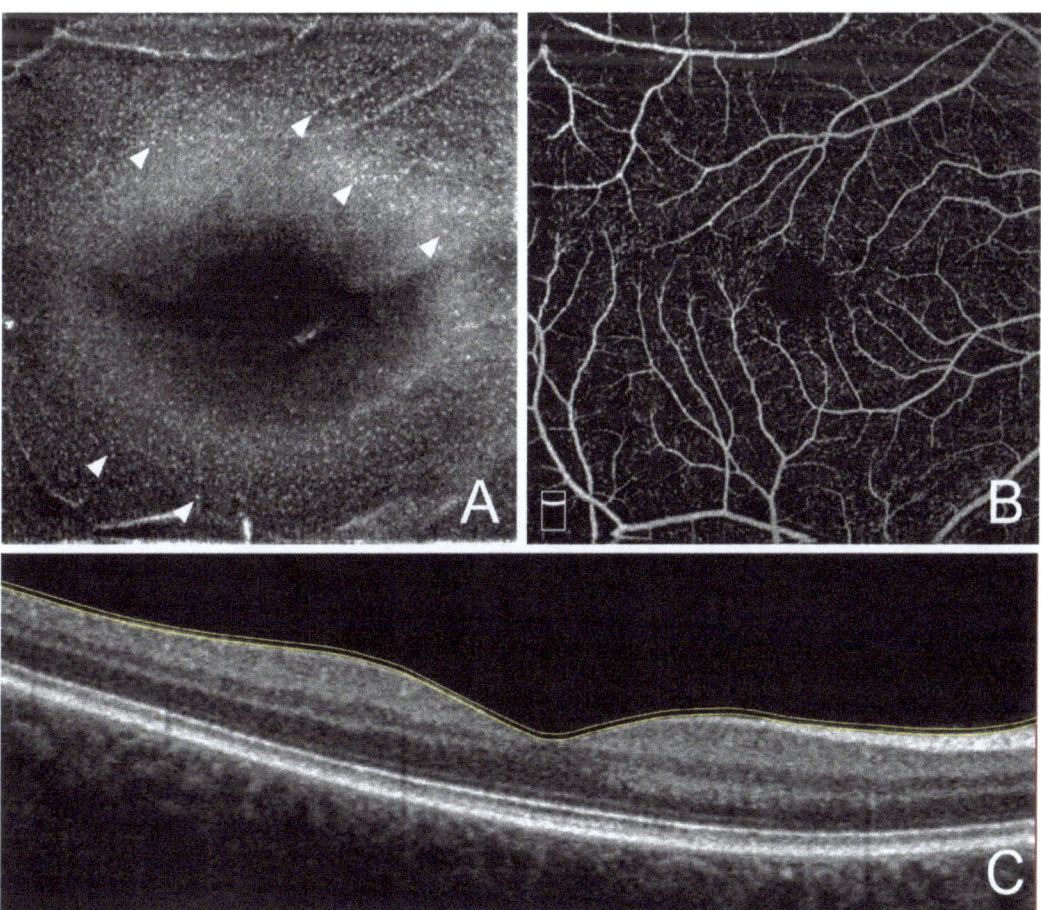

Figure 1. Representative example of visualization of retinal macrophage-like cells using 9-μm structural en face projection between two segmentation lines of the inner limiting membrane with −9 μm and 0 μm offset. (**A**) Structural en face optical coherence tomography angiography (OCTA) projection. Arrowheads indicate individual macrophage-like cells. (**B**) En face OCTA projection of superficial capillary plexus slab. (**C**) Cross-sectional OCT scan trough the center of the macula. Yellow lines represent segmentation lines of inner limiting membrane with 0 and −9 μm offset.

Statistical analysis was performed in MedCalc 18.4.1 (MedCalc Software, Ostend, Belgium). The Kolmogorov–Smirnov test was used to check normality. The paired t-test was used to compare MLC density between the affected and fellow eyes of RVO patients as well as MLC density between the affected and unaffected area within BRVO eyes. The Wilcoxon test was used to compare MLC density between ischemic and non-ischemic RVO eyes as well as between central RVO (CRVO) and BRVO eyes. To define the factors associated with the density of MLC, the correlation coefficient was calculated for the density of MLC and age, clinical, retinal structural, and vascular parameters. Receiver operating characteristic (ROC) analysis was performed to evaluate MLC as a biomarker for the presence of subfoveal fluid. To assess the interrater repeatability of MLC density calculation, the intraclass correlation coefficient was calculated; $p < 0.05$ was considered statistically significant.

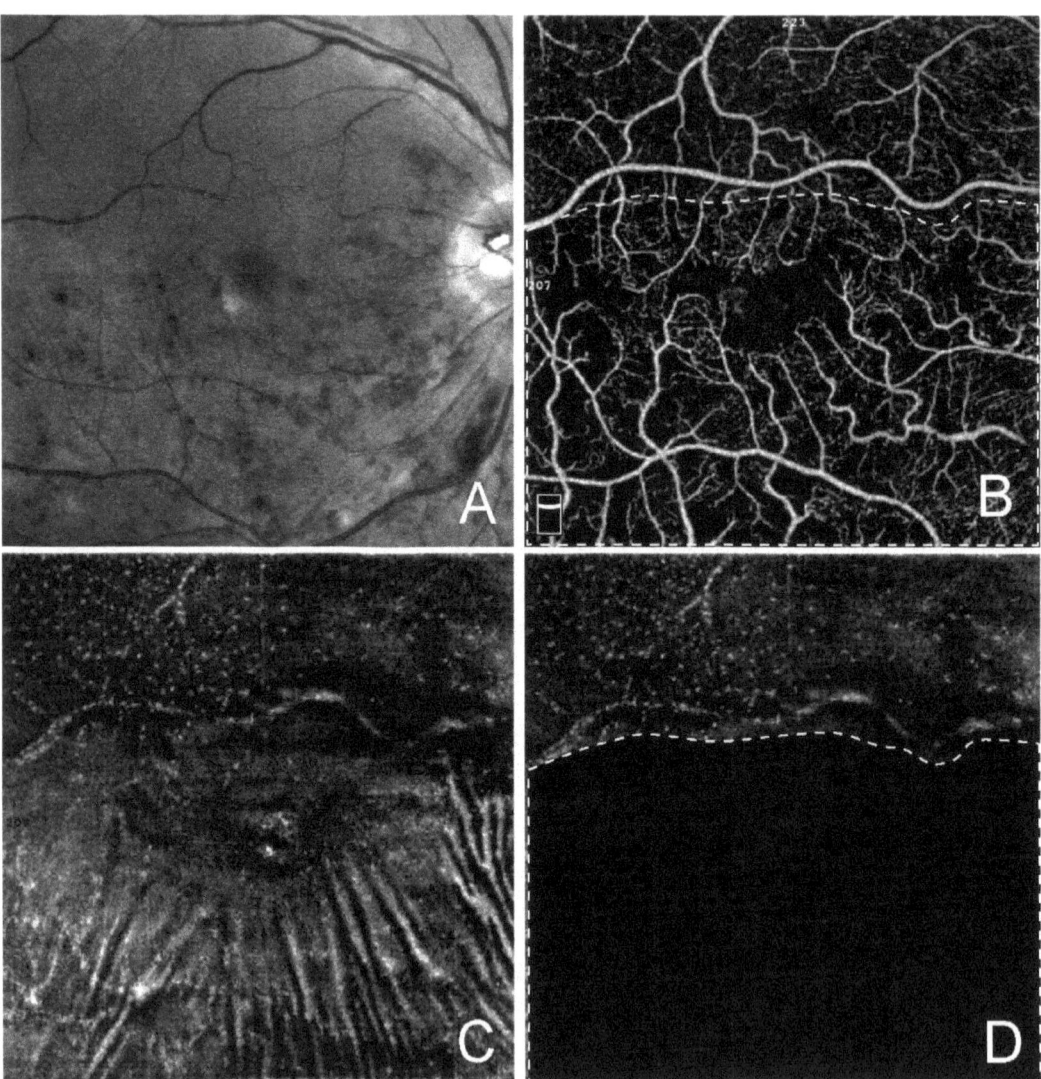

Figure 2. Counting of retinal macrophage-like cells in branch retinal vein occlusions. (**A**) Green scanning laser ophthalmoscopy showing area of occlusion. (**B**) En face optical coherence tomography angiography (OCTA) projection in the eye with branch retinal vein occlusion (BRVO). The yellow dashed line delineates the area of BRVO. (**C**) Structural en face OCTA projection displaying MLC. (**D**) Structural en face OCTA projection with the area affected by RVO masked to calculate MLC in unaffected area. The yellow dashed line delineates the area of BRVO.

3. Results

Thirty-six eyes of 36 patients (21 males and 15 females, mean age 48.9 ± 9.8 years) were included. The mean LogMAR best-corrected visual acuity (BCVA) was 0.51 ± 0.27 (20/63 Snellen equivalent). The mean period after RVO onset was 25 days (ranging from

5 days to 3 months). There were twenty-eight BRVO and eight CRVO cases. Twelve BRVO and two CRVO cases were considered ischemic based on the FA data. The mean CRT and SCT was 466.3 ± 193.0 μm and 345.5 ± 105.4 μm, respectively. The mean area of the macula involved in RVO was 17.6 ± 9.8 mm^2.

The density of MLC in the affected eye was statistically significantly higher than in the fellow eye, 8.5 ± 5.5 and 4.0 ± 3.6 cells/mm^2, respectively ($p < 0.001$). This difference remained statistically significant in CRVO and BRVO separately ($p < 0.05$) (Figure 3). There was a strong correlation of MLC density between both eyes of each patient (r = 0.76, $p < 0.001$).

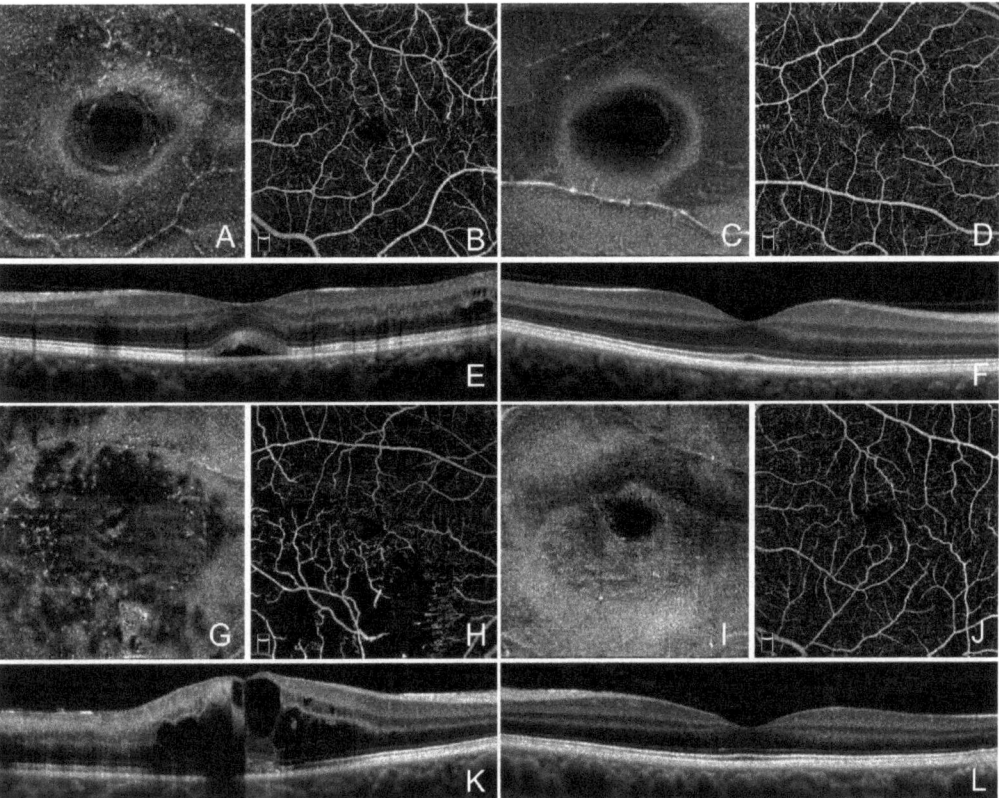

Figure 3. Optical coherence tomography angiography imaging of retinal macrophage-like cells in retinal vein occlusion with and without subfoveal fluid. (**A**) Structural en face optical coherence tomography angiography (OCTA) projection in the RVO eye with macular edema and subfoveal fluid. (**B**) En face OCTA projection of superficial capillary plexus slab. (**C**) Structural en face OCTA projection in the fellow unaffected eye. (**D**) En face OCTA projection of superficial capillary plexus slab in the fellow unaffected eye. (**E**) Cross-sectional OCT image showing macular edema and subfoveal fluid in the RVO eye. (**F**) Cross-sectional OCT image showing normal macula in the fellow eye. (**G**) Structural en face OCTA projection in the RVO eye with macular edema and no subfoveal fluid. (**H**) En face OCTA projection of superficial capillary plexus slab. (**I**) Structural en face OCTA projection in the fellow unaffected eye. (**J**) En face OCTA projection of superficial capillary plexus slab in the fellow unaffected eye. (**K**) Cross-sectional OCT image showing macular edema without subfoveal fluid in the RVO eye. (**L**) Cross-sectional OCT image showing normal macula in the fellow eye.

Although the density of MLC was higher in non-ischemic RVO compared to ischemic RVO eyes, this difference was not statistically significant ($p = 0.38$). The mean density of MLC within the affected area of BRVO eyes was statistically significantly lower compared to that of the unaffected region, 6.3 ± 5.3 and 10.5 ± 6.2 cells/mm^2 ($p = 0.009$), respectively. The intraclass correlation coefficient values for MLC density in affected and fellow eyes were 0.94 (95% confidence interval (CI) 0.93–0.97) and 0.98 (95% CI 0.97–0.99), respectively. Age, time after occlusion, gender, BCVA, CRT, SCT, the area of the affected region, and vessel density in SCP or DCP had no association with MLC density in the affected eye ($p > 0.05$) (Table 1).

Table 1. Correlation analysis for macrophage-like cells density and various parameters in eyes with retinal vein occlusion.

	MLC Density of RVO Eye	
	r	p-Value
Age	−0.13	0.53
Time after occlusion	0.14	0.55
BCVA	−0.21	0.11
CRT	0.09	0.68
SCT	0.02	0.92
Area of the affected region	0.12	0.55
Vessel density in SCP	−0.06	0.76
Vessel density in DCP	−0.03	0.87

BCVA, best-corrected visual acuity; CRT, central retinal thickness; DCP, deep capillary plexus; MLC, macrophage-like cells; RVO, retinal vein occlusion; SCP, superficial capillary plexus; SCT, subfoveal choroidal thickness.

Twelve eyes (four CRVO and eight BRVO) had subfoveal fluid. Eyes with subfoveal fluid had statistically significantly higher density of MLC than the eyes without subfoveal fluid, 12.6 ± 6.3 and 6.9 ± 4.0 cells/mm^2, respectively ($p = 0.009$) (Figure 4). ROC analysis showed the area under the ROC curve 0.83, sensitivity 88.9%, and specificity 66.7% for MLC as a biomarker for the presence of subfoveal fluid. Regarding the density of MLC in the fellow eye, there was a statistically significant difference between RVO eyes with and without subfoveal fluid, 5.8 ± 5.0 and 3.0 ± 2.3 cells/mm^2, respectively ($p = 0.04$).

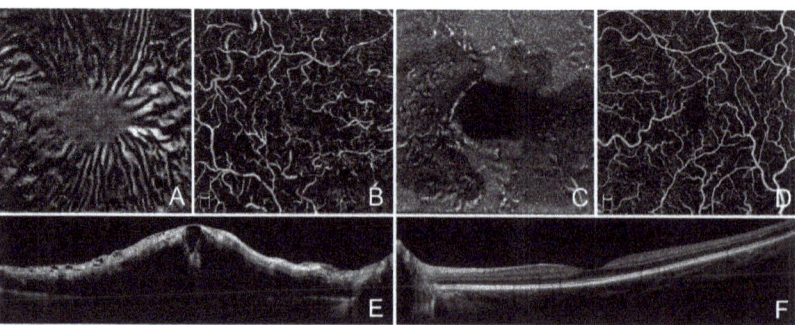

Figure 4. Optical coherence tomography angiography imaging of retinal macrophage-like cells in central retinal vein occlusion. (A) Structural en face optical coherence tomography angiography

(OCTA) projection displaying macrophage-like cells. (**B**) En face OCTA projection of superficial capillary plexus slab. (**C**) Structural en face OCTA projection in fellow unaffected eye. (**D**) En face OCTA projection of superficial capillary plexus slab. (**E**) Cross-sectional OCT image showing severe macular edema in the affected eye. (**F**) Cross-sectional OCT image showing normal macula in the fellow eye.

4. Discussion

In this study, we showed that MLC on the inner retinal surface more densely populate the macula in eyes with RVO compared to the healthy unaffected eyes of unilateral RVO patients. The density of MLC in RVO eyes varies significantly between individuals but has a strong correlation with the density of MLC in the fellow eye of each patient. Although these cells disappear from affected areas in eyes with BRVO, they seem to not be related to the ischemic status of RVO eyes. Moreover, apart from the presence of subfoveal fluid, MLC show no correlation with various clinical and OCT characteristics of RVO.

Retinal macrophage-like cells were first described on the inner limiting membrane using clinical OCT and image averaging by Castanos and coauthors [7]. This finding was later confirmed by adaptive optics imaging [8]. Both these studies demonstrated dendriform morphology and motility of the cells. Retinal cells, macrophages, glial cells, hyalocytes, and leukocytes may look like motile randomly distributed cells. However, leukocytes are normally absent in the healthy retina, while the cells on the inner limiting membrane are present in a high number in healthy eyes [7,8]. All other possible candidates for these cells have macrophage origin. It is possible, even without histopathological confirmation, to describe the cells under study as macrophage-like cells [9]. This term also allows us to define a particular cellular pool on the inner limiting membrane imaged with clinical OCT.

Changes of MLC in various posterior eye segment disorders have been proposed. However, MLC have only been studied in diabetic retinopathy where they demonstrated growth of the population during the conversion of non-proliferative retinopathy to PDR [10]. MLC have also shown increased density in the acute stage of multiple evanescent white dots syndrome [11]. Another feature registered in PDR was the accumulation of these cells along the large retinal vessels avoiding avascular regions. This may suggest the involvement of these cells in both vascular remodeling and in retinal ischemia. In our study, the density of MLC in the non-affected area was higher than in the affected area within the OCTA scan of BRVO patients. This phenomenon may indicate the migration of those cells from ischemia regions to normal areas, possibly due to the oxygen saturation gradient. Another explanation may be the recruitment of new MLC in uninvolved areas through the inflammatory pathways. The results of this study show that ischemia reduces the density of MLC. However, the ischemia in BRVO is a local factor, while inflammation is general (since the mediators of inflammation are distributed in the vitreous and affect the entire posterior eye pole). Therefore, MLC depopulation may be observed only over affected areas, while increase of MLC density may be seen over all non-involved regions. In general, the increase of MLC population appears to prevail over ischemic effects as is seen in CRVO cases, which demonstrate an increase of MLC population despite the absence of non-involved retina. We also cannot exclude that both migration and recruitment of MLC are operating simultaneously during RVO.

RVO are associated with overexpression, not only of VEGF, but also of many proinflammatory cytokines, including IL-6, IL-8, PIGF, MCP-1, ICAM-1, all of which increase retinal vessel permeability, leukocytes rolling and slow down the blood flow [3,6,12–14]. Activation of inflammatory signaling pathways may explain the relatively poor response to intravitreal anti-VEGF therapy in some cases of RVO. Such cases may benefit from corticosteroids therapy. However, identification of RVO cases where inflammation plays a leading role remains challenging. Inflammation biomarkers in RVO include subfoveal fluid and intraretinal hyperreflective foci [12,15], both of which have an association with MCP-1. MCP-1 is, in turn, responsible for the recruitment of monocytes and macrophages [16].

MCP-1 was shown to be significantly overexpressed in RVO. We therefore may expect activation of the MLC pool in this condition.

The problem with studying molecular signaling pathways in RVO mostly results from the invasive character of the procedures required to obtain aqueous humor or vitreous tape. Therefore, direct measuring of the intraocular level of different inflammatory factors in RVO is not appropriate outside of clinical studies. This highlights the importance of studying clinical biomarkers indicating the role of inflammation in each particular RVO case.

In this study, we found a significant increase of MLC population in eyes with RVO compared to fellow unaffected eyes. As was previously shown in eyes with diabetic retinopathy, MLC in RVO eyes avoided the retinal regions which have decreased perfusion or non-perfused areas. However, the density of MLC was still higher in RVO eyes. We may therefore conclude that MLC not only migrate from the area affected by the occlusion to unaffected areas, but also that some cells may be recruited to the inner retinal surface as was seen in multiple evanescent white dots syndrome [11]. The density of MLC does not correlate with the area of the occlusion or vessel density in SCP or DCP and therefore cannot be used as a biomarker for the ischemic status of the RVO. No other parameters of the RVO showed correlation with MLC density, including CRT, SCT or visual acuity. Only the presence of subfoveal fluid demonstrated an association with the density of MLC in RVO eyes. Subfoveal retinal fluid is a known biomarker of inflammation in RVO which was shown to be correlated with the levels of IL-6 and MCP-1 [12,17]. The high density of MLC in newly diagnosed RVO, taken together with other inflammatory biomarkers, may indicate the potential benefit of corticosteroids in the treatment of RVO. One confirmation for this suggestion can be obtained by monitoring changes in MLC density under the application of topical non-steroidal anti-inflammatory drugs.

Since the high density of the MLC in both affected and fellow eyes was associated with subfoveal fluid in RVO eyes and had a high interindividual difference, we suggest that baseline density of the MLC may indicate a predisposition to the activation of inflammatory pathways in RVO. In other words, if a patient had a high density of MLC, the inflammation may play a greater role in RVO, if any occurs in that patient. We suggest that these cells may participate in inflammatory pathways of RVO patients. Indeed, there are no known factors which could predict predominantly inflammatory status of RVO in each case. This status seems to be a unique characteristic of every affected eye, as is MLC density.

The limitations of these study are the strict exclusion criteria. Firstly, we avoided any cases with vitreoretinal interface abnormalities, including any stage of posterior vitreous detachment, since there are no data on the effects of changes of posterior vitreous on visualization of MLC. This resulted in inclusion of relatively young patients. The mean age of our study group was 49 years while the mean age of RVO patients in other studies is about 65 years. The effect of intraretinal hemorrhages and cotton-wool spots as factors distorting the retinal surface and potentially limiting MLC visualization also remains unknown. However, it would not change the main conclusion that MLC density increases in RVO and is associated with subfoveal fluid. Secondly, the consequence of applying strict inclusion criteria is the low number of cases included. Therefore, further studies with a larger and more diverse population of unilateral RVO patients is required. Thirdly, MLC of the foveal region were not identifiable on the structural en face OCT projections as was previously mentioned [7]. Finally, studies which measure vitreous and aqueous levels of proinflammatory mediators with regard to the density of MLC, as well as dynamic changes of MLC with the course of the disease are required. We did not include the control group in our study since interindividual difference in the fellow eyes of RVO patient was quite high (from 0.41 to 11.5 cells/mm^2) and until now, there are no known factors defining the MLC density in healthy patients.

In conclusion, this study revealed the potential role of MLC of the inner retinal surface as a novel biomarker in RVO possibly indicating the activation of inflammatory pathways. MLC density increases in eyes with BRVO and CRVO and is associated with the accumulation of subfoveal fluid, a known biomarker of inflammation in RVO.

Author Contributions: Conceptualization, D.S.M. and Y.V.V.; methodology, D.S.M.; software, Y.V.V.; validation, M.A.B., A.S.V. and A.N.K.; formal analysis, Y.V.V.; investigation, D.S.M. and Y.V.V.; resources, A.N.K.; data curation, A.N.K.; writing—original draft preparation, M.A.B. and A.S.V.; writing—review and editing, D.S.M.; visualization, D.S.M. and A.S.V.; supervision, A.N.K.; project administration, D.S.M. All authors have read and agreed to the published version of the manuscript.

Funding: This research received no external funding.

Institutional Review Board Statement: The study was conducted in accordance with the Declaration of Helsinki and approved by the Local Ethics Committee of Military Medical Academy (an extract from protocol #232 from 18 February 2020).

Informed Consent Statement: Informed consent was obtained from all subjects involved in the study.

Data Availability Statement: The primary data are available from Dmitrii S. Maltsev via email glaz.med@yandex.ru.

Conflicts of Interest: The authors declare no conflict of interest.

References

1. Kolar, P. Risk Factors for Central and Branch Retinal Vein Occlusion: A Meta-Analysis of Published Clinical Data. *J. Ophthalmol.* **2014**, *2014*, 724780. [CrossRef] [PubMed]
2. Park, S.P.; Ahn, J.K.; Mun, G.H.; Hyeong, G. Aqueous vascular endothelial growth factor levels are associated with serous macular detachment secondary to branch retinal vein occlusion. *Retina* **2010**, *30*, 281–286. [CrossRef] [PubMed]
3. Noma, H.; Funatsu, H.; Mimura, T.; Tatsugawa, M.; Shimada, K.; Eguchi, S. Vitreous inflammatory factors and serous macular detachment in branch retinal vein occlusion. *Retina* **2012**, *32*, 86–91. [CrossRef] [PubMed]
4. Do, J.R.; Park, S.J.; Shin, J.P.; Park, D.H. Assessment of Hyperreflective Foci after Bevacizumab or Dexamethasone Treatment According to Duration of Macular Edema in Patients with Branch Retinal Vein Occlusion. *Retina* **2021**, *41*, 355–365. [CrossRef] [PubMed]
5. Chen, L.; Yuan, M.; Sun, L.; Chen, Y. Choroidal thickening in retinal vein occlusion patients with serous retinal detachment. *Graefes Arch. Clin. Exp. Ophthalmol.* **2021**, *259*, 883–889. [CrossRef] [PubMed]
6. Noma, H.; Mimura, T.; Shimada, K. Role of inflammation in previously untreated macular edema with branch retinal vein occlusion. *BMC Ophthalmol.* **2014**, *14*, 67. [CrossRef] [PubMed]
7. Castanos, M.V.; Zhou, D.B.; Linderman, R.E.; Allison, R.; Milman, T.; Carroll, J.; Migacz, J.; Rosen, R.B.; Chui, T.Y. Imaging of Macrophage-Like Cells in Living Human Retina Using Clinical OCT. *Invest. Ophthalmol. Vis. Sci.* **2020**, *61*, 48. [CrossRef] [PubMed]
8. Hammer, D.X.; Agrawal, A.; Villanueva, R.; Saeedi, O.; Liu, Z. Label-free adaptive optics imaging of human retinal macrophage distribution and dynamics. *Proc. Natl. Acad. Sci. USA* **2020**, *117*, 30661–30669. [CrossRef] [PubMed]
9. Rathnasamy, G.; Foulds, W.S.; Ling, E.A.; Kaur, C. Retinal microglia—A key player in healthy and diseased retina. *Prog. Neurobiol.* **2019**, *173*, 18–40. [CrossRef] [PubMed]
10. Ong, J.X.; Nesper, P.L.; Fawzi, A.A.; Wang, J.M.; Lavine, J.A. Macrophage-Like Cell Density Is Increased in Preöliferative Diabetic Retinopathy Characterized by Optical Coherence Tomography Angiography. *Invest. Ophthalmol. Vis. Sci.* **2021**, *62*, 2. [CrossRef] [PubMed]
11. Maltsev, D.S.; Kulikov, A.N.; Vasiliev, A.S. Optical Coherence Tomography Imaging of Retinal Macrophage-Like Cells in Patients with Multiple Evanescent White Dot Syndrome. *Retin. Cases Brief Rep.* **2022**; *ahead of print*. [CrossRef]
12. Koss, M.; Pfister, M.; Rothweiler, F.; Rejdak, R.; Ribeiro, R.; Cinatl, J.; Schubert, R.; Kohnen, T.; Kocha, F.H. Correlation from undiluted vitreous cytokines of untreated central retinal vein occlusion with spectral domain optical coherence tomography. *Open Ophthalmol. J.* **2013**, *7*, 11–17. [CrossRef] [PubMed]
13. Pfister, M.; Rothweiler, F.; Michaelis, M.; Cinatl, J., Jr.; Schubert, R.; Koch, F.H.; Koss, M.J. Correlation of inflammatory and proangiogenic cytokines from undiluted vitreous samples with spectral domain OCT scans, in untreated branch retinal vein occlusion. *Clin. Ophthalmol.* **2013**, *7*, 1061–1067. [CrossRef] [PubMed]
14. Yong, H.; Qi, H.; Yan, H.; Wu, Q.; Zuo, L. The correlation between cytokine levels in the aqueous humor and the prognostic value of anti-vascular endothelial growth factor therapy for treating macular edema resulting from retinal vein occlusion. *Graefes Arch. Clin. Exp. Ophthalmol.* **2021**, *259*, 3243–3250. [CrossRef] [PubMed]
15. Ogino, K.; Murakami, T.; Tsujikawa, A.; Miyamoto, K.; Sakamoto, A.; Ota, M.; Yoshimura, N. Characteristics of optical coherence tomographic hyperreflective foci in retinal vein occlusion. *Retina* **2012**, *32*, 77–85. [CrossRef] [PubMed]

16. Singh, S.; Anshita, D.; Ravichandiran, V. MCP-1: Function, regulation, and involvement in disease. *Int. Immunopharmacol.* **2021**, *101*, 107598. [CrossRef] [PubMed]
17. Noma, H.; Funatsu, H.; Mimura, T. Vascular endothelial growth factor and interleukin-6 are correlated with serous retinal detachment in central retinal vein occlusion. *Curr. Eye Res.* **2012**, *37*, 62–67. [CrossRef] [PubMed]

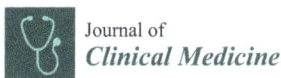

Article

Iris Racemose Hemangioma Assessment with Swept Source Optical Coherence Tomography Angiography: A Feasibility Study and Stand-Alone Comparison

Filippo Confalonieri [1,2,3,*,†], Huy Bao Ngo [1,†], Helga Halldorsdottir Petersen [1], Nils Andreas Eide [1] and Goran Petrovski [1,2,4,*]

1. Department of Ophthalmology, Oslo University Hospital, Kirkeveien 166, 0450 Oslo, Norway
2. Center for Eye Research and Innovative Diagnostics, Department of Ophthalmology, Institute for Clinical Medicine, University of Oslo, Kirkeveien 166, 0450 Oslo, Norway
3. Department of Biomedical Sciences, Humanitas University, Via Rita Levi Montalcini 4, Pieve Emanuele, 20090 Milan, Italy
4. Department of Ophthalmology, University of Split School of Medicine and University Hospital Centre, 21000 Split, Croatia

* Correspondence: filippo.confalonieri01@gmail.com (F.C.); goran.petrovski@medisin.uio.no (G.P.)
† These authors contributed equally to this work.

Abstract: Purpose: To evaluate arteriovenous malformations (AVM) with swept-source (SS) optical coherence tomography (OCT) angiography (OCTA) in iris racemose hemangioma and compare it with traditional intravenous iris fluorescein angiography (IVFA). Methods: A cross-sectional observational clinical study was conducted on patients with iris racemose hemangioma with the ZEISS PLEX Elite 9000 SS OCT & OCTA. Results: Three eyes of three patients were imaged. Iris racemose hemangiomas demonstrated a tortuous, well-defined, and continuous course of the AVM. The ZEISS PLEX Elite 9000 SS OCT & OCTA allowed for a detailed visualization of the ARM and was superior to IVFA in depicting small caliber, fine vessels. Conclusions: SS-OCTA may provide a dye-free, no-injection, cost-effective method comparable to spectral domain OCTA and IVFA for diagnosing and monitoring iris racemose hemangiomas for growth and vascularity.

Keywords: iris racemose hemangioma; iris arteriovenous malformation; iris arteriovenous aneurysm; Swept Source Optical Coherence Tomography (SS-OCT); OCT angiography (OCTA)

1. Introduction

The iris racemose hemangioma, also known as iris arteriovenous malformation (AVM) and AV aneurysm, is a benign vascular lesion [1]. Its fundamental pathophysiology is an artery that joins directly to a vein, bypassing the capillary network. A true AVM of the iris is rare, and little has been published about this entity [2].

Traditionally, intravenous iris fluorescein angiography (IVFA) has been regarded as the diagnostic procedure of choice for iris racemose hemangioma. IVFA shows a hyperfluorescent lesion that is rapidly filling in, and shown nearly no mid-to-late phase leaking. Additionally, intervening iris hypoperfusion can be seen. Iris indocyanine green angiography can be utilized to better penetrate through the iris pigmentation in individuals with darker irides [2,3].

Spectral domain (SD) optical coherence tomography angiography (OCTA) has previously been shown to be a useful tool in physiologic iris vascular imaging [4]. Iris racemose hemangioma has previously been shown to have distinct features on SD-OCTA only in one descriptive, noncomparative case series [5].

The ZEISS PLEX Elite 9000 Swept-Source (SS) OCT & OCTA is an evolution of the previous SD-OCTA technology [6] which generates high-resolution three-dimensional maps of the retinal and choroidal microvasculature. SS-OCTA has previously been established as an

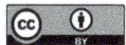

effective, non-invasive tool in the management of corneal and iris neovascularization [7,8]. To our knowledge, no validation report exists on SS-OCTA capability to image iris racemose hemangioma, which we hereby report and discuss the results of by comparing them to traditional IVFA imaging capabilities.

2. Materials and Methods

This is a retrospective, comparative, observational case series of 3 consecutive unilateral iris racemose hemangiomas seen at the Department of Ophthalmology of the Oslo University Hospital (OUH), Oslo, Norway from October 2020 to February 2022. Institutional review board approval from the OUH was not necessary, but written consent was obtained from all patients and approval from the data protection officer at OUH were obtained.

All patients underwent comprehensive ophthalmic examination including slit lamp evaluation with gonioscopy, and anterior segment (AS) photography, dilated funduscopic examination, ultrasound biomicroscopy (UBM), posterior segment OCT, AS OCT, IVFA and OCTA. The latter was performed using a ZEISS PLEX Elite 9000 SS OCT & OCTA, (Carl Zeiss Meditec AG Goeschwitzer Str. 51-52 07745 Jena, Germany) [6]. For AS SS-OCTA, a volume cube scan protocol was used to scan the lesion (3 × 3 mm; AngioRetina); however, the positioning and focus settings were adjusted manually to allow visualization of the AS, and to obtain a precise focus of the OCT B-scan.

Patient demographics (age, ethnicity, and sex) were recorded. Data regarding clinical features included the affected eye, best corrected visual acuity (BCVA), iris color, iris racemose hemangioma location, type, and size (number of clock hours), presence of iris or ciliary body mass, and other concomitant ocular lesions. Imaging features were recorded from AS photography, AS SS-OCT, SS-OCT, OCTA, IVFA, and ocular ultrasound. The imaging results of the vascular course analysis obtained with AS SS-OCT were then qualitatively compared to that obtained with IVFA.

3. Results

The mean age at the first referral was 62.6 years (range, 59–69 years), and all patients were Caucasian with measured BCVA in the involved eye equal to 20/20 (n = 2) and 20/32 (n = 1). The patients were both male (n = 2) and female (n = 1) and they were all referred with the diagnosis of a pigmented iris lesion. The eyes studied were both right (n = 2) and left (n = 1). The iris color was blue in all cases and no concomitant iris or ciliary body masses were found. Both at the slit lamp and at the UBM imaging the lesions appeared structurally ill defined. Specifically, by slit lamp biomicroscopy, the iris racemose hemangiomas were barely noticeable within the iris stroma as a relatively long, dark-red vessel with a tortuous course, buried within the normal stromal tissue without solid tumor in the iris or ciliary body. The hemangioma was located temporally in the right (n = 2) or nasal in the left (n = 1) eye and demonstrated up to 4 clock hours of involvement. AS-OCT showed cystic lesions in the iris stroma in all cases, which likely correspond to the large vascular lumen. All lesions were classified as complex type due to intertwining convolutions, and not a simple loop. Table 1 summarizes the features of the lesions.

3.1. Patient 1

A 59-year-old male was referred for increased intraocular pressure (IOP) in the left eye and an asymptomatic abnormal iris pigmentation in the right eye. The iris lesion in the right eye was diagnosed as complex iris racemose hemangioma; no treatment was required, and the patient was followed-up. Figure 1 shows the multimodal imaging pertinent to the iris lesion. The structural AS-OCT shows hyporeflective cystic cavities representing the lumen of the racemose hemangioma of the iris. These structures appear localized in the anterior iris stroma and have variable dimensions determined by the direction of the vessels in relation to the cross section of the AS-OCT. Figure 2 compares the late phase IVFA with the iris OCTA, showing that the convoluted vascular network from 7 to 8 o'clock is equally discernible with both of the imaging techniques and nearly no leakage is present at IVFA.

Table 1. The demographics, clinical and SS-OCTA imaging features of the patients having iris racemose hemangioma.

Demographics	Patient 1	Patient 2	Patient 3
Age	59	69	60
Ethnicity	Caucasian	Caucasian	Caucasian
Sex	Male	Female	Male
Referral diagnosis	Pigmented iris lesion	Pigmented iris lesion	Pigmented iris lesion
Involved eye	Right eye	Right eye	Left eye
BCVA	20/20	20/32	20/20
Iris color	Blue	Blue	Blue
Clock hour	7–8	6–10	10–12
Concomitant iris or ciliary body mass	no	no	no
Visibility UBM	Indistinct	Indistinct	Indistinct
Visibility at the slit lamp	Red lesion	Red indistinct lesion	Red indistinct lesion
Visibility at AS-OCT	Cystic lesions	Cystic lesions	Cystic lesions
Visibility at SS-OCTA	Well defined vascular network	Well defined vascular network	Well defined vascular network
Visibility at IVFA	Well defined vascular network without leakage	Well defined vascular network without leakage	Well defined vascular network without leakage
Vascular course	Convoluted	Convoluted at the pupil margin	Convoluted at the pupil margin
Hemangioma type characterization	Complex	Complex	Complex

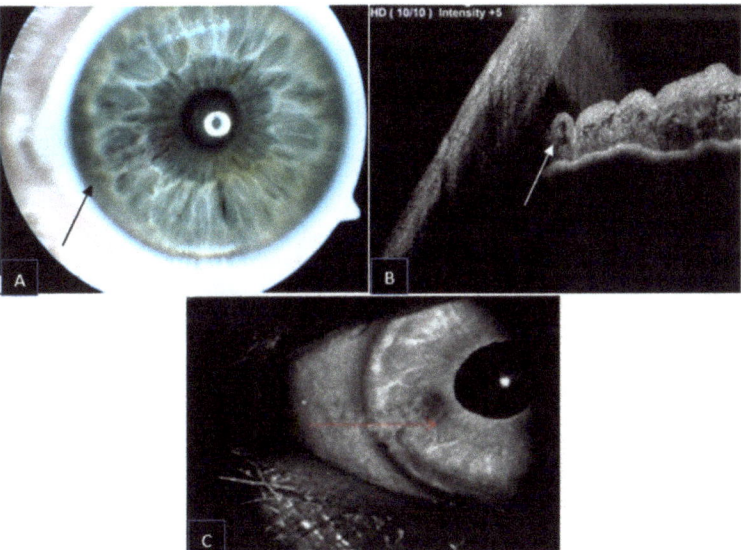

Figure 1. Iris racemose hemangioma appearance on slit lamp photography ((A); black arrow) with a corresponding AS-OCT ((B); white arrow) and infrared photograph ((C); red arrow). The arrows indicate the inferior border of the lesion.

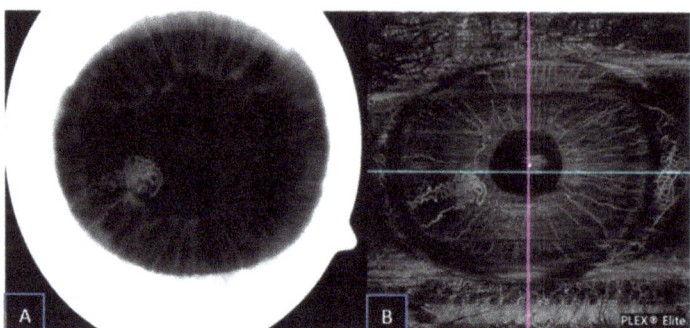

Figure 2. Iris racemose hemangioma under late-phase IVFA (**A**) and corresponding SS-OCTA (**B**) imaging.

3.2. Patient 2

A 69-year-old female was referred for herpes zoster ophthalmicus in the area of the right ophthalmic branch of the trigeminal nerve. Incidentally, after the resolution of the eczematous lesion, dry age-related macular degeneration was diagnosed and an abnormal, asymptomatic iris pigmentation in the right eye was noted. The iris lesion in the right eye was diagnosed as complex iris racemose hemangioma, no treatment was required, and the patient was followed-up. Figure 3 shows the multimodal imaging pertinent to the iris lesion. The racemose hemangioma of the iris is shown as hyporeflective cystic cavities on the structural AS-OCT. These structures appear deep in the iris stroma. Since the structural AS-OCT scan is acquired in correspondence of a horizontal running, relatively non-convoluted large vessel, these cystic spaces look quite different than the corresponding image in the previous case. Figure 4 compares the late phase IVFA with the iris OCTA, showing that the convoluted vascular network from 6 to 10 o'clock is equally discernible with both the imaging techniques and nearly no leakage is present at IVFA.

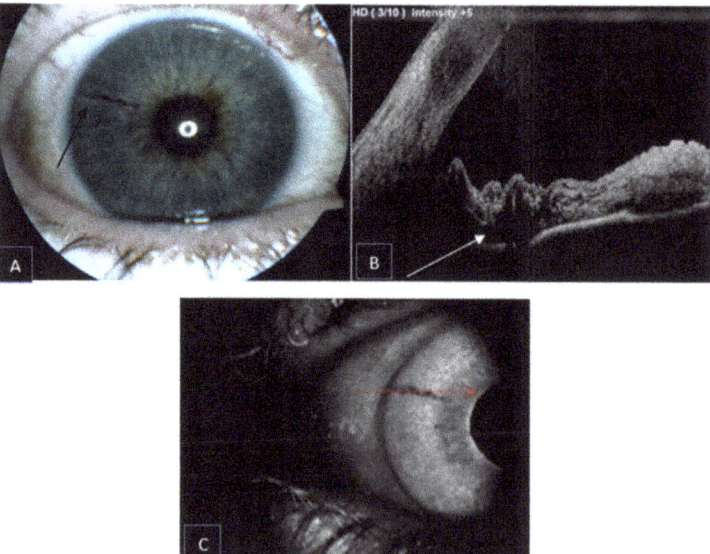

Figure 3. Iris racemose hemangioma appearance on slit lamp photography ((**A**); black arrow) with a corresponding AS-OCT ((**B**); white arrow) and infrared photograph ((**C**); red arrow). The arrows indicate the superior border of the lesion.

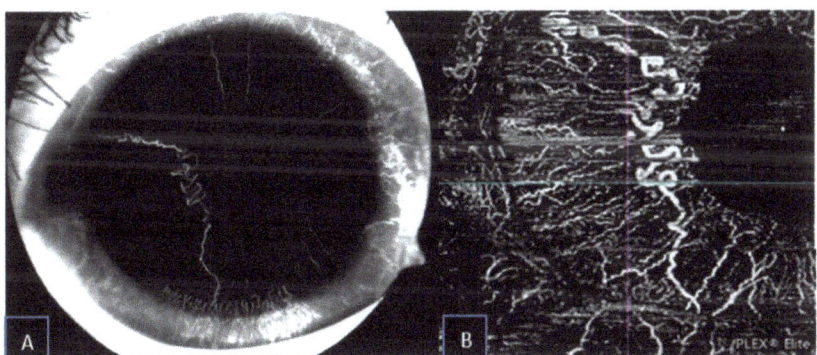

Figure 4. Iris racemose hemangioma under late-phase IVFA (**A**) and corresponding SS-OCTA (**B**) imaging.

3.3. Patient 3

A 60-year-old male was referred for an asymptomatic iris pigmented lesion in the left eye noted right after bilateral refractive lens exchange surgery. The iris lesion in the left eye was diagnosed as complex iris racemose hemangioma, no treatment was required, and the patient was followed-up. The structural AS-OCT shows two hyporeflective cystic cavities representing the lumen of the racemose hemangioma of the iris forming a loop. The septum between the two cavities represents the vessel wall that folds back in on itself. The slab represents the area of OCTA flow acquisition, and it shows no specific signal inside the cystic cavities, probably due to the disruption of laminar flow inside the vascular malformation. Figure 5 shows the multimodal imaging pertinent to the iris lesion. Figure 6 compares the late phase IVFA with the iris OCTA, showing that the convoluted vascular network from 6 to 10 o'clock is equally discernible with both the imaging techniques and nearly no leakage is present at IVFA.

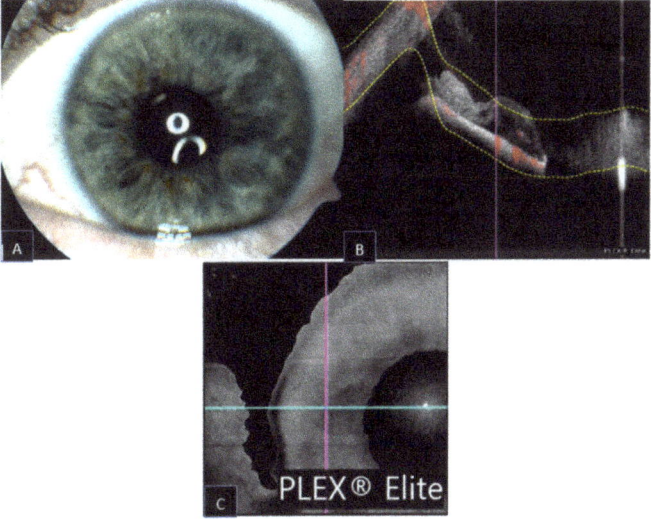

Figure 5. Iris racemose hemangioma appearance on slit lamp photography (**A**) and a corresponding AS-OCT with superimposed flow signal (**B**) and infrared photograph (**C**) with the blue line corresponding to the cross-sectional OCT image plane acquisition.

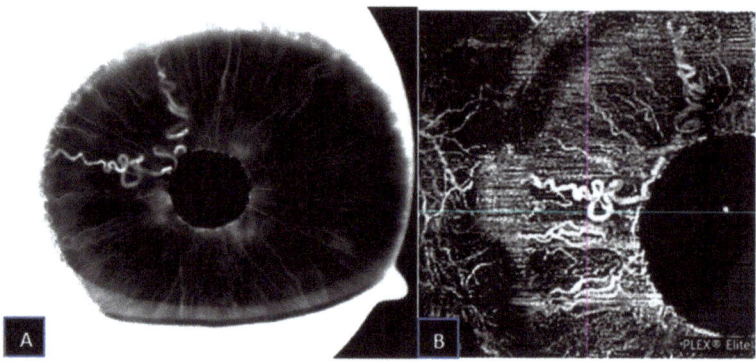

Figure 6. Iris racemose hemangioma under late-phase IVFA (**A**) and corresponding SS-OCTA (**B**) imaging.

All the iris racemose hemangiomas showed a clear structural resolution by SS-OCTA imaging, comparable to the resolution obtained with IVFA. The fine caliber vessels of the irides studied were better discernible by SS-OCTA imaging than by IVFA.

No associated vascular malformation was detected on magnetic resonance imaging (MRI) of the head and orbits in the three patients studied.

4. Discussion

AS SD-OCTA has been demonstrated to be a useful and reliable tool for the vascular imaging of both normal irides and benign or malignant lesions of the iris, with possible applications in vascular conjunctival lesions, as well [4,5,9–11].

Using AS SD-OCTA, Skalet et al. found that iris melanomas contain higher intertumoral vascular density than benign iris nevi [9]. Chien et al. employed SD-OCTA to identify extensive vasculature within conjunctival racemose hemangioma, which was not visible on FA [11]. Kang et al. showed iris microhemangiomatosis by SD-OCTA, outlining small vascular lesions with flow signal from the posterior iris stroma [10]. Furthermore, Chien et al. [5] showed that SD-OCTA clearly depicts the looping course of iris racemose hemangiomas and can highlight the fine details of radial iris vessels, indistinguishable by IVFA [5]. The same result of superiority in the resolution of the vessels by SD-OCTA over IVFA was described by Zett et al. in normal iris [12].

SS-OCTA has recently emerged as an imaging technology, and it has been described to be able to better define the iris vessels in normal pigmented iris than SD-OCTA [13].

To our knowledge, this is the first study to report the outcome of racemic iris hemangiomas when imaged with SS-OCTA.

On SS-OCTA imaging, all our studied iris racemose hemangiomas displayed a sharp delineation, comparable to the resolution attained with IVFA in large caliber vessels and superior in small caliber vessels. By using SS-OCTA, the normal fine caliber vessels of the irides studied could also be more clearly delineated than by IVFA, which is consistent with the previous findings conducted with SD-OCTA [5]. These findings suggest that OCTA in general, and possibly SS-OCTA more than SD-OCTA, might be able to detect smaller caliber, abnormal vessels when they are not yet detectable on slit lamp examination or by IVFA. The application of SS-OCTA can find wider applications in other neovascular diseases involving the iris, such as that of early imaging of iris neovascularization in neovascular glaucoma—a pathologic process that has just been recently investigated for the first time using SS-OCTA [14].

The patients enrolled in this study had lightly pigmented irides. The iris color affects the ability to detect flow signals by OCTA, and flow is most effectively detected in irides that are lightly pigmented [9]. This means that the same resolution of the vascular lesions might not be attainable in darkly pigmented irides, even though the higher transmittance of the signal and higher resolution found with fine vessels in SS-OCTA imaging suggests that this technique would anyway be capable of better image iris vessels compared to IVFA.

Even though this study aims at highlighting the potential of the recently introduced SS-OCTA technology, it is crucial to understand that each strategy has a number of drawbacks. The light penetrance of deeper tissue and vascular leakage, which can hide microvascular features, restricts the use of IVFA. On the other hand, the limitations of SS-OCTA and OCTA technology in general, are due to the motion artifacts and its inability to recognize specific flow patterns, in particular, vascular leakage. Since iris racemose hemangiomas do not leak at IVFA, as opposed to iris neovascularization, which demonstrates a specifically modest dye leakage, IVFA may be still superior to differentiate iris vascular diseases in circumstances when they are difficult to distinguish. On the contrary, the fine, clinically invisible iris vessels can be detected by OCTA in the very early stages, as well as in the regressed stage of iris neovascularization [15]. In addition, leakage IVFA may be superior in differentiating iris racemose hemangioma from other vascular or solid tumors of the iris that display a pathologic vessel wall structure, such as malignant neoplasms [16].

The main drawback of our research is the lack of direct comparison between the information derived from SS-OCTA and SD-OCTA to determine if there is an actual clinical advantage. Further studies are required to determine the clinical advantage of SS-OCTA in iris vascular imaging over other imaging techniques.

5. Conclusions

SS-OCTA may provide a dye-free, no-injection, cost-effective method that is comparable and complementary to SD-OCTA and IVFA for diagnosing and monitoring iris racemose hemangiomas for growth and vascularity.

Author Contributions: For Conceptualization, all authors; methodology, F.C., H.B.N. and G.P.; investigation, H.B.N., N.A.E. and H.H.P.; resources, G.P.; data curation, H.B.N.; writing—original draft preparation, F.C.; writing—review and editing, all authors; supervision, G.P. All authors have read and agreed to the published version of the manuscript.

Funding: This research received no external funding.

Institutional Review Board Statement: The study was conducted in accordance with the Declaration of Helsinki, and approved by the Institutional Review Board of the Oslo University Hospital.

Informed Consent Statement: Patient consent was gathered according to the local regulations of the Ethics Committee of the Oslo University Hospital, Oslo, Norway.

Data Availability Statement: Not applicable.

Acknowledgments: We acknowledge support from the Open Access Publication Fund of the University of Oslo.

Conflicts of Interest: The authors declare no conflict of interest.

References

1. Prost, M. Arteriovenous Communication of the Iris. *Br. J. Ophthalmol.* **1986**, *70*, 856–859. [CrossRef] [PubMed]
2. Shields, J.A.; Streicher, T.F.E.; Spirkova, J.H.J.; Stubna, M.; Shields, C.L. Arteriovenous Malformation of the Iris in 14 Cases. *Arch. Ophthalmol.* **2006**, *124*, 370–375. [CrossRef] [PubMed]
3. Iris Arteriovenous Malformation—EyeWiki. Available online: https://eyewiki.aao.org/Iris_Arteriovenous_Malformation (accessed on 24 September 2022).
4. Allegrini, D.; Montesano, G.; Pece, A. Optical Coherence Tomography Angiography in a Normal Iris. *Ophthalmic Surg. Lasers Imaging Retin.* **2016**, *47*, 1138–1139. [CrossRef] [PubMed]
5. Chien, J.L.; Sioufi, K.; Ferenczy, S.; Say, E.A.T.; Shields, C.L. Optical Coherence Tomography Angiography Features of Iris Racemose Hemangioma in 4 Cases. *JAMA Ophthalmol.* **2017**, *135*, 1106–1110. [CrossRef] [PubMed]
6. Rosenfeld, P.J.; Durbin, M.K.; Roisman, L.; Zheng, F.; Miller, A.; Robbins, G.; Schaal, K.B.; Gregori, G. ZEISS Angioplex™ Spectral Domain Optical Coherence Tomography Angiography: Technical Aspects. *Dev. Ophthalmol.* **2016**, *56*, 18–29. [CrossRef] [PubMed]
7. Shiozaki, D.; Sakimoto, S.; Shiraki, A.; Wakabayashi, T.; Fukushima, Y.; Oie, Y.; Usui, S.; Sato, S.; Sakaguchi, H.; Nishida, K. Observation of Treated Iris Neovascularization by Swept-Source-Based En-Face Anterior-Segment Optical Coherence Tomography Angiography. *Sci. Rep.* **2019**, *9*, 10262. [CrossRef] [PubMed]

8. Ang, M.; Cai, Y.; Tan, A.C.S. Swept Source Optical Coherence Tomography Angiography for Contact Lens-Related Corneal Vascularization. *J. Ophthalmol.* **2016**, *2016*, e9685297. [CrossRef] [PubMed]
9. Skalet, A.H.; Li, Y.; Lu, C.D.; Jia, Y.; Lee, B.; Husvogt, L.; Maier, A.; Fujimoto, J.G.; Thomas, C.R.; Huang, D. Optical Coherence Tomography Angiography Characteristics of Iris Melanocytic Tumors. *Ophthalmology* **2017**, *124*, 197–204. [CrossRef] [PubMed]
10. Kang, A.S.; Welch, R.J.; Sioufi, K.; Say, E.A.T.; Shields, J.A.; Shields, C.L. Optical Coherence Tomography Angiography of Iris Microhemangiomatosis. *Am. J. Ophthalmol. Case Rep.* **2017**, *6*, 24–26. [CrossRef] [PubMed]
11. Chien, J.L.; Sioufi, K.; Shields, C.L. Optical Coherence Tomography Angiography of Conjunctival Racemose Hemangioma. *Ophthalmology* **2017**, *124*, 449. [CrossRef] [PubMed]
12. Zett, C.; Stina, D.M.R.; Kato, R.T.; Novais, E.A.; Allemann, N. Comparison of Anterior Segment Optical Coherence Tomography Angiography and Fluorescein Angiography for Iris Vasculature Analysis. *Graefe Arch. Clin. Exp. Ophthalmol.* **2018**, *256*, 683–691. [CrossRef] [PubMed]
13. Ang, M.; Devarajan, K.; Tan, A.C.; Ke, M.; Tan, B.; Teo, K.; Sng, C.C.A.; Ting, D.S.; Schmetterer, L. Anterior Segment Optical Coherence Tomography Angiography for Iris Vasculature in Pigmented Eyes. *Br. J. Ophthalmol.* **2021**, *105*, 929–934. [CrossRef] [PubMed]
14. Akagi, T.; Fujimoto, M.; Ikeda, H.O. Anterior Segment Optical Coherence Tomography Angiography of Iris Neovascularization After Intravitreal Ranibizumab and Panretinal Photocoagulation. *JAMA Ophthalmol.* **2020**, *138*, e190318. [CrossRef] [PubMed]
15. Roberts, P.K.; Goldstein, D.A.; Fawzi, A.A. Anterior Segment Optical Coherence Tomography Angiography for Identification of Iris Vasculature and Staging of Iris Neovascularization: A Pilot Study. *Curr. Eye Res.* **2017**, *42*, 1136–1142. [CrossRef] [PubMed]
16. Shields, J.A.; Bianciotto, C.; Kligman, B.E.; Shields, C.L. Vascular Tumors of the Iris in 45 Patients: The 2009 Helen Keller Lecture. *Arch. Ophthalmol.* **2010**, *128*, 1107–1113. [CrossRef] [PubMed]

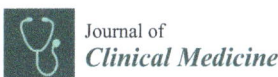

Article

Structural Features of Patients with Drusen-like Deposits and Systemic Lupus Erythematosus

Marc Kukan [1], Matthew Driban [2], Kiran K. Vupparaboina [2], Swen Schwarz [1], Alice M. Kitay [1], Mohammed A. Rasheed [3], Catharina Busch [4], Daniel Barthelmes [1,5], Jay Chhablani [2] and Mayss Al-Sheikh [1,*]

1. Department of Ophthalmology, University Hospital Zurich, University of Zurich, Frauenklinikstrasse 24, 8091 Zurich, Switzerland
2. UPMC Eye Center, University of Pittsburgh, Pittsburgh, PA 15213, USA
3. School of Optometry and Vision Science, University of Waterloo, Waterloo, ON N2L 3G1, Canada
4. Department of Ophthalmology, University Hospital Leipzig, 04103 Leipzig, Germany
5. Save Sight Institute, The University of Sydney, Sydney, NSW 2000, Australia
* Correspondence: mayss.al-sheikh@usz.ch or mayss.alsheikh@gmail.com

Abstract: Background: The relevance of drusen-like deposits (DLD) in patients with systemic lupus erythematosus (SLE) is to a large extent uncertain. Their genesis is proposed to be correlated to immune-complex and complement depositions in the framework of SLE. The intention of this study was to determine potential morphological differences in the choroid and retina as well as potential microvascular changes comparing two cohorts of SLE patients divergent in the presence or absence of DLD using multimodal imaging. Methods: Both eyes of 16 SLE patients with DLD were compared to an age- and sex-matched control-group consisting of 16 SLE patients without detectable DLD. Both cohorts were treated with hydroxychloroquine (HCQ) and did not differ in the treatment duration or dosage. Using spectral-domain optical coherence tomography (SD-OCT) choroidal volume measures, choroidal vascularity indices (CVI) and retinal layer segmentation was performed and compared. In addition, by the exploitation of optical coherence tomography angiography vascular density, perfusion density of superficial and deep retinal capillary plexuses and the choriocapillaris were analyzed. For the choroidal OCT-scans, a subset of 51 healthy individuals served as a reference-group. Results: CVI measures revealed a significant reduction in eyes with DLD compared to healthy controls (0.56 (0.54–0.59) versus 0.58 (0.57–0.59) ($p = 0.018$) and 0.56 (0.54–0.58) versus 0.58 (0.57–0.60) ($p < 0.001$)). The photoreceptor cell layer presented significant thinning in both eyes of subjects with DLD compared to control subjects without DLD (68.8 ± 7.7 µm vs. 77.1 ± 7.3 µm for right eyes, $p = 0.008$, and 66.5 ± 10.5 µm vs. 76.1 ± 6.3 µm for left eyes, $p = 0.011$). OCTA scans revealed no significant changes, yet there could be observed numerically lower values in the capillary plexuses of the retina in eyes with DLD than in eyes without DLD. Conclusions: Our results illustrated significant alterations in the choroidal and retinal analyzes, suggesting a correlation between DLD and the progression of inflammatory processes in the course of SLE leading to retinal degeneration. For this reason, DLD could serve as a biomarker for a more active state of disease.

Keywords: drusen-like deposits; systemic lupus erythematosus; optical coherence tomography; choroidal vascularity index; optical coherence tomography angiography

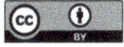

1. Introduction

Systemic lupus erythematosus (SLE) is an autoimmune disease presenting itself in a heterogenous way with a multitude of clinical manifestations ranging from renal, cardiovascular, to ocular damage [1]. It is characterized by an elaborate set of immunologic processes, in particular the loss of immune tolerance and subsequent dysregulation by production of autoantibodies, formation of immunocomplexes, and activation of the complement system [1,2]. As the disease develops, systemic inflammation progresses leading to increasing organ destruction in a chronic relapsing course [2].

The etiology is yet unknown; the classification of SLE is based on criteria defined by the American College of Rheumatology (ACR) including various clinical and immunologic manifestations [1]. Although ocular involvement is not outlined in the diagnostic assessment [3], it can occur in up to 30% of SLE patients including conditions as keratoconjunctivitis, retinopathy, and optic neuritis among other ocular manifestations [1]. In the majority of cases, retinopathy and visual impairment manifests in already well-advanced disease states [4]. More rarely, choroidopathy has been detected [5], conceivably because of the limited technical possibilities to analyze the deeper more hidden part of the visual organ in the past.

Nowadays, more advanced optical coherence tomography (OCT) techniques enable us to perform in-depth evaluations of the retina as well as the choroid [6].

The involvement of the choriocapillaris has currently been subject of interest in SLE patients [6–8], as it appears to be influenced by disease activity [6]. The choroidal thickness seems to decrease in patients due to vasculitis and deposition of complement factors leading to a reduction in blood flow [6]. An upcoming method to examine the choroid, the choroidal vascularity index (CVI), is suggested to advance previous analyses of choroidal thickness by providing more stable results due to being less susceptible to physiological elements [9]. It could therefore be a potential new player in the evaluation of disease progression in SLE.

In recent years, the assessment of drusen-like deposits (DLD) has emerged without a considerable number of studies concerning this matter yet. Located between the Bruch membrane and the retinal pigment epithelium (RPE), there are differing hypotheses proposed regarding the potential value of DLD in disease process. Baglio et al. have found that DLD, detected by indocyanine green angiography (ICGA), only occur in SLE patients with lupus nephritis and having the anatomical commonalities of choroid and glomeruli in mind, stated that they could be an early marker for renal involvement [7]. Invernizzi et al., however, which made use of OCT, did not fully support that assumption, as they found DLD occurring in SLE patients without lupus nephritis as well [3]. They postulated it was more likely that the deposits are associated with complement pathway dysregulations taking place in the eye and in other capillary systems. On the other hand, the authors had discovered that the number, size, and distribution was significantly higher in SLE patients with renal involvement, correlating to the results found by Baglio et al. In conclusion, they claimed that DLD could be a marker for disease activity, as their presumed genesis accompanies the known pathophysiology of SLE and increases when renal involvement is present [3]. Former studies support this argumentation, as they found the presence of similar lesions as DLD to increase the threat of vision loss [10,11].

Ocular manifestations, as DLD and choroidal alterations, can be present without any noticeable symptoms and may therefore hold the opportunity to serve as a marker for further disease progression [4,10]

In this study, we aim to assess the morphological features in patients with SLE and drusen-like deposits using non-invasive imaging modalities and to compare them to age- and sex-matched group with SLE but without DLD and to a group of healthy subjects.

2. Methods

2.1. Study Design

Within the frame of a large-scale monitoring of patients treated with hydroxychloroquine (HCQ) at the Departments of Ophthalmology, University Hospital Zurich, from January 2012 to December 2020, patient data was extracted to be analyzed in a retrospective observational comparative cohort study. The trial is compliant with international norms as it was approved by the Institutional review board of Swiss ethics/BASEC (No. 2019-00972). A written informed consent was obtained from all patients participating.

2.2. Patient Inclusion and Exclusion Criteria

Subjects had to meet the following inclusion criteria: male or female patients with a confirmed diagnosis of systemic lupus erythematosus at an age ≥ 18 years were included from the HCQ clinic during regular screening exam. Furthermore, drusen-like deposits, defined as an accumulating precipitation leading to a detectable detachment of the RPE from the Bruch membrane, had to be verifiable in OCT (Figure 1). Patients were regularly seen in the course of routine HCQ-toxicity-screening including regular OCT-scans. A sufficient OCT and OCTA image quality had to be ensured to qualify for further analysis.

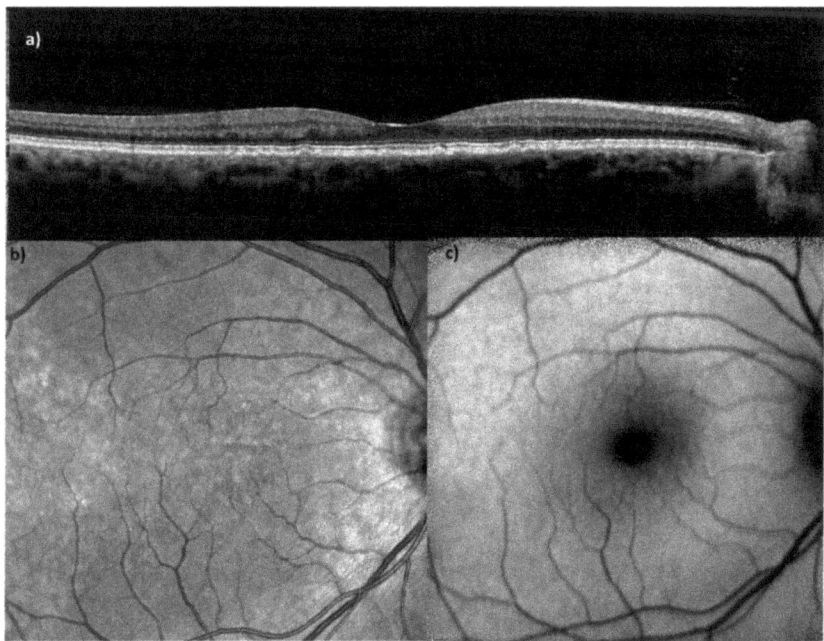

Figure 1. Multimodal imaging of a SLE patient with drusen-like deposits. (**a**) Illustrates an optical coherence tomography scan, (**b**) a near-infrared (NIR) image, and (**c**) a fundus autofluorescence image.

Evidence of other ocular or systemic diseases other than SLE, current or previous macular and retinal diseases, myopia > -3 diopters, and significant lens opacities were the exclusion criteria.

2.3. Data Collection

A cohort of 16 SLE-patients with documented drusen-like deposits were analyzed and compared to a control group including 16 SLE-patients without DLD, which were matched for age, sex, ethnicity, smoking status, dosage, and HCQ-treatment duration. HCQ-dosage data was collected by examination of the prescription on each consultation, which was cross checked by taking the patient's medication history. Concerning the risk profile, an incidental significant difference in the prevalence of cardiovascular disease could be detected. Both the right and the left eye were scanned in the first exam and the last follow-up in order to identify potential alterations over time. The cohorts were further set against a healthy control group without retinopathy, systemic diseases involving the retina, or HCQ-intake. The probands were selected out of a pool of patients consulting our clinic due to various complaints and conditions, without influence to retinal structures, as for example conjunctivitis, complications concerning contact lenses, or cataract.

Spectral-domain optical coherence tomography (SD-OCT) enabled us to thoroughly analyze and assess differences in the retinal layers. An OCT scan and other imaging modalities of a SLE patient with DLD is illustratively demonstrated in Figure 1. The equipment was fully integrated with the analytical software, HEYEX 2, provided by Heidelberg Engineering (Heidelberg, Germany), which carried out an automatic segmentation. First, using ETDRS thickness maps, according to the ETDRS grid as shown in Figure 2, the software application automatically segmented the retinal layers into retinal nerve fiber layer (RNFL), ganglion cell layer (GCL), inner plexiform layer (IPL), inner nuclear layer (INL), outer plexiform layer (OPL), outer nuclear layer (ONL), and retinal pigment epithelium (RPE) (Figure 2). Thereafter, manual correction of potential artifacts risen from the automatic segmentation process was performed. Subsequently, the gathered data was compared to a healthy control group. For all layers analyzed, the thinnest and the thickest section in the centerfield of the ETDRS grid was determined, described as "Center Min" and "Center Max", respectively.

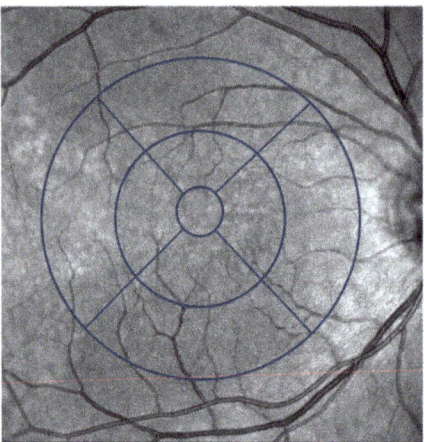

Figure 2. Grid for retinal layer thickness measurement. Retinal layer thickness was measured according to the ETDRS grid that was divided into a central area including the fovea with a diameter of 1mm, an inner ring with a diameter of 3mm, and an outer ring with 6 mm.

Choroidal vascularity index (CVI) for the volume scans was calculated based on a previously reported algorithm. In brief, it involves shadow compensation, localization, and binarization of the choroid [12], as visualized in Figure 3. Shadow compensation reduces noise and increases the contrast enhancement of B-scans [13]. Choroidal segmentation was accomplished by identification of choroidal inner and outer boundaries shown as RPE-Bruch's membrane and choroid-scleral interface, respectively. This was followed by binarization of choroidal vessels, wherein lumen of choroidal vessels was shown as dark areas and stromal areas were marked as bright areas. The ratio of choroidal luminal area to total choroidal area was defined as CVI.

Imaging by optical coherence tomography angiography (OCTA) was executed by PLEX Elite 9000 device, software version 2.0.1.47652 (Carl Zeiss Meditec Inc., Dublin, CA, USA). Centered on the fovea, images with the dimensions of 3 × 3 mm and 6 × 6 mm were obtained by a well-trained, certified ophthalmologist, whereas only the 3 × 3 mm-frames are presented in this study. Scans with a signal strength of 8 out of 10 or higher were included, as signal strength has been shown to influence quantitative measurements in OCTA [14]. Quantitative parameters of the 3 × 3-mm scans were automatically generated; layers of the superficial, deep retinal capillary plexuses and choriocapillaris were obtained using layer segmentation produced by the instrument software and prototype analysis vascular density quantification software (Macular Density v. 0.7.1, ARI Network Hub, Carl Zeiss Meditec Inc., Dublin, CA, USA) supplied by the manufacturer. The analyzed region of interest was the innermost ring of the ETDRS grid (inner ring, iR), with an inner diameter of 1 mm and an outer diameter of 3 mm, centered on the fovea.

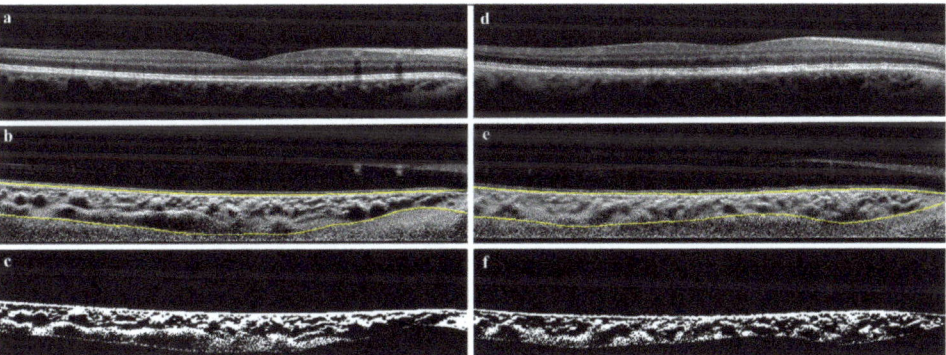

Figure 3. Choroidal vascularity index (CVI). CVI data was generated from OCT cross-sections (**a,d**) through automatic segmentation (**b,e**) and binarization (**c,f**). Pictured is a SLE patient without DLD (**left column**) and a SLE patient with DLD (**right column**).

2.4. Statistical Analysis

Data was analyzed using Stata16 (StataCorp (2019) Stata Statistical Software: Release 16, College Station, TX, USA). Summary statistics included mean and standard deviation for continuous variables and frequencies with percentages for categorical variables. Clinical and OCT/OCTA data were reported as proportions, mean and standard deviation, or median and interquartile range for skewed data. Patients were divided into separate cohorts including SLE with DLD, SLE without DLD, and healthy controls. Data was compared between cohorts using chi-squared and Kruskal–Wallis tests. Statistical significance was defined as a p-value < 0.050.

3. Results

The demographics of the participants are illustrated in Table 1. There were no significant differences in the distribution of age, gender, ethnicity, or smoking status ($p > 0.050$). At the outset, the mean age in the study group was 41.2 ± SD (22–61) years, as compared to the control group without DLD 40.6 ± SD (20–61) years and the reference group of healthy people 57.7 ± SD (24–93) years. The majority of participants were female, as 12 out of 16 accounted for 66.7% of subjects in the study group and 11 out of 16, i.e., 68.8%, subjects in the control group were female. Regarding ethnicity, 13 patients of the DLD group were Caucasian and 3 were Asian; in the matched control group 10 were Caucasian, 5 were Asian, and 1 patient belonged to a different ethnic group. In the first group, five participants were smokers, four non-smokers, one person quit, and three had an unknown smoking status. The second group showed a similar tendency, with eight smokers, five non-smokers, one person who quit, and two individuals with an unknown smoking status.

Both SLE-patients with DLD and patients without DLD were treated with HCQ. As demonstrated in Table 2, no significant disparities in HCQ dose or treatment duration were found ($p > 0.050$). The median daily dose amounted to 200 mg in both groups with a mean cumulative dose of 567.6 g in the study group and 486.6 g in the control group. The dosage, measured in milligrams HCQ per kilograms bodyweight, was on average 3.8 mg/kg in probands with DLD and 4.3 mg/kg in probands without DLD. Treatment duration ran for 7.4 years and for 5.3 years in the case and the control group, respectively.

Table 1. Baseline demographics. SD, standard deviation.

	Eyes with DLD (n = 16)	Eyes without DLD (n = 16)	Healthy Control Group (n = 51)
Age, years, mean (SD)			
First Exam	41.2 (12.3)	40.6 (12.3)	57.7 (18.3)
Sex, n (%)			
Male	4 (33.3)	5 (31.3)	24 (47.1)
Female	12 (66.7)	11 (68.8)	27 (52.9)
Ethnicity, n (%)			
Caucasian	13 (81.3)	10 (62.5)	
Asian	3 (18.8)	5 (31.3)	
Other	0 (0.0)	1 (6.3)	
Smoking Status, n (%)			
Yes	5 (38.5)	8 (50.0)	
No	4 (30.8)	5 (31.3)	
Quit	1 (7.7)	1 (6.3)	
Unknown	3 (23.1)	2 (12.6)	

Table 2. HCQ treatment characteristics and prevalence of relevant comorbidities. Significant differences shown in bold type. SD, standard deviation.

	Eyes with DLD (n = 16)	Eyes without DLD (n = 16)	p-Value
HCQ Treatment			
Daily Dose, mg (range)	200 (200–200)	200 (200–400)	0.260
Cumulative Dose, g (range)	567.6 (450.5–899.8)	486.6 (322.4–1026.5)	0.429
Dosage, mg/kg (range)	3.8 (2.8–5.1)	4.3 (2.7–5.3)	0.612
Treatment Duration, years (range)	7.4 (4.7–12.3)	5.3 (2.5–8.3)	0.188
Comorbidity, n (%)			
Cardiovascular Disease	10 (62.5)	3 (18.8)	**0.036**
Renal Involvement	3 (18.8)	2 (12.5)	0.678
GFR 1, mean (SD)	88.1 (33.7)	101.4 (18.0)	0.321
GFR 2, mean (SD)	90.6 (32.7)	96.4 (31.4)	0.856

In regard to the comorbidities, there could be found a significant difference in the prevalence of cardiovascular diseases with 10 out of 16 subjects (62.5%) in the study group versus 3 out of 16 subjects (18.8%) in the control group. The distribution of renal involvement was homologous in both groups.

Table 3 compares choroid volume, bright and dark region volumes, as well as CVI. Information for eyes of SLE patients with DLD and SLE patients without DLD are demonstrated. The dataset was compared to a heathy control group.

Patients with DLD revealed significantly lower values concerning the CVI than eyes of the healthy subjects, serving as a reference 0.56 (0.54–0.59) versus 0.58 (0.57–0.59) (p = 0.018) and 0.56 (0.54–0.58) versus 0.58 (0.57–0.60) (p < 0.001) for OD and OS, respectively. No significant difference in CVI could be observed comparing eyes of patients with DLD to eyes of patients without DLD.

The choroid volumes, the bright region volumes, and the dark region volumes showed no significant alteration in comparison of the three demonstrated groups.

In addition to the analysis of the choroid, the retinal thickness of the different retinal layers was measured as shown in Table 4.

The ganglion cell layer was significantly greater in eyes with DLD compared to eyes without DLD in the area with the highest measured thickness (36.9 ± 9.2 μm versus 28.6 ± 12.3 μm, p = 0.029).

Table 3. Choroid volume analysis and choroidal vascularity indices. Significant differences shown in bold type.

		Eyes with DLD (n = 16)	Eyes without DLD (n = 16)	Healthy Control Group (n = 51)
Bright Region Volume WSR, mm^3, mean (range)	OD	0.62 (0.54–0.76)	0.49 (0.35–1.06)	0.77 (0.48–0.90)
	OS	0.57 (0.46–0.72)	0.49 (0.39–1.18)	0.57 (0.49–0.81)
Dark Region Volume, mm^3, mean (range)	OD	0.26 (0.24–0.32)	0.22 (0.15–0.42)	0.31 (0.21–0.36)
	OS	0.25 (0.21–0.31)	0.20 (0.16–0.50)	0.24 (0.19–0.32)
CVI WSR Proposed, mean (range)	OD	0.35 (0.28–0.43)	0.26 (0.20–0.63)	0.44 (0.29–0.52)
	OS	0.32 (0.25–0.40)	0.28 (0.21–0.67)	0.34 (0.26–0.48)
Bright Region Volume WSR, mm^3, mean (range)	OD	**0.56 (0.54–0.59)**	0.57 (0.52–0.58)	**0.58 (0.57–0.59)**
	OS	**0.56 (0.54–0.58)**	0.56 (0.55–0.58)	**0.58 (0.57–0.60)**

OD oculus dexter, OS oculus sinister, CVI choroidal vascularity index, WSR with shadow removal.

Table 4. Retinal layer analysis. Significant differences shown in bold type. SD, standard deviation.

		Eyes with DLD		Eyes without DLD	
		OD	OS	OD	OS
Retina, μm	Center Min ± SD	222.6 ± 20.2	224.3 ± 14.0	205.1 ± 59.4	217.3 ± 25.4
	Center Max ± SD	318.4 ± 24.9	321.8 ± 17.7	291.2 ± 82.5	313.8 ± 27.1
Ganglion Cell Layer, μm	Center Min ± SD	1.4 ± 1.5	0.8 ± 1.5	1.1 ± 1.2	1.3 ± 1.2
	Center Max ± SD	**36.9 ± 9.2**	37.9 ± 11.0	**28.6 ± 12.3**	32.5 ± 10.5
Outer Nuclear Layer, μm	Center Min ± SD	55.3 ± 14.9	50.7 ± 13.9	51.6 ± 19.3	54.5 ± 17.1
	Center Max ± SD	117.8 ± 12.4	117.1 ± 14.7	102.4 ± 32.3	108.5 ± 17.1
Retinal Pigment Epithelium, μm	Center Min ± SD	11.4 ± 1.9	11.4 ± 2.6	11.6 ± 3.5	12.5 ± 2.2
	Center Max ± SD	28.1 ± 6.9	36.1 ± 23.1	23.6 ± 6.7	25.6 ± 4.2
Outer Retinal Layers, μm	Center Min ± SD	81.0 ± 5.5	81.5 ± 5.3	79.8 ± 21.9	84.4 ± 5.7
	Center Max ± SD	98.4 ± 7.8	104.6 ± 18.4	95.9 ± 26.5	101.7 ± 8.6
Photoreceptor Cell Layer, μm	Center Min ± SD	69.7 ± 5.8	69.5 ± 4.5	72.7 ± 5.5	71.9 ± 5.3
	Center Max ± SD	**68.8 ± 7.7**	**66.5 ± 10.5**	**77.1 ± 7.3**	**76.1 ± 6.3**

OD oculus dexter, OS oculus sinister.

The outer retinal layers and the photoreceptor cell layer demonstrated a significant thinning in eyes with DLD in contrast to eyes without DLD, opposing to the previously described tendency of thicker layers in the study subjects. The thinnest area of the ORL at last follow-up in the left eye showed a significant difference between the cohorts (81.0 ± 6.6 μm versus 84.5 ± 2.8 μm, $p = 0.012$). Concordantly, the layer of the photoreceptor cells presented significant thinning in both right and left eyes of study subjects compared to control subjects (68.8 ± 7.7 μm versus 77.1 ± 7.3 μm, $p = 0.008$ and 66.5 ± 10.5 μm versus 76.1 ± 6.3 μm, $p = 0.011$, respectively).

Table 5 shows the summarized data collected by optical coherence tomography angiography. The inner ring, in accordance to the ETDRS grid, was analyzed regarding the vessel density and perfusion density of the superficial and deep capillary plexus and regarding the choriocapillaris.

Table 5. Vascular analysis using OCTA. SD, standard deviation.

		Eyes with DLD	Eyes without DLD	p-Value
3×3 Mean Inner Ring, mm/mm^2, mean (SD)	Vessel Density Superficial	16.4 (2.4)	17.6 (1.1)	0.248
	Vessel Density Deep	12.7 (3.3)	13.1 (1.6)	0.847
	Perfusion Density Superficial	0.37 (0.05)	0.39 (0.02)	0.501
	Perfusion Density Deep	0.27 (0.07)	0.28 (0.04)	0.773
	Choriocapillaris Area	1.6 (0.0)	1.6 (0.0)	1.000
	Choriocapillaris % Area	18.1 (5.1)	18.1 (4.3)	0.700

While there were subtle numerical differences, with a tendency of decreased values in eyes with DLD when compared to eyes without DLD, there could not be found any significant changes.

4. Discussion

In this study, we investigated morphological alterations in the retina and choroid as well as changes in vasculature depending on the presence of drusen-like deposits in patients with systemic lupus erythematosus. For this purpose, the choroidal volumes, choroidal vascularity indices, retinal layers, and optical coherence tomography angiography images of SLE patients with documented DLD were compared to sex- and age-matched controls and a subset of healthy individuals.

Eyes of SLE patients showed an overall reduction in choroid volumes compared to healthy subjects and a noticeable tendency could be observed with greater volumes held by eyes with DLD than eyes without DLD. Furthermore, DLD eyes revealed a significant decrease in CVI. The retinal layer analysis demonstrated a trend leaning to a thickness increase of the retinal segments in the study subjects. Conversely, the photoreceptor cell layer illustrated a significant thinning in patients with DLD. Evaluating the OCTA analysis, there was an overall leaning to lower values in the capillary plexuses of the retina in eyes with DLD.

In our investigations, the choroid volumes tended to be greater in patients with DLD than in patients without; still, when set against healthy subjects, a general decrease was observed. Altinkaynak et al., who examined the choroidal thickness in SLE patients, detected a thinner choroidal layer and stated that this could be a consequence of vasculitis and immune-deposits leading to a decrease in blood flow with following atrophy in the choroid [6]. This could be an explanation for the tendency of lower choroid volumes in diseased patients in our cohort but does not explain why eyes with DLD show higher values than eyes without DLD. More clarification in this regard can be brought by Invernizzi et al., who found thicker CTs in patients with SLE compared to controls and proposed that this finding was due to the known relationship between choroidal thickness and systemic inflammatory conditions in SLE. They suggest that DLD could be a factor for active disease and that an active inflammatory state is the cause for the thicker CTs [3]. While atrophy through capillary luminal obstruction leads to a thinning, as shown by Altinkaynak et al., where an inclusion criterion was an inactive state of SLE, active inflammation leads to thicker choroids, i.e., through inflammatory cell infiltration [3,6,7].

In the present study, CVI was significantly lower in patients with DLD in comparison to healthy controls. On the first glance, this seems not to be concomitant with the detected higher choroid volumes. However, if considering that CVI as opposed to the absolute volume measures is a relative value resulting from the division of the luminal area to the total choroidal area, consisting of the luminal and the stromal area, there is a possible explanation. SLE is an inflammatory disease affecting primarily the capillary systems and the connective tissue [3,15]. As inflammation progresses with activation of inflammatory cytokines, antibody, and cell infiltration, the stromal area expands by accumulation, simultaneously a vascular occlusion by deposition of immunocomplexes and complement factors lead to a decreasing diameter of the vascular lumen of the choroid [6,16]. In conclusion, the CVI can decrease without a decline of the absolute choroidal volume values. To our knowledge, there is only one other study examining the CVI in SLE patients with the juvenile type, who found no significant difference between diseased and healthy probands. They justified their results by concurrent inflammatory deposition in the stroma and vasodilation [15], though it can be assumed that patients with juvenile SLE do not show much degenerative changes in the vasculature yet.

Consistent with the results from Dias-Santos et al. [17], we observed that the photoreceptor cell layer was significantly thinner in SLE patients with DLD compared to patients without DLD. As a tissue with high metabolic needs, the function of the cones and rods is directly dependent on the neighboring nourishing choriocapillaris [6,17,18]. As described above, SLE can involve the choroidal structures and blood flow and thus, leading to ischemia and atrophy in the retinal segments they supply with oxygen and nutrients [17]. In this context, our results could suggest that DLD, as a possible expression of choroidopathy, could be a sign of advancing disease [8].

Our results show that retinal layers and the retina itself are thicker in SLE patients with DLD compared to patients without. This comparison is the first to our knowledge. When assuming that DLD are a sign of advancing disease, this finding stands in contrast with the known literature. Previous studies mostly state a thinning of the retinal layers in patients diagnosed with SLE compared to healthy controls nota bene [17,19,20]. Liu et al. reason, that this thinning is due to vasculitis with subsequent atrophy in the ganglion cell layer [20]. Dias-Santos et al. suggest there is retinal neurodegeneration taking place in the course of SLE disease progression. However, the authors observed that the layer increases in thickness as SLE advances, justifying this with neuronal remodeling [17]. Investigated and discussed in more detail by Jones et al., who examined the development of neurodegeneration in the retina, illustrated that after initial retinal damage, as for example in retinis pigmentosa or AMD, cell death with loss of neurons, reactive unstructured neuritogenesis, reformation of new synaptic connections, and glial reaction come to pass [21]. This remodeling is seen as a part of the degenerative process and could be affecting most of the retinal layers [21]. Furthermore, in a histopathological examination of a SLE patient, an infiltration of macrophages into the retina could be proven [22]. Those inflammatory and degenerative processes in SLE could, to a certain extent, be a possible explanation on why thicker retinal layers could be measured in the current study.

Drusen-like deposits seem to differ from AMD-derived drusen regarding the pathogenesis. Drusen develop by a progredient accumulation of lipoproteins, especially in the macular Bruch membrane [23]. As further proteins and lipids precipitate, conductivity of the membrane becomes poorer leading to oxidative stress and subsequent inflammation mostly manifesting with advanced age. This process is additionally promoted by different genetical and environmental parameters [23,24].

The mechanism of formation of DLD is not fully clear; it is assumed that depositions of immunocomplexes and alteration of the complement system are playing a major role [3,6]. Further points to reinforce this assumption is the age of manifestation, as DLD appear to occur in diseases affecting younger patients, seen in SLE in the present study [1] and other diseases, where the complement system is involved [25,26]. In addition, the distribution differs from drusen; while drusen do not spare the fovea, DLD are observed to mainly present in a perifoveal arrangement leaving the centerfield out [3]. Once more, this is supported by observations in diseases other than SLE, where immunocomplex and complement activation are implicated [25]. The fact that drusen-like deposits and similar lesions are detected in SLE as well as in primarily renal diseases strongly suggest a shared susceptibility to similar pathophysiologic triggers due to the anatomical and functional resemblance of the glomerular system and the Bruch membrane-RPE complex [7]. In addition, in patients with lupus nephritis, the manifestation of DLD was significantly more pronounced [3], further indicating a prognosticating value of these ocular lesions for disease severity and progression. Another aspect to be mentioned is that so-called silent lupus nephritis was frequently detected by renal biopsies but did not show any alteration in conventional urinalysis or laboratory findings [27], thus assigning OCT a leading role as a possible screening method to identify patients at risk for renal and visual impairment.

In regard to the OCTA analysis, the present study showed no significant results, yet an apparent reduction in the VD and PD of both superficial and deep retinal capillary plexuses of patients with DLD. This finding goes in line with the earlier literature, as the studies we investigated all showed a decrease in retinal microvascular density in SLE patients [19,28–32]. An altered capillary blood flow causes microangiopathy and subsequently, if left untreated, vasoocclusion with retinal damage and threat to visual acuity [28,31]. Microangiopathy is the most common etiology of lupus retinopathy, which in turn is the most common cause for visual impairment in SLE patients and is furthermore associated with poorer survival prognosis [4,29]. VD measurement is suggested to serve as a potential biomarker for SLE disease activity, as they exhibit a significant negative correlation to each other [29,30]. A possible explanation for the non-significant results in the current study could be provided by the suggested protective effect of HCQ concerning the VD, as Conigliaro et al. found a positive correlation between superficial and deep retinal vessel densities and HCQ intake [32]. All of our enrolled SLE patients were administered to lower dosages of HCQ than in the study from Conigliaro et al. [32].

Limitations to our study include the limited number of probands enrolled. Furthermore, retinal layers and OCTA images had no control group consisting of healthy individuals, who could serve as reference. No involvement or correlation of disease-activity scores such as the systemic lupus erythematosus disease activity index (SLEDAI), which could possibly deliver more validity to our statements, were included. In addition, a correlation analysis between DLD and systemic alterations, according to the individual classification criteria of the ACR, was not pursued; however, this would be an interesting point to investigate in more detail in future research.

In conclusion, SLE patients with DLD seem to be in a more active state of disease as compared to patients without such lesions. Supported by our study results, the choroid volumes tend to be greater and the CVI to be lesser in patients with present DLD as a likely consequence of an active inflammatory state including vasculitis, immunocomplex, and complement depositions in the capillary systems, all characteristics in the pathophysiology of SLE. Subsequently, as our findings illustrate degenerative processes in the retina follow with a thinning of the photoreceptor cell layer and a decrease in retinal blood flow.

Author Contributions: Conceptualization, M.K., D.B., J.C. and M.A.-S.; Data curation, M.K., K.K.V., S.S., A.M.K., M.A.R. and M.A.-S.; Formal analysis, M.D., K.K.V., S.S., A.M.K., M.A.R. and C.B.; Investigation, M.D. and J.C.; Methodology, M.A.-S.; Project administration, M.K. and S.S.; Writing—original draft, M.K.; Writing—review & editing, M.D., C.B., D.B., J.C. and M.A.-S. All authors have read and agreed to the published version of the manuscript.

Funding: This research received no external funding. Mayss Al-Sheikh received protected research time through career development program for young researchers from the University of Zurich—Filling the gap program.

Institutional Review Board Statement: The trial was approved by the Institutional review board of Swiss ethics/BASEC (No. 2019-00972).

Informed Consent Statement: Informed consent was obtained from all subjects involved in the study.

Data Availability Statement: Full access to the data is possible by the corresponding author.

Conflicts of Interest: The authors declare no conflict of interest.

References

1. Fortuna, G.; Brennan, M.T. Systemic Lupus Erythematosus. Epidemiology, Pathophysiology, Manifestations, and Management. *Dent. Clin. N. Am.* **2013**, *57*, 631–655. [CrossRef]
2. Leffler, J.; Bengtsson, A.A.; Blom, A.M. The Complement System in Systemic Lupus Erythematosus: An Update. *Ann. Rheum. Dis.* **2014**, *73*, 1601–1606. [CrossRef]
3. Invernizzi, A.; dell'Arti, L.; Leone, G.; Galimberti, D.; Garoli, E.; Moroni, G.; Santaniello, A.; Agarwal, A.; Viola, F. Drusen-like Deposits in Young Adults Diagnosed With Systemic Lupus Erythematosus. *Am. J. Ophthalmol.* **2017**, *175*, 68–76. [CrossRef]
4. Stafford-Brady, F.J.; Urowitz, M.B.; Gladman, D.D.; Easterbrook, M. Lupus Retinopathy. Patterns, Associations, and Prognosis. *Arthritis Rheum.* **1988**, *31*, 1105–1110. [CrossRef] [PubMed]
5. Kemeny-Beke, A.; Szodoray, P. Ocular Manifestations of Rheumatic Diseases. *Int. Ophthalmol.* **2020**, *40*, 503–510. [CrossRef] [PubMed]
6. Altinkaynak, H.; Duru, N.; Uysal, B.S.; Erten, Ş.; Kürkcüoğlu, P.Z.; Yüksel, N.; Duru, Z.; Çağıl, N. Choroidal Thickness in Patients with Systemic Lupus Erythematosus Analyzed by Spectral-Domain Optical Coherence Tomography. *Ocul. Immunol. Inflamm.* **2016**, *24*, 254–260. [CrossRef] [PubMed]
7. Baglio, V.; Gharbiya, M.; Balacco-Gabrieli, C.; Mascaro, T.; Gangemi, C.; di Franco, M.; Pistolesi, V.; Morabito, S.; Pecci, G.; Pierucci, A. Choroidopathy in Patients with Systemic Lupus Erythematosus with or without Nephropathy. *J. Nephrol.* **2011**, *24*, 522–529. [CrossRef] [PubMed]
8. Nguyen, Q.D.; Uy, H.S.; Akpek, E.K.; Harper, S.L.; Zacks, D.N.; Foster, C.S. Choroidopathy of Systemic Lupus Erythematosus. *Lupus* **2000**, *9*, 288–298. [CrossRef]
9. Iovino, C.; Pellegrini, M.; Bernabei, F.; Borrelli, E.; Sacconi, R.; Govetto, A.; Vagge, A.; Di Zazzo, A.; Forlini, M.; Finocchio, L.; et al. Choroidal Vascularity Index: An in-Depth Analysis of This Novel Optical Coherence Tomography Parameter. *J. Clin. Med.* **2020**, *9*, 595. [CrossRef]
10. Leys, A.; Vanrenterghem, Y.; Van Damme, B.; Snyers, B.; Pirson, Y.; Leys, M. Fundus Changes in Membranoproliferative Glomerulonephritis Type II. A Fluorescein Angiographic Study of 23 Patients. *Graefe's Arch. Clin. Exp. Ophthalmol. = Albr. von Graefes Arch. fur Klin. und Exp. Ophthalmol.* **1991**, *229*, 406–410. [CrossRef]
11. Leys, A.; Michielsen, B.; Leys, M.; Vanrenterghem, Y.; Missotten, L.; Van Damme, B. Subretinal Neovascular Membranes Associated with Chronic Membranoproliferative Glomerulonephritis Type II. *Graefe's Arch. Clin. Exp. Ophthalmol. = Albr. von Graefes Arch. fur Klin. und Exp. Ophthalmol.* **1990**, *228*, 499–504. [CrossRef] [PubMed]
12. Goud, A.; Singh, S.R.; Sahoo, N.K.; Rasheed, M.A.; Vupparaboina, K.K.; Ankireddy, S.; Lupidi, M.; Chhablani, J. New Insights on Choroidal Vascularity: A Comprehensive Topographic Approach. *Investig. Ophthalmol. Vis. Sci.* **2019**, *60*, 3563–3569. [CrossRef] [PubMed]
13. Vupparaboina, K.K.; Dansingani, K.K.; Goud, A.; Rasheed, M.A.; Jawed, F.; Jana, S.; Richhariya, A.; Freund, K.B.; Chhablani, J. Quantitative Shadow Compensated Optical Coherence Tomography of Choroidal Vasculature. *Sci. Rep.* **2018**, *8*, 6461. [CrossRef] [PubMed]
14. Al-Sheikh, M.; Falavarjani, K.G.; Akil, H.; Sadda, S.R. Impact of Image Quality on OCT Angiography Based Quantitative Measurements. *Int. J. Retin. Vitr.* **2017**, *3*, 4–9. [CrossRef]
15. Ağın, A.; Kadayıfçılar, S.; Sönmez, H.E.; Baytaroğlu, A.; Demir, S.; Sağ, E.; Özen, S.; Eldem, B. Evaluation of Choroidal Thickness, Choroidal Vascularity Index and Peripapillary Retinal Nerve Fiber Layer in Patients with Juvenile Systemic Lupus Erythematosus. *Lupus* **2019**, *28*, 44–50. [CrossRef] [PubMed]
16. Nakamura, A.; Yokoyama, T.; Kodera, S.; Zhang, D.; Hirose, S.; Shirai, T.; Kanai, A. Ocular Fundus Lesions in Systemic Lupus Erythematosus Model Mice. *Jpn. J. Ophthalmol.* **1998**, *42*, 345–351. [CrossRef]
17. Dias-Santos, A.; Tavares Ferreira, J.; Pinheiro, S.; Cunha, J.P.; Alves, M.; Papoila, A.L.; Moraes-Fontes, M.F.; Proença, R. Neurodegeneration in Systemic Lupus Erythematosus: Layer by Layer Retinal Study Using Optical Coherence Tomography. *Int. J. Retin. Vitr.* **2020**, *6*, 1–11. [CrossRef] [PubMed]
18. Dias-Santos, A.; Tavares Ferreira, J.; Pinheiro, S.; Paulo Cunha, J.; Alves, M.; Papoila, A.; Moraes-Fontes, M.F.; Proença, R. Choroidal Thickness Changes in Systemic Lupus Erythematosus Patients. *Clin. Ophthalmol.* **2019**, *13*, 1567–1578. [CrossRef]
19. Işık, M.U.; Akmaz, B.; Akay, F.; Güven, Y.Z.; Solmaz, D.; Gercik, Ö.; Kabadayı, G.; Kurut, İ.; Akar, S. Evaluation of Subclinical Retinopathy and Angiopathy with OCT and OCTA in Patients with Systemic Lupus Erythematosus. *Int. Ophthalmol.* **2021**, *41*, 143–150. [CrossRef] [PubMed]
20. Liu, G.Y.; Utset, T.O.; Bernard, J.T. Retinal Nerve Fiber Layer and Macular Thinning in Systemic Lupus Erythematosus: An Optical Coherence Tomography Study Comparing SLE and Neuropsychiatric SLE. *Lupus* **2015**, *24*, 1169–1176. [CrossRef] [PubMed]
21. Jones, B.W.; Pfeiffer, R.L.; Ferrell, W.D.; Watt, C.B.; Marmor, M.; Marc, R.E. Retinal Remodeling in Human Retinitis Pigmentosa. *Exp. Eye Res.* **2016**, *150*, 149–165. [CrossRef] [PubMed]
22. Cao, X.; Bishop, R.J.; Forooghian, F.; Cho, Y.; Fariss, R.N.; Chan, C.-C. Autoimmune Retinopathy in Systemic Lupus Erythematosus: Histopathologic Features. *Open Ophthalmol. J.* **2009**, *3*, 20–25. [CrossRef] [PubMed]
23. Khan, K.N.; Mahroo, O.A.; Khan, R.S.; Mohamed, M.D.; McKibbin, M.; Bird, A.; Michaelides, M.; Tufail, A.; Moore, A.T. Differentiating Drusen: Drusen and Drusen-like Appearances Associated with Ageing, Age-Related Macular Degeneration, Inherited Eye Disease and Other Pathological Processes. *Prog. Retin. Eye Res.* **2016**, *53*, 70–106. [CrossRef] [PubMed]
24. Cheung, L.K.; Eaton, A. Age-Related Macular Degeneration. *Pharmacotherapy* **2013**, *33*, 838–855. [CrossRef]
25. Lally, D.R.; Baumal, C. Subretinal Drusenoid Deposits Associated with Complement-Mediated IgA Nephropathy. *JAMA Ophthalmol.* **2014**, *132*, 775–777. [CrossRef] [PubMed]

26. Duvall-Young, J.; MacDonald, M.K.; McKechnie, N.M. Fundus Changes in (Type II) Mesangiocapillary Glomerulonephritis Simulating Drusen: A Histopathological Report. *Br. J. Ophthalmol.* **1989**, *73*, 297–302. [CrossRef]
27. Ishizaki, J.; Saito, K.; Nawata, M.; Mizuno, Y.; Tokunaga, M.; Sawamukai, N.; Tamura, M.; Hirata, S.; Yamaoka, K.; Hasegawa, H.; et al. Low Complements and High Titre of Anti-Sm Antibody as Predictors of Histopathologically Proven Silent Lupus Nephritis without Abnormal Urinalysis in Patients with Systemic Lupus Erythematosus. *Rheumatology* **2015**, *54*, 405–412. [CrossRef] [PubMed]
28. Bao, L.; Zhou, R.; Wu, Y.; Wang, J.; Shen, M.; Lu, F.; Wang, H.; Chen, Q. Unique Changes in the Retinal Microvasculature Reveal Subclinical Retinal Impairment in Patients with Systemic Lupus Erythematosus. *Microvasc. Res.* **2020**, *129*, 103957. [CrossRef]
29. Arfeen, S.A.; Bahgat, N.; Adel, N.; Eissa, M.; Khafagy, M.M. Assessment of Superficial and Deep Retinal Vessel Density in Systemic Lupus Erythematosus Patients Using Optical Coherence Tomography Angiography. *Graefe's Arch. Clin. Exp. Ophthalmol.* **2020**, *258*, 1261–1268. [CrossRef] [PubMed]
30. Ermurat, S.; Koyuncu, K. Evaluation of Subclinical Retinal Microvascular Changes in Systemic Lupus Erythematosus Patients Using Optical Coherence Tomography Angiography and Its Relationship with Disease Activity. *Lupus* **2022**, *31*, 541–554. [CrossRef] [PubMed]
31. Pichi, F.; Woodstock, E.; Hay, S.; Neri, P. Optical Coherence Tomography Angiography Findings in Systemic Lupus Erythematosus Patients with No Ocular Disease. *Int. Ophthalmol.* **2020**, *40*, 2111–2118. [CrossRef] [PubMed]
32. Conigliaro, P.; Cesareo, M.; Chimenti, M.S.; Triggianese, P.; Canofari, C.; Aloe, G.; Nucci, C.; Perricone, R. Evaluation of Retinal Microvascular Density in Patients Affected by Systemic Lupus Erythematosus: An Optical Coherence Tomography Angiography Study. *Ann. Rheum. Dis.* **2019**, *78*, 287–288. [CrossRef] [PubMed]

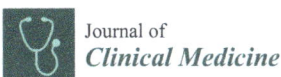

Article

Two Year Functional and Structural Changes—A Comparison between Trabeculectomy and XEN Microstent Implantation Using Spectral Domain Optical Coherence Tomography

Caroline Bormann [1,*], Catharina Busch [1], Matus Rehak [2], Manuela Schmidt [1], Christian Scharenberg [3], Focke Ziemssen [1] and Jan Darius Unterlauft [1,4]

[1] Department of Ophthalmology, University of Leipzig, Liebigstrasse 10-14, 04103 Leipzig, Germany
[2] Department of Ophthalmology, University of Giessen, Friedrichstrasse 18, 35392 Giessen, Germany
[3] Augenärzte am Kurpark, Soltauer Straße 6a, 21335 Lüneburg, Germany
[4] Department of Ophthalmology, Inselspital, University of Bern, Freiburgstrasse 18, 3010 Bern, Switzerland
* Correspondence: caroline.bormann@medizin.uni-leipzig.de; Tel.: +49-341-9721825

Abstract: The aim of this study was to analyze retinal nerve fiber layer (RNFL) thickness after trabeculectomy (TE) versus XEN microstent implantation (XEN) in primary open-angle glaucoma (POAG) cases naïve to prior incisional glaucoma surgery. We examined 119 consecutive glaucoma patients retrospectively, who received a TE or XEN for medically uncontrolled POAG. Intraocular pressure (IOP), amount of IOP-lowering medication, mean deviation of standard automated perimetry and peripapillary RNFL thickness were evaluated during the first 24 months after surgery. Fifty eyes were treated with TE and 69 eyes with XEN. Mean IOP decreased from 25.1 ± 0.8 to 13.3 ± 0.6 mm Hg ($p < 0.01$) and mean number of IOP-lowering eye drops from 3.2 ± 0.2 to 0.4 ± 0.1 ($p < 0.01$) 24 months after TE. In 69 eyes undergoing XEN, mean IOP dropped from 24.8 ± 0.6 to 15.0 ± 0.4 mm Hg ($p < 0.01$) and medication from 3.0 ± 0.1 to 0.6 ± 0.1 ($p < 0.01$) during the 24 months follow-up. Mean deviation of standard automated perimetry remained stable in TE (8.5 ± 0.7 to 8.1 ± 0.8 dB; $p = 0.54$) and XEN group (11.0 ± 0.5 to 11.5 ± 0.5 dB; $p = 0.12$) after 24 months, while mean RNFL thickness further deteriorated in the TE (-2.28 ± 0.65 µm/year) and XEN (-0.68 ± 0.34 µm/year) group. Postoperative RNFL loss develops after TE and XEN despite effective and significant lowering of IOP and amount of IOP-lowering medication. RNFL loss was more pronounced in the first year after glaucoma surgery.

Keywords: glaucoma surgery; RNFL thickness; optical coherence tomography; primary open-angle glaucoma

1. Introduction

Glaucoma is one of the most common causes of irreversible blindness worldwide with an estimated prevalence of up to 111.8 million in 2040 [1,2]. This chronic disease damages the nerve fiber layer due to apoptosis of retinal ganglion cells. This leads to visual field defects and loss of visual acuity or complete blindness in the final disease stages [3,4].

The most important risk factor for the development and progression of glaucoma is the intraocular pressure (IOP), which can be influenced therapeutically [5]. Unalterable risk factors are myopia, higher age, positive family history and ethnic background [6].

The pathologically transformed trabecular meshwork leading to chronically increased IOP seems to play a major role during development and progression of primary open angle glaucoma (POAG) [7]. The treatment of glaucoma aims at delaying progression by lowering IOP, either through medication and/or surgery, if the IOP cannot be lowered sufficiently by medication alone [5,8].

Trabeculectomy (TE) is considered the gold standard for surgical glaucoma treatment and is effective in many different glaucoma entities [9]. Furthermore, in recent years,

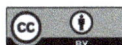

minimally invasive glaucoma surgery (MIGS) techniques were developed to reduce surgical trauma and complications compared to TE [10]. One of these is the XEN45 Gel Stent, (XEN, Allergan, Irvine, CA, USA), which consists of a flexible tube of 6 mm length and 500 μm thickness with an internal lumen of 45 μm diameter. The stent connects the anterior chamber with the subconjunctival/subtenonal space and has a comparable effect on IOP as TE. The few studies that compared TE and XEN did not find any differences in the risk for failure or the safety profiles [11,12].

Historically, visual field defects are an important marker for disease progression and thereby effectiveness of glaucoma surgery over time, but visual field testing is highly subjective and strongly depending on patient cooperation. Additionally, in the early disease stages visual field defects are hardly measurable at all. Today, modern imaging techniques, such as optical coherence tomography (OCT) are able to visualize the optic nerve and to measure the thickness of the peripapillary retinal nerve fiber layer (RNFL) automatically in order to detect possible disease progression.

The aim of this study was to compare the efficacy of TE and XEN in POAG cases. We therefore performed a retrospective, monocentric single surgeon trial over a 24-month follow-up period and analyzed postoperative changes in visual acuity, visual field defects and peripapillary RNFL thickness using OCT techniques.

2. Materials and Methods

This study was designed as a retrospective, monocentric, comparative cohort study. All POAG patients were treated with TE or XEN (XEN, Allergan, Irvine, CA, USA) at the Department of Ophthalmology of the University Clinic Leipzig, Germany between October 2017 and March 2019. All surgical procedures were performed by the same surgeon (JDU). Requirements for inclusion in the study were pseudophakia, an age of at least 40 years, an IOP repeatedly documented above target pressure and thus not sufficiently controllable by medical treatment, no prior incisional glaucoma surgery and verified presence of POAG.

The diagnosis of POAG was based on the following criteria: presence of typical glaucomatous optic disc changes, history of an IOP of 21 mm Hg or above without therapy and the absence of clinical signs raising suspicion towards any other glaucoma entity (increased iris transillumination, PEX material, etc.) or optic neuropathies of non-glaucomatous origin. Additionally, the indication to perform surgery required a progressive POAG in form of increasing scotomas or an increase in mean defect (2 dB/year) despite maximum tolerable IOP-lowering medication. Progression was verified by three repeated visual field tests during the last 12 months before surgery. Exclusion criteria were the presence of any other glaucoma entities other than POAG. In the regular cases of patients in need of glaucoma surgery on both eyes, only data originating from the first eye undergoing surgery was included in this analysis.

For all surgical procedures, written informed consent was obtained from all patients. The study was approved by the local ethics committee (209/18-ek) and was registered with the German Clinical Trial Register (DRKS, trial number: DRKS00020800), which is part of the WHO registry network. All procedures were conducted according to the Declaration of Helsinki.

The indication for glaucoma surgery was usually set during an ambulant examination in the outpatient care department of the eye clinic. Additionally, a full ophthalmologic examination was performed on the day of admission to the hospital, in order to confirm the indication for surgery. The examination included taking patients ophthalmologic and general medical history, best corrected visual acuity (BCVA) using Snellen charts (transformed to logMAR for statistical analysis), examination of anterior and posterior eye segments including a close evaluation of the optic disc to verify existence of glaucomatous changes, Goldmann applanation tonometry, visual field assessment using standard automated perimetry (Twinfield 2, Oculus Optikgeräte GmbH, Wetzlar, Germany; 24-2 test strategy, 55 target points), measurement of the retinal nerve fiber layer (RNFL) thickness using optical coherence tomography (OCT; Spectralis, Heidelberg Engineering GmbH,

Heidelberg, Germany). The mean global RNFL thickness was assessed using the circular peripapillary scan with 3.5 mm diameter centered around the optic nerve head. For further RNFL analysis, the Garway-Heath sector analysis tool was used.

The decision between TE and XEN was based on the following assumptions. XEN is considered a minimally invasive glaucoma surgery (MIGS) technique. The XEN is implanted using an ab interno approach, which bares the risk of causing damage to the crystalline lens with consecutive opacification and was therefore implanted only into already pseudophakic eyes. Additionally, the XEN does not comprise a valve mechanism and therefore bares (in theory) a higher risk for expulsive hemorrhages. TE was introduced more than 60 years ago and experience with this technique is more extensive than with XEN. Due to these reasons, TE was undertaken in eyes in need of a more aggressive/safer IOP reduction. Cases not falling into these lastly described categories and fulfilling the above-mentioned inclusion criteria were treated by XEN.

The XEN- and TE- techniques have already been described in detail before [11]. In short: TE was performed using a fornix-based conjunctival approach and a scleral flap of 4×4 mm. A 3×3 mm sponge soaked with mitomycin C (concentration 0.2 mg/mL, produced by) was applied for 2 minutes. The adaptation of the scleral flap was performed using 2–4 10/0 sutures (non-absorbable). To adapt the conjunctiva to the limbus, 4 absorbable single button sutures were used. Depending on postoperative visible bleb function, IOP and conjunctival scar formation we decided about suture lysis and/or application of subconjunctival 5-Fluorouracil (5-FU). For XEN implantation the anterior chamber was filled with a dispersive viscoelastic agent and the conjunctiva was prepared with an injection of up to 0.1 mL mitomycin C (concentration 0.1 mg/mL). Then, the XEN was inserted into the eyes anterior chamber via a side port incision opposite to the planned implantation site (Figure 1). Afterwards the outer orifice was detached from adherent Tenon's capsule using a 30 G needle.

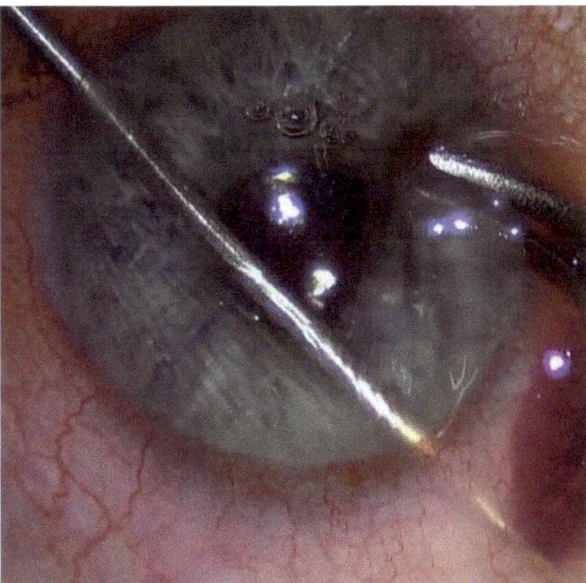

Figure 1. Intraoperative picture during XEN implantation with the injector inserted through a side port incision temporal-inferiorly and the injector tip directed so that the tip becomes visible approximately 2 mm behind the corneal limbus underneath the conjunctiva.

Postoperative treatment was similar in both treatment groups and included antibiotic (gentamicin; QID for 1 week), cycloplegic (atropine 1%; BID for 1 week) and steroid eye drops (prednisolone acetate 1%; QID for 4 weeks, titrated thereafter depending on clinical assessment). Depending on the IOP and the morphology of the bleb we decided about a secondary needling procedure with 0.1 mL of 5-FU (50 mg/mL). If necessary, a laser suture lysis was performed no longer than 12 weeks after TE.

Before surgery and during the follow-up period, the following data was collected: age, gender, side of surgery (left or right eye), IOP, BCVA, number of IOP-lowering drugs, mean deviation (MD) of standard automated perimetry and mean peripapillary RNFL thickness. Follow-up examinations were scheduled 6, 12 and 24 months after surgery. Clinical success was evaluated following the recommendations published by the World Glaucoma Association (Guidelines on Design and Reporting of Glaucoma Surgical Trials). For complete success, IOP had to be decreased >20% compared to baseline without the additional use of any IOP-lowering drugs and the resulting IOP had to be <21 mm Hg. For qualified success, IOP had to be lowered by >20% compared to baseline with the additional use of IOP-lowering drugs, if the preoperative number of drugs was not exceeded. To meet the success criteria, no additional surgical intervention was allowed during the 24-month follow-up after TE or XEN except laser suture lysis (TE group) or needling procedures with 5-FU (in both groups). All cases not meeting these criteria were considered as unsuccessful.

Data acquisition and statistical analysis were performed using Excel (Version 2007, Microsoft; Redmond, DC, USA) and SPSS (IBM Version 22.0; Chicago, IL, USA). For patient age, IOP, number of IOP-lowering drugs, visual acuity, mean defect of standard automated perimetry and RNFL thickness the mean and standard error of the mean were calculated. The Wilcoxon test was used for within-group comparisons and the Mann-Whitney-U test for between-group comparisons. In both cases, $p < 0.05$ was set to indicate statistical significance.

3. Results

In total, 119 eyes of 119 POAG patients were included in this study. Fifty eyes were treated with TE and 69 eyes underwent a XEN. For all 119 eyes, a full 24-month post-surgical follow-up could be obtained. Patient demographics such as age, gender, side of surgery, IOP and number of IOP-lowering drugs before surgery did not differ significantly for both groups. However, visual acuity and mean deviation of visual field showed statistically significant differences with eyes being more affected by POAG in the XEN group (for details see Table 1).

Table 1. Baseline characteristics of all eyes included and treated with either TE or XEN. n.a.: not applicable; IOP: intraocular pressure; RNFL: retinal nerve fiber layer.

	TE	XEN	Mann-Whitney-U Test $p =$
Age [years]	73.9 ± 1.3	75.5 ± 0.8	0.29
Gender	28 female 22 male	44 female 25 male	0.39
$n =$	50	69	n.a.
Laterality	28 left (56%) 22 right (44%)	28 left (41%) 41 right (59%)	0.10
IOP [mm Hg]	25.1 ± 0.8	24.8 ± 0.6	0.92
Medication [n]	3.2 ± 0.2	3.0 ± 0.1	0.25
Visual acuity [logMAR]	0.13 ± 0.02	0.24 ± 0.03	**<0.01**
Mean visual field defect [dB]	8.5 ± 0.7	11.0 ± 0.5	**<0.01**
Mean RNFL thickness [μm]	67.8 ± 2.6	60.2 ± 1.8	0.12

3.1. IOP

The IOP was similar in both groups initially (TE: 25.1 ± 0.8 mm Hg; XEN: 24.8 ± 0.6 mm Hg). In the TE group, IOP decreased to 13.5 ± 0.6 mm Hg ($p < 0.01$) and 13.3 ± 0.6 mm Hg ($p < 0.01$) 12 and 24 months after surgery, corresponding to a 44% IOP reduction compared to baseline. During the same time IOP dropped to 15.2 ± 0.4 mm Hg ($p < 0.01$) and 15.0 ± 0.4 mm Hg ($p < 0.01$) in the XEN group (Table 2 and Figure 2A), respectively. This relates to an IOP-reduction of 36% and 37% from baseline. The IOP differed significantly between the two groups for all three follow-up examinations at 6 ($p = 0.01$), 12 ($p < 0.01$) and 24 months ($p < 0.01$) after surgery (Table 2).

3.2. IOP-Lowering Medication

The mean number of IOP-lowering medication was significantly reduced from 3.2 ± 0.2 to 0.5 ± 0.1 ($p < 0.01$) and 0.4 ± 0.1 ($p < 0.01$) 12 and 24 month after TE and from 3.0 ± 0.1 to 0.6 ± 0.1 ($p < 0.01$) and 0.6 ± 0.1 ($p < 0.01$) 12 and 24 month after XEN (Table 2 and Figure 2B). There was no statistically significant difference between the two groups for any of the follow-up examinations though (Table 2).

3.3. Success Levels

The exact percentages of eyes reaching success levels A to D 24 months after surgery are presented in Table 3. Although there is no statistically significant difference in eyes reaching lower success levels A and B between both treatment groups, a significant difference was found for higher success levels C and D, with higher success rates in the TE group.

Table 2. Baseline and follow-up results for IOP, prescribed medication, visual acuity and mean MD in the TE and XEN group together with the results of statistical analysis. IOP: intraocular pressure, n.a.: not applicable, MD: mean defect, RNFL: retinal nerve fiber layer.

			TE	Comparison to Baseline (Wilcoxon-Test) $p =$	XEN	Comparison to Baseline (Wilcoxon-Test) $p =$	Intergroup Comparison (Mann-Whitney-U Test) $p =$
IOP [mm Hg]		baseline	25.1 ± 0.8	n.a.	24.8 ± 0.6	n.a.	0.92
		6 months	13.6 ± 0.7	<0.01	15.3 ± 0.4	<0.01	0.01
		12 months	13.5 ± 0.6	<0.01	15.2 ± 0.4	<0.01	<0.01
		24 months	13.3 ± 0.6	<0.01	15.0 ± 0.4	<0.01	<0.01
medication		baseline	3.2 ± 0.2	n.a.	3.0 ± 0.1	n.a.	0.25
		6 months	0.3 ± 0.1	<0.01	0.7 ± 0.1	<0.01	0.08
		12 months	0.5 ± 0.1	<0.01	0.6 ± 0.1	<0.01	0.29
		24 months	0.4 ± 0.1	<0.01	0.6 ± 0.1	<0.01	0.27
visual acuity [logMAR]		baseline	0.13 ± 0.02	n.a.	0.24 ± 0.03	n.a.	<0.01
		6 months	0.16 ± 0.03	0.06	0.23 ± 0.03	0.51	0.15
		12 months	0.17 ± 0.03	0.01	0.22 ± 0.03	0.18	0.67
		24 months	0.22 ± 0.06	0.04	0.22 ± 0.03	0.17	0.75
MD [dB]		baseline	8.5 ± 0.7	n.a.	11.0 ± 0.5	n.a.	<0.01
		6 months	7.85 ± 0.8	0.17	11.63 ± 0.5	0.07	0.15
		12 months	8.0 ± 0.7	0.41	11.3 ± 0.5	0.15	<0.01
		24 months	8.1 ± 0.8	0.54	11.5 ± 0.5	0.12	<0.01
RNFL thickness [μm]		baseline	67.8 ± 2.6	n.a.	60.2 ± 1.8	n.a.	0.12
		6 months	64.3 ± 2.6	<0.01	60.5 ± 1.9	0.38	<0.01
		12 months	62.9 ± 2.6	<0.01	59.3 ± 1.8	0.22	0.01
		24 months	63.2 ± 2.6	<0.01	58.9 ± 1.8	0.06	0.04

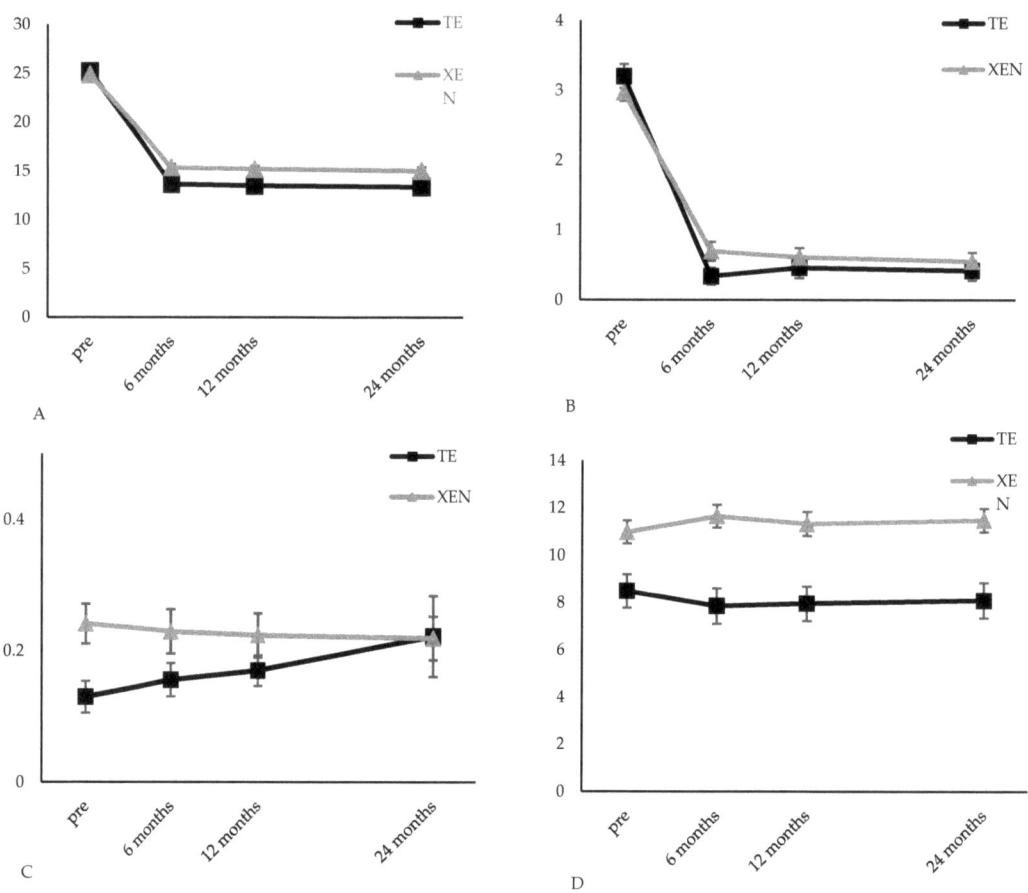

Figure 2. Results for IOP (**A**), glaucoma medication (**B**), visual acuity (**C**) and mean defect of standard automated visual field tests (**D**) development during the first 24 months after TE or XEN. pre: preoperative.

Table 3. Percentage of eyes in the TE- and XEN-groups reaching complete or qualified success levels A-D 24 months after surgery.

		TE	XEN	$p =$ (Mann-Whitney-U Test)
A (<21 mm Hg)	complete	80.0%	71.0%	0.89
	qualified	92.0%	91.3%	0.27
B (<18 mm Hg)	complete	80.0%	65.2%	0.14
	qualified	92.0%	82.6%	0.08
C (<15 mm Hg)	complete	72.0%	43.5%	**0.01**
	qualified	76.0%	52.2%	**0.01**
D (<12 mm Hg)	complete	44.0%	23.2%	**0.03**
	qualified	44.0%	24.6%	**0.02**

3.4. Visual Acuity, Visual Field

The mean BCVA worsened significantly from 0.13 ± 0.02 logMAR before surgery to 0.17 ± 0.03 logMAR ($p = 0.01$) and 0.22 ± 0.06 logMAR ($p = 0.04$) 12 and 24 months after TE. In the XEN group, the mean BCVA was 0.24 ± 0.03 logMAR at baseline and remained stable with 0.22 ± 0.03 logMAR ($p = 0.18$) and 0.22 ± 0.03 logMAR ($p = 0.17$) 12 and 24 months after surgery (Table 2 and Figure 2C). The intergroup comparison showed a statistically significant difference of mean BCVA at baseline ($p < 0.01$), so further postoperative analysis was not conducted. In the TE group, MD did not change significantly over the 24 months follow-up (12 months: 8.0 ± 0.7 dB, $p = 0.41$; 24 months: 8.1 ± 0.8, $p = 0.54$). During the same time, changes in MD did not reveal differences of statistical significance with 11.3 ± 0.5 dB ($p = 0.15$) and 11.5 ± 0.5 dB ($p = 0.12$) in the XEN group (Table 2, Figure 2D).

3.5. RNFL Thickness

The mean RNFL thickness did not differ significantly at baseline with 67.8 ± 2.6 µm in the TE group and 60.2 ± 1.8 µm in the XEN group ($p = 0.12$). During postsurgical follow-up, the global mean RNFL-thickness only decreased significantly in the TE group. Mean RNFL thickness decreased to 62.9 ± 2.6 µm ($p < 0.01$) and to 63.2 ± 2.6 µm ($p < 0.01$) 12 and 24 months after TE (Figure 3A), corresponding to a −4.56 ± 1.30 µm mean global RNFL loss after 24 months. Statistical analysis showed a trend towards a significant reduction in mean RNFL thickness at 24 months after XEN (58.9 ± 1.8 µm; $p = 0.06$; Figure 3B) with a mean global RNFL loss of −1.35 ± 0.67 µm for the same period. Comparison of mean RNFL thickness values revealed statistically significant differences between the two groups and loss was more pronounced in the TE group 12 ($p = 0.01$) and 24 months ($p = 0.04$) after surgery (Table 2). Additionally, the comparison of 12- and 24 months results showed that the mean global RNFL loss was most pronounced in the first year with almost no changes of global RNFL in the second year of follow-up. Further statistical analysis for the significant RNFL-decrease in the TE group revealed, that a high surgical IOP-reduction was correlated with a lower RNFL-loss (12 months: $r = -0.472$, $p < 0.01$; 24 months: $r = -0.443$, $p < 0.01$).

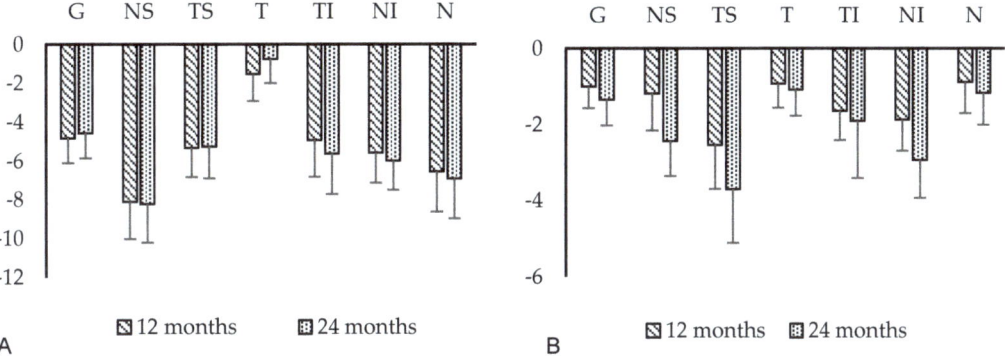

Figure 3. Development of postoperative global and sectoral (Garway-Heath) RNFL loss 12 and 24 months after TE (**A**) and XEN (**B**). G: global; NS: nasal−superior; TS: temporal−superior; T: temporal; TI: temporal−inferior; NI: nasal−inferior; N: nasal.

3.6. Garway-Heath-Sector Analysis

However, postoperative RNFL thickness changes were not distributed evenly around the optic nerve head. The exact pattern of postoperative RNFL loss is depicted in Figure 3A,B and Figure 4. The analysis of the six Garway-Heath sectors revealed that RNFL loss was most pronounced in the inferior and superior sectors with different results for compared to baseline values before surgery was statistically significant in the nasal superior sector in the TE-group (−8.22 ± 1.98 µm, $p < 0.01$) and temporal superior sector in the XEN group (−3.71 ± 1.41 µm, $p = 0.01$) during the postsurgical period. Lowest RNFL loss was seen in the temporal sector with −0.76 ± 1.23 µm in the TE group and −1.09 ± 0.68 µm in the XEN group during 24 months of follow-up.

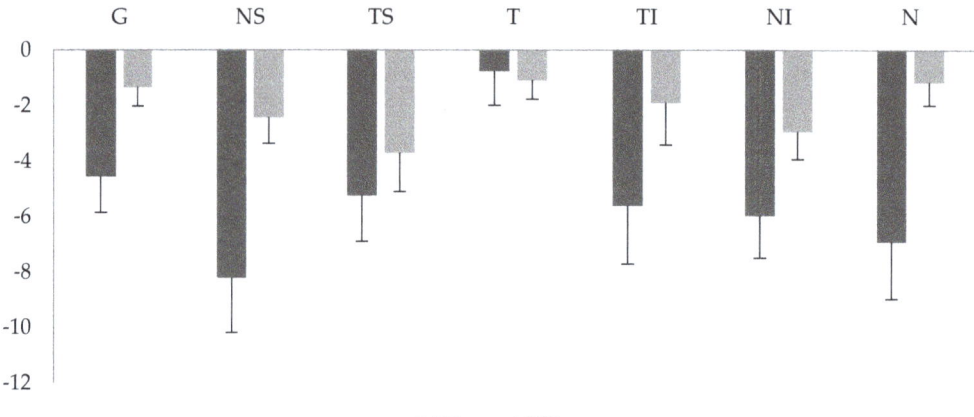

Figure 4. Development of postoperative global and sectoral (Garway-Heath) RNFL loss compared between TE and XEN groups 24 months after surgery. G: global; NS: nasal−superior; TS: temporal−superior; T: temporal; TI: temporal−inferior; NI: nasal−inferior; N: nasal.

4. Discussion

Our study shows an effective and significant decrease in mean IOP and number of IOP-lowering medication 2 years after TE or XEN in POAG eyes naïve to prior surgical glaucoma treatment. In addition, postsurgical follow-up showed a global RNFL loss, which was more pronounced during the first than the second year after glaucoma surgery. This suggests a possible association with perioperative factors, but there were no abnormalities of postoperative IOP spikes, hypotonia or cases of pronounced vision loss in the early postoperative period in these cohorts.

TE has been the standard surgical procedure to lower IOP and the number of necessary IOP-lowering drugs and thus decelerating disease progression in various types of glaucoma. The efficacy was proven multiple times by different single- and multicenter trials before and is nowadays widely accepted [13,14]. Kirwan et al. demonstrated the effectivity of TE using a multicenter trial conducted in the UK including 428 eyes with POAG. They showed a postoperative reduction in mean IOP (from 23.0 ± 5.5 mm Hg to 12.4 ± 4.0 mm Hg) and IOP-lowering eye drops (from 2.5 ± 0.9 to 0.1 ± 0.4) for a 24 months follow-up period [15]. Equally, the effectivity of the XEN was also demonstrated in different types of glaucoma by a number of single and multicenter trials in recent years [16,17]. Reitsamer et al. presented a successful reduction in mean IOP from 21.4 ± 3.4 mm Hg to 15.2 ± 4.2 mm Hg and IOP-lowering medication from 2.7 ± 0.9 to 1.1 ± 1.2 24 months after implantation in 202 POAG eyes treated with XEN [18].

The results of our study also demonstrated an effective IOP reduction after TE or XEN, which was comparable to the above-mentioned trials. Mean IOP decreased significantly from 25.1 ± 0.8 to 13.3 ± 0.6 mm Hg after TE and from 24.8 ± 0.6 to 15.0 ± 0.4 mm Hg after XEN during the 24-month follow-up period. The resulting IOP difference between the two groups was statistically significant at 24 months after surgery. Additionally, the mean number of IOP-lowering medication was significantly reduced ($p < 0.01$) in the two groups during follow-up. Similar to already published data, IOP reduction and higher success levels were more pronounced in eyes undergoing a TE compared to a XEN [19–21].

During the 24-month follow-up, mean MD remained stable in both treatment groups. No differences of statistical significance could be found comparing MD values measured before as well as 12 and 24 months after TE or XEN. Our findings are in line with studies also reporting no changes of visual field function after glaucoma surgery [22,23]. Schargus et al. also revealed stable visual field indices during the first 24 months after TE or XEN or XEN combined with cataract surgery in POAG eyes naïve to glaucoma surgery [20]. Kim et al.

demonstrated stable visual field indices although further statistically significant RNFL decrease during the first 12 months after TE or Ahmed valve implantation [24]. A lack of direct correlation between defect depth and RNFL thickness could also be due to the decreasing relevance and informative value of OCT examination with progressive damage.

Despite the successful reduction in IOP and medication as well as visual field stabilization, a further deterioration of peripapillary RNFL could be found in both of our presented treatment groups. This effect was however more pronounced in eyes undergoing TE compared to XEN. Already published data concerning RNFL development after glaucoma surgery using OCT techniques are somehow contradictive. This may partially be due to different patient characteristics, included disease stages, surgical methods and initial global RNFL. Some authors stated no significant changes of RNFL thickness after TE in short follow-up periods of 6 to 12 months [22,25,26]. However, other studies showed significant RNFL changes for 12 to 18 months after different glaucoma surgeries [23,24,27]. Kim et al. found a significant RNFL thinning 12 months after TE or Ahmed valve implantation. They speculated that RNFL thinning may reflect the resolution of RNFL-swelling due to higher preoperative IOP (IOP > 37 mm Hg) [24]. Ch'ng et al. observed a transient increase in peripapillary RNFL 1 month after filtering surgery [28]. Our results show further RNFL-reduction after TE although reaching lower mean IOP levels and higher percentages of surgical success compared to our XEN group. Mean reduction in global RNFL thickness around the optic nerve head was -4.8 ± 1.3 µm/year in the TE group and -1.4 ± 0.7 µm/year in the XEN group during the first follow up year. These findings are in line with those published by Chua et al., who found a mean reduction in RNFL thickness of -4.2 ± 0.3 µm/year in 105 eyes 12 months after TE [27]. Interestingly, the amount of RFNL thickness loss was higher in the first than in the second year after surgery. One reason for the more pronounced RNFL reduction in the first year might be the elevated preoperative IOP, which may already have damaged the retinal ganglion cells up until the point of surgery. Possibly, the initiated apoptosis up until the point of operation continues thereafter and global RNFL thinning is seen only months later using OCT. Additionally, mean global RNFL decreased only significantly in the TE-group from 67.8 ± 2.6 µm to 63.2 ± 2.6 µm ($p < 0.01$) over 24 months. The reasons for this might be the major intraoperative trauma, more inflammation and intraoperative IOP-changes related to apoptosis of retinal ganglion cells in the TE group. Additionally, mean global RNFL thickness was lower in the XEN group than in the TE group at baseline, which might have an effect on further development during follow-up. In summary, TE as well as XEN could decelerate the progression of glaucoma. However, both techniques were not able to stop disease progression and RNFL decrease completely. In addition, the amount of RFNL thickness loss was higher in the first than in the second postoperative year, suggesting a time dependent course of postoperative RNFL loss. Furthermore, long-time follow-up investigations would definitely be interesting and necessary to evaluate the further clinical course after glaucoma surgery.

The pattern of occurring postoperative RNFL loss was also of interest in this study. Analysis of the six sectors described by Garway-Heath showed that further postoperative RNFL loss was pronounced superiorly and inferiorly. These (superior and inferior) poles are known to be most susceptible to glaucoma damage. A closer look revealed that in the TE-group RNFL loss was most pronounced in nasal inferior sector and in the XEN-group in the temporal superior sector. Damage occurring at the temporal side of the optic nerve head was minimal in both groups during the postoperative follow-up, because the major preoperative damage was already in this sector.

Major limitations of the present study are its retrospective as well as the non-blinded and non-randomized design. Additionally, the mode of IOP measurements might have been biased, because it did not follow a strict workflow schedule (non-blinded, not repeated multiple times). Visual field examinations often showed a higher variability; so "false-negative" results are possible. Furthermore, due to the strict inclusion criteria the study population is rather small in order to compare two different glaucoma surgeries. In the future, multicenter studies with longer follow-up times, fixed follow-up intervals and larger cohorts are necessary. Additionally, including OCT monitoring into prospective studies would be profitable to evaluate the patterns of postoperative RNFL loss not only in the long term but also during the first year after surgery. Comparing these loss patterns between different surgical procedures may enhance clinical decisions.

5. Conclusions

Postoperative RNFL loss develops following certain patterns. The amount and pattern of RNFL loss differs between eyes undergoing TE or XEN, and seems to be independent from a reduction in IOP, IOP lowering medication and postoperatively reached success levels, at least during the first year after surgery.

Author Contributions: Conceptualization: J.D.U. and C.B. (Caroline Bormann); methodology: J.D.U. and C.B. (Caroline Bormann); software: J.D.U.; validation, formal analysis, J.D.U. and C.B. (Caroline Bormann); investigation: C.B. (Catharina Busch), M.R., M.S. and C.S.; resources: J.D.U. and M.R.; data curation: J.D.U. and C.B. (Caroline Bormann); writing—original draft preparation: C.B. (Caroline Bormann) and J.D.U.; writing—review and editing: C.B. (Catharina Busch), J.D.U. and F.Z.; visualization: J.D.U.; supervision: J.D.U.; project administration: J.D.U.; All authors have read and agreed to the published version of the manuscript.

Funding: The publication was partially funded by the Library of the University of Leipzig.

Institutional Review Board Statement: The study was conducted in accordance with the Declaration of Helsinki, and approved by the Institutional Ethics Committee of the University of Leipzig (209/18-ek).

Informed Consent Statement: Informed consent was obtained from all subjects involved in the study.

Data Availability Statement: Datasets generated during the current study are available from the corresponding author upon reasonable request.

Conflicts of Interest: F.Z.: Consultant: Alimera Sciences, Allergan/Abbvie, Bayer, Boehringer-Ingelheim, Novartis, NovoNordisk, MSD, Oxurion, Roche/Genentech; Speaker: Alimera, Allergan/Abbvie, Bayer, BDI, CME Health, Gerling, Novartis, ODOS, Roche, Research: Bayer, BMBF, Clearside, DFG, Kodiak, Iveric, Ophtea, Novartis, Regeneron. All other authors declare no conflict of interest.

References

1. Tham, Y.C.; Li, X.; Wong, T.Y.; Quigley, H.A.; Aung, T.; Cheng, C.Y. Global prevalence of glaucoma and projections of glaucoma burden through 2040: A systematic review and meta-analysis. *Ophthalmology* **2014**, *11*, 2081–2090. [CrossRef]
2. Flaxman, S.R.; Bourne, R.R.A.; Resnikoff, S.; Ackland, P.; Braithwaite, T.; Cicinelli, M.V.; Das, A.; Jonas, J.B.; Keeffe, J.; Kempen, J.H.; et al. Global causes of blindness and distance vision impairment 1990–2020: A systematic review and meta-analysis. *Lancet Glob Health* **2017**, *12*, e1221–e1234. [CrossRef]
3. Quigley, H.A. Ganglion cell death in glaucoma: Pathology recapitulates ontogeny. *Aust. N. Z. J. Ophthalmol.* **1995**, *23*, 85–91. [CrossRef] [PubMed]
4. Levkovitch-Verbin, H. Retinal ganglion cell apoptotic pathway in glaucoma: Initiating and downstream mechanisms. *Prog. Brain Res.* **2015**, *220*, 37–57.
5. Heijl, A.; Leske, M.C.; Bengtsson, B.; Hyman, L.; Bengtsson, B.; Hussein, M. Early Manifest Glaucoma Trial Group. Reduction of intraocular pressure and glaucoma progression: Results from the Early Manifest Glaucoma Trial. *Arch. Ophthalmol.* **2002**, *120*, 1268–1279. [CrossRef]
6. Schuster, A.K.; Erb, C.; Hoffmann, E.M.; Dietlein, T.; Pfeiffer, N. The Diagnosis and Treatment of Glaucoma. *Dtsch. Arztebl. Int.* **2020**, *13*, 225–234. [CrossRef]
7. Tektas, O.Y.; Lutjen-Drecoll, E. Structural changes of the trabecular meshwork in different kinds of glaucoma. *Exp. Eye Res.* **2009**, *88*, 769–775. [CrossRef]
8. Schmidl, D.; Schmetterer, L.; Garhofer, G.; Popa-Cherecheanu, A. Pharmacotherapy ofglaucoma. *J. Ocul. Pharmacol. Ther.* **2015**, *31*, 63–77. [CrossRef] [PubMed]
9. Razeghinejad, M.R.; Spaeth, G.L. A history of the surgical management of glaucoma. *Optom. Vis. Sci.* **2011**, *88*, E39–E47. [CrossRef]
10. Lavia, C.; Dallorto, L.; Maule, M.; Ceccarelli, M.; Fea, A.M. Minimally-invasive glaucoma surgeries (MIGS) for open angle glaucoma: A systematic review and meta-analysis. *PLoS ONE* **2017**, *12*, e0183142. [CrossRef]

11. Theilig, T.; Rehak, M.; Busch, C.; Bormann, C.; Schargus, M.; Unterlauft, J.D. Comparing the efficacy of trabeculectomy and XEN gel microstent implantation for the treatment of primary open-angle glaucoma: A retrospective monocentric comparative cohort study. *Sci. Rep.* **2020**, *1*, 19337. [CrossRef]
12. Schlenker, M.B.; Gulamhusein, H.; Conrad-Hengerer, I.; Somers, A.; Lenzhofer, M.; Stalmans, I.; Reitsamer, H.; Hengerer, F.H.; Ahmed, I.I.K. Efficacy, Safety, and Risk Factors for Failure of Standalone Ab Interno Gelatin Microstent Implantation versus Standalone Trabeculectomy. *Ophthalmology* **2017**, *11*, 1579–1588. [CrossRef]
13. Edmunds, B.; Thompson, J.R.; Salmon, J.F.; Wormald, R.P. The National Survey of Trabeculectomy. II. Variations in operative technique and outcome. *Eye* **2001**, *15*, 441–448. [CrossRef] [PubMed]
14. Fontana, H.; Nouri-Mahdavi, K.; Lumba, J.; Ralli, M.; Caprioli, J. Trabeculectomy with mitomycin C: Outcomes and risk factors for failure in phakic open-angle glaucoma. *Ophthalmology* **2006**, *113*, 930–936. [CrossRef]
15. Kirwan, J.F.; Lockwood, A.J.; Shah, P.; Macleod, A.; Broadway, D.C.; King, A.J.; McNaught, A.I.; Agrawal, P. Trabeculectomy Outcomes Group Audit Study Group. Trabeculectomy in the 21st century: A multicenter analysis. *Ophthalmology* **2013**, *12*, 2532–2539. [CrossRef]
16. Karimi, A.; Lindfield, D.; Turnbull, A.; Dimitriou, C.; Bhatia, B.; Radwan, M.; Gouws, P.; Hanifudin, A.; Amerasinghe, N.; Jacob, A. A multi-centre interventional case series of 259 ab-interno Xen gel implants for glaucoma, with and without combined cataract surgery. *Eye* **2019**, *3*, 469–477. [CrossRef]
17. Schargus, M.; Theilig, T.; Rehak, M.; Busch, C.; Bormann, C.; Unterlauft, J.D. Outcome of a single XEN microstent implant for glaucoma patients with different types of glaucoma. *BMC Ophthalmol.* **2020**, *1*, 490. [CrossRef] [PubMed]
18. Sheybani, A.; Lenzhofer, M.; Hohensinn, M.; Reitsamer, H.; Ahmed, I.I. Phacoemulsification combined with a new ab interno gel stent to treat open-angle glaucoma: Pilot study. *J. Cataract. Refract. Surg.* **2015**, *9*, 1905–1909. [CrossRef]
19. Wagner, F.M.; Schuster, A.K.; Emmerich, J.; Chronopoulos, P.; Hoffmann, E.M. Efficacy and safety of XEN®-Implantation vs. trabeculectomy: Data of a "real-world" setting. *PLoS ONE* **2020**, *4*, e0231614. [CrossRef]
20. Schargus, M.; Busch, C.; Rehak, M.; Meng, J.; Schmidt, M.; Bormann, C.; Unterlauft, J.D. Functional Monitoring after Trabeculectomy or XEN Microstent Implantation Using Spectral Domain Optical Coherence Tomography and Visual Field Indices-A Retrospective Comparative Cohort Study. *Biology* **2021**, *4*, 273. [CrossRef]
21. Edmunds, B.; Thompson, J.R.; Salmon, J.F.; Wormald, R.P. The National Survey of Trabeculectomy. III. Early and late complications. *Eye* **2002**, *16*, 297–303. [CrossRef] [PubMed]
22. Gietzelt, C.; von Goscinski, C.; Lemke, J.; Schaub, F.; Hermann, M.M.; Dietlein, T.S.; Cursiefen, C.; Heindl, L.M.; Enders, P. Dynamics of structural reversal in Bruch's membrane opening-based morphometrics after glaucoma drainage device surgery. *Graefes Arch. Clin. Exp. Ophthalmol.* **2020**, *6*, 1227–1236. [CrossRef]
23. Gietzelt, C.; Lemke, J.; Schaub, F.; Hermann, M.M.; Dietlein, T.S.; Cursiefen, C.; Enders, P.; Heindl, L.M. Structural Reversal of Disc Cupping After Trabeculectomy Alters Bruch Membrane Opening-Based Parameters to Assess Neuroretinal Rim. *Am. J. Ophthalmol.* **2018**, *194*, 143–152. [CrossRef] [PubMed]
24. Kim, W.J.; Kim, K.N.; Sung, J.Y.; Kim, J.Y.; Kim, C.S. Relationship between preoperative high intraocular pressure and retinal nerve fibre layer thinning after glaucoma surgery. *Sci. Rep.* **2019**, *9*, 13901. [CrossRef] [PubMed]
25. Sanchez, F.G.; Sanders, D.S.; Moon, J.J.; Gardiner, S.K.; Reynaud, J.; Fortune, B.; Mansberger, S.L. Effect of Trabeculectomy on OCT Measurements of the Optic Nerve Head Neuroretinal Rim Tissue. *Ophthalmol. Glaucoma* **2020**, *1*, 32–39. [CrossRef] [PubMed]
26. Waisbourd, M.; Ahmed, O.M.; Molineaux, J.; Gonzalez, A.; Spaeth, G.L.; Katz, L.J. Reversible structural and functional changes after intraocular pressure reduction in patients with glaucoma. *Graefes Arch. Clin. Exp. Ophthalmol.* **2016**, *6*, 1159–1166. [CrossRef]
27. Chua, J.; Kadziauskienė, A.; Wong, D.; Ašoklis, R.; Lesinskas, E.; Quang, N.D.; Chong, R.; Tan, B.; Girard, M.J.A.; Mari, J.M.; et al. One year structural and functional glaucoma progression after trabeculectomy. *Sci. Rep.* **2020**, *1*, 2808. [CrossRef] [PubMed]
28. Ch'ng, T.W.; Gillmann, K.; Hoskens, K.; Rao, H.L.; Mermoud, A.; Mansouri, K. Effect of surgical intraocular pressure lowering on retinal structures—nerve fibre layer, foveal avascular zone, peripapillary and macular vessel density: 1 year results. *Eye* **2020**, *3*, 562–571. [CrossRef]

Article

Association of Fundus Autofluorescence Abnormalities and Pachydrusen in Central Serous Chorioretinopathy and Polypoidal Choroidal Vasculopathy

Timothy Y. Y. Lai [1,2,*], Ziqi Tang [1], Adrian C. W. Lai [2,3], Simon K. H. Szeto [1], Ricky Y. K. Lai [2] and Carol Y. Cheung [1]

1. Department of Ophthalmology & Visual Sciences, The Chinese University of Hong Kong, Hong Kong, China
2. 2010 Retina & Macula Centre, Tsim Sha Tsui, Kowloon, Hong Kong, China
3. Faculty of Medicine & Health, UNSW Sydney, Kensington, NSW 2052, Australia
* Correspondence: tyylai@cuhk.edu.hk

Abstract: A specific form of drusen, known as pachydrusen, has been demonstrated to be associated with pachychoroid eye diseases, such as central serous chorioretinopathy (CSC) and polypoidal choroidal vasculopathy (PCV). These pachydrusen have been found in up to 50% of eyes with CSC and PCV and may affect the disease progression and treatment response. This study aims to investigate the association between pachydrusen and changes in fundus autofluorescence (FAF) in eyes with CSC and PCV. A total of 65 CSC patients and 32 PCV patients were evaluated. Pachydrusen were detected using both color fundus photography and spectral-domain optical coherence tomography. The relationships between pachydrusen and FAF changes were then investigated. The prevalence of pachydrusen in CSC and PCV eyes was 16.7% and 61.8%, respectively. The mean age of patients with pachydrusen was significantly older than those without pachydrusen (CSC: 56.3 vs. 45.0 years, $p < 0.001$; PCV: 68.8 vs. 59.5 years, $p < 0.001$). No significant difference was found in the mean subfoveal choroidal thickness between eyes with or without pachydrusen. Eyes with pachydrusen were significantly associated with more extensive FAF changes in both CSC and PCV ($p < 0.001$ and $p = 0.037$, respectively). The study demonstrated that pachydrusen are more prevalent in PCV than CSC. Increasing age and more extensive abnormalities in FAF are associated with the presence of pachydrusen, suggesting that dysfunction of retinal pigment epithelial cells is associated with pachydrusen.

Keywords: pachychoroid; pachydrusen; drusen; central serous chorioretinopathy; polypoidal choroidal vasculopathy; optical coherence tomography; fundus autofluorescence; neovascular age-related macular degeneration

1. Introduction

Pachychoroid eye diseases are eye conditions that are associated with localized thickening of choroid with dilated or congested choroidal veins, reduced or absent choriocapillaris, causing progressive dysfunction of the retinal pigment epithelia (RPE), and may lead to macular neovascularization [1,2]. Conditions classified in this spectrum of pachychoroid eye diseases include pachychoroid pigment epitheliopathy, central serous chorioretinopathy (CSC), polypoidal choroidal vasculopathy (PCV), focal choroidal excavation, pachychoroid neovasculopathy, and peripapillary pachychoroid syndrome [1,2].

One of the clinical features more commonly detected in patients with pachychoroid eye diseases is a specific type of drusen known as pachydrusen [3,4]. These pachydrusen are larger than 125 μm, more asymmetrical in shape with irregular outer contour, have a diffuse and more widespread distribution over the posterior pole that spares the central macula, and can occur in multiple groups of several deposits or in isolation [3]. Pachydrusen can be diagnosed using multimodal imaging including color fundus photographs, spectral-domain optical coherence tomography (OCT) and enhanced depth imaging OCT [3]. The prevalence of pachydrusen in patients with pachychoroid eye diseases appear to vary among different eye conditions and ethnic groups, with reported rates of 6.8% to 60% in eyes with CSC [5–8], and 14.1% to 56% in eyes with PCV [8–11]. With the use of multimodal imaging including indocyanine green angiography (ICGA) and OCT B-scans and en face images, it has been demonstrated that the majority of pachydrusen are located over pachyvessels (dilated Haller vessels) and concentrated within areas of geographic filling delay of choriocapillaris [5,12]. These pachydrusen are known to be of specific prognostic significance, as they have been demonstrated to be associated with progression to PCV but not to typical neovascular age-related macular degeneration (AMD) [13,14].

Fundus autofluorescence (FAF) is a non-invasive imaging technique that makes use of light stimulation of lipofuscin in the RPE, and changes in the levels of FAF emitted have the potential to assess the RPE functional activity [15]. Several studies have evaluated the changes in FAF in eyes with pachychoroid diseases and have demonstrated various severity of FAF abnormalities due to RPE dysfunction [16–22]. However, the association between pachydrusen and functional imaging using FAF has not been evaluated previously. We postulated that pachydrusen might be associated with the dysfunction of RPE demonstrated by FAF. The aim of this study is to evaluate the prevalence of pachydrusen and to assess the association between FAF changes and pachydrusen in eyes with CSC and PCV.

2. Materials and Methods

2.1. Study Design

This was a retrospective study of consecutive patients with newly diagnosed treatment-naïve CSC or PCV referred for fluorescein angiography (FA) and ICGA performed in the 2010 Retina and Macula Centre, Hong Kong from January 2013 to December 2018. The inclusion criteria of the study included: CSC or PCV diagnosed based on existing definitions [1,2]; and no prior treatment for macular or retinal diseases including anti-vascular endothelial growth factor (anti-VEGF) injection, verteporfin photodynamic therapy and thermal laser photocoagulation. Exclusion criteria included: high myopia (spherical equivalent refractive error < -6 diopters); other co-existing retinal or macular diseases such as epiretinal membrane, macular hole, diabetic retinopathy, retinal vascular occlusion, posterior uveitis, retinal detachment; and media opacity affecting ophthalmic imaging quality. The study was conducted in accordance with the Declaration of Helsinki.

2.2. Imaging and Image Analyses

All patients underwent fundus photography, FAF, FA, and ICGA using the flash-based TRC-50DX retinal camera (Topcon, Tokyo, Japan). Spectral-domain OCT scans were obtained using with the Cirrus HD-OCT 4000 (Carl Zeiss Meditec, Dublin, CA, USA) with the enhanced depth imaging (EDI) mode. Subfoveal choroidal thickness (SFCT) was measured using the horizontal and vertical OCT B-scan EDI images at the fovea with the caliper measurement tool within the OCT system software. SFCT was measured from the outer surface of the RPE band to the inner surface of the choroidal-scleral interface at the fovea [11]. Pachydrusen were diagnosed based on the following criteria: drusen diameter > 125 µm; irregular outer contours of the drusen; and drusen occurring in isolation or in groups [3,5]. The area of pachydrusen (mm^2) was measured, as in the fundus photographs, using an imaging software (ImageJ version 1.53a, National Institutes of Health, Bethesda, MD, USA) [23]. The area of FAF abnormality was measured based on the sum of all sites of FAF abnormalities in the FAF images and was classified as <2 disc areas or $\geq$2 disc areas.

2.3. Statistical Analyses

All data were entered into a computer spreadsheet software (Mircosoft Excel for Mac version 16.54, Mircosoft Corp, Redmond, WA, USA) and statistical analyses were carried out using a statistical module (StatPlus:mac Pro Core version 5.9.80, AnalystSoft Inc., Walnut, CA, USA) running within the spreadsheet software. Descriptive data were summarized as mean ± standard deviation (SD) or percentages. Comparisons between eyes with or without pachydrusen were performed using two-tailed t-test (for continuous variables) or chi-squared test (for categorical variables). A p-value of ≤ 0.05 was considered as statistically significant.

3. Results
3.1. Patient Demongraphics

A total of 72 eyes of 65 CSC patients and 34 eyes of 32 PCV patients was included. Seven patients had bilateral CSC and two patients had bilateral PCV. For the 65 CSC patients, the mean ± SD age was 46.7 ± 8.8 years (range, 29 to 69 years) and there were 50 (76.9%) males and 15 (23.1%) females. For the 32 PCV patients, the mean ± SD age was 65.0 ± 8.2 years (range, 44 to 82 years) and there were 23 (71.9%) males and 9 (28.1%) females.

3.2. Eyes with Central Serous Chorioretinopathy

Pachydrusen were found in 12 (16.7%) of the 72 eyes with CSC and the mean ± SD area of pachydrusen was 0.20 ± 0.26 mm^2. The mean ± SD age of 10 CSC patients with pachydrusen was significantly older than the 55 CSC patients without pachydrusen, with 56.3 ± 7.8 years and 45.0 ± 7.8 years, respectively (two-tailed t-test, $p < 0.001$) (Table 1). For the seven patients with bilateral CSC, five (71.4%) had no pachydrusen in both eyes, one (14.3%) had pachydrusen in one eye, and one (14.3%) had pachydrusen in both eyes. The mean ± SD SFCT for all CSC eyes was 359.2 ± 42.9 µm. There was no significant difference between the mean ± SD SFCT of CSC eyes with or without pachydrusen (two-tailed t-test, $p = 0.38$). FAF abnormalities were found in 71 (98.6%) of 72 eyes with CSC, with 37 (51.4%) eyes having < 2 disc areas of FAF abnormality, and 34 (47.2%) eyes having $\geq$ 2 disc areas of FAF abnormality. Eyes with pachydrusen were found to have significantly more extensive area of FAF abnormality with $\geq$ 2 disc areas than eyes without pachydrusen (chi-squared test, $p < 0.001$). An example of a CSC eye with pachydrusen and FAF abnormalities is displayed in Figure 1.

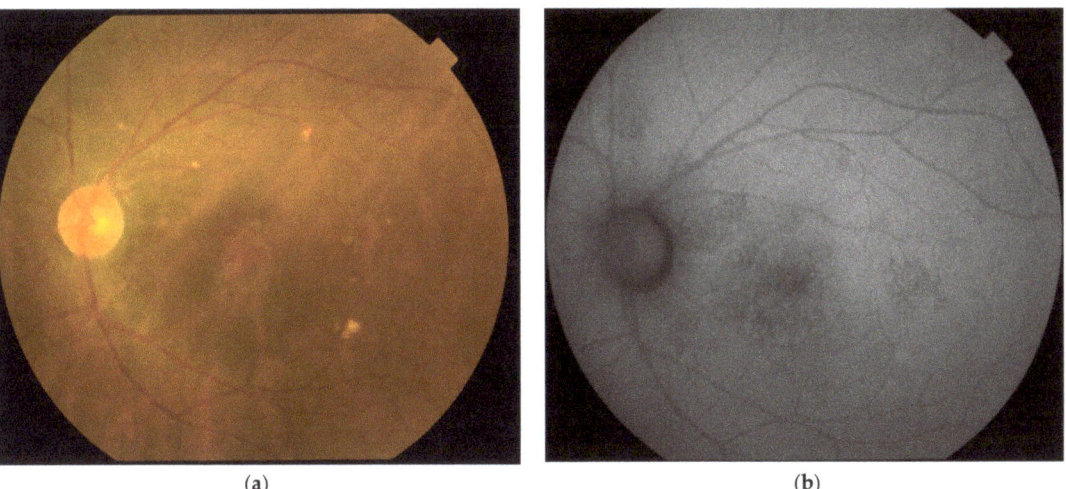

Figure 1. (a) Fundus photograph of a 69-year-old patient with central serous chorioretinopathy showing multiple pachydrusen in the inferiotemporal and temporal macula occurring as a cluster and scattered in the superior macula around the vascular arcade; (b) fundus autofluorescence showing mixed increased and reduced autofluorescence of $\geq$2 disc areas scattered in the macula due to widespread dysfunction of the retinal pigment epithelium.

Table 1. Characteristics of CSC eyes with or without pachydrusen.

Characteristics	All CSC Eyes (n = 72)	With Pachydrusen (n = 12)	Without Pachydrusen (n = 60)	p Value
Mean ± SD age (years)	46.7 ± 8.8	56.3 ± 7.8	45.0 ± 7.8	<0.001 [1]
Mean ± SD SFCT (μm)	359.2 ± 42.9	348.5 ± 33.8	361.8 ± 44.8	0.38 [2]
FAF abnormality				
None	1 (1.4%)	0 (0.0%)	1 (1.7%)	
<2 disc areas	37 (51.4%)	0 (0.0%)	37 (61.7%)	<0.001 [3]
≥2 disc areas	34 (47.2%)	12 (100.0%)	32 (36.7%)	

SD: standard deviation; CSC: central serous chorioretinopathy; SFCT: subfoveal choroidal thickness; FAF: fundus autofluorescence. [1] two-tailed *t*-test between patients with pachydrusen vs. without pachydrusen. [2] two-tailed *t*-test between eyes with pachydrusen vs. without pachydrusen. [3] chi-square test between eyes with pachydrusen vs. without pachydrusen.

3.3. Eyes with Polypoidal Choroidal Vasculopathy

Pachydrusen was found in 21 (61.8%) of the 34 eyes with PCV and the mean ± SD area of pachydrusen was 0.32 ± 0.60 mm². Similar to CSC, the mean age of the 19 PCV patients with pachydrusen was significantly older than the 13 PCV patients without pachydrusen, with 68.8 years and 59.5 years, respectively (two-tailed *t*-test, $p < 0.001$) (Table 2). For the two patients with bilateral PCV, both patients had pachydrusen in both eyes. The mean ± SD SFCT for all PCV eyes was 264.5 ± 68.0 μm. No significant difference between the mean ± SD SFCT of PCV eyes with or without pachydrusen was observed (two-tailed *t*-test, $p = 0.88$). FAF abnormalities were found in all 33 (100%) eyes with PCV, with 5 (14.7%) eyes having < 2 disc areas of FAF abnormality and 29 (85.3%) eyes having ≥ 2 disc areas of FAF abnormality. The proportion of eyes with FAF abnormality of ≥ 2 disc areas was significantly higher in eyes with PCV than CSC (chi-squared test, $p = 0.001$). There was also a significant association between the presence of pachydrusen and ≥ 2 disc areas extent of FAF abnormality (chi-squared test, $p = 0.037$). An example of a PCV eye with pachydrusen and FAF abnormalities is displayed in Figure 2.

Table 2. Characteristics of PCV eyes with or without pachydrusen.

Characteristics	All PCV eyes (n = 34)	With Pachydrusen (n = 21)	Without Pachydrusen (n = 13)	p Value
Mean ± SD age (years)	65.0 ± 8.2	68.8 ± 7.2	59.5 ± 6.6	< 0.001 [1]
Mean ± SD SFCT (μm)	264.5 ± 68.0	262.8 ± 70.0	267.0 ± 68.7	0.88 [2]
FAF abnormality				
<2 disc areas	5 (14.7%)	1 (4.8%)	4 (30.8%)	0.37 [3]
≥2 disc areas	29 (85.3%)	20 (95.2%)	9 (69.2%)	

SD: standard deviation; CSC: central serous chorioretinopathy; SFCT: subfoveal choroidal thickness; FAF: fundus autofluorescence. [1] two-tailed *t*-test between patients with pachydrusen vs. without pachydrusen. [2] two-tailed *t*-test between eyes with pachydrusen vs. without pachydrusen. [3] chi-square test between eyes with pachydrusen vs. without pachydrusen.

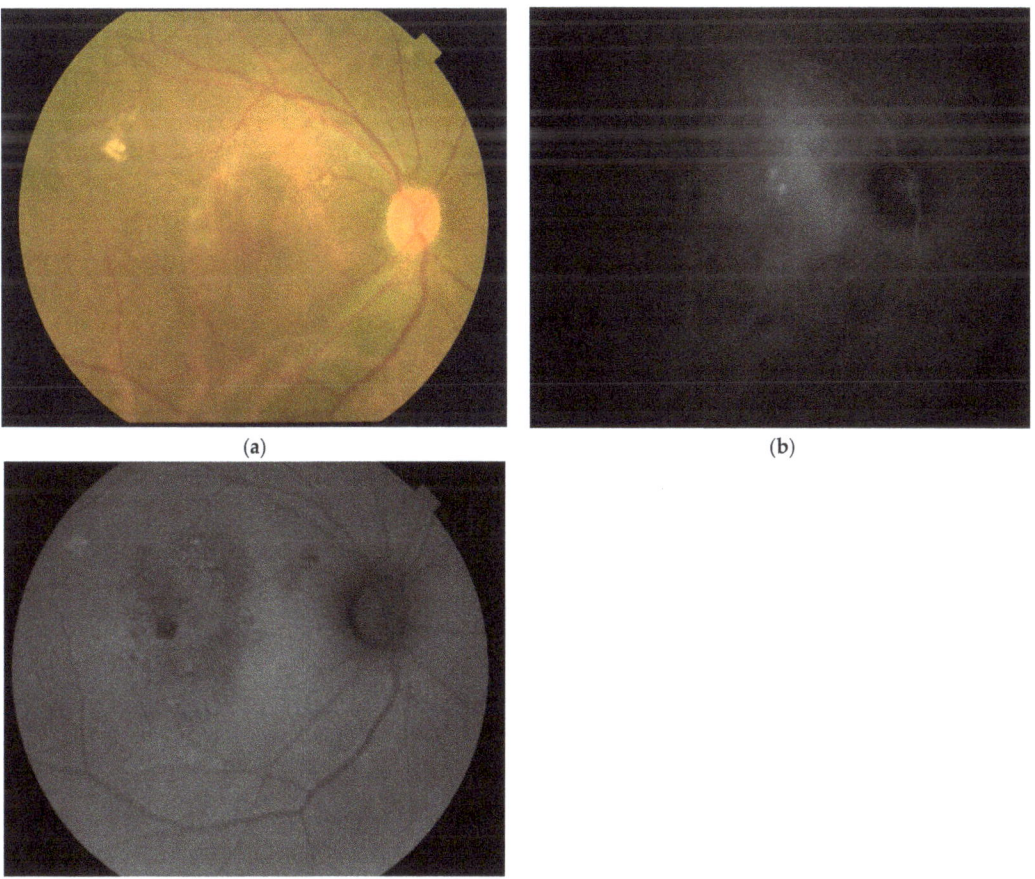

Figure 2. (**a**) Fundus photo of a 65-year-old patients with polypoidal choroidal vasculopathy showing multiple pachydrusen occurring as a cluster in the superiotemporal macula with a few small isolated drusen in the superionasal retina; (**b**) indocyanine green angiography showing multiple polypoidal lesions at the macula with dilated choroidal vasculature and choroidal hyperpermeability; (**c**) fundus autofluorescence showing mixed autofluorescence abnormalities with increase and reduced autofluorescence of ≥2 disc areas scattered in the central macula with a ring of increased autofluorescence highlighting the polypoidal lesions.

4. Discussion

In this study, we evaluated the prevalence of pachydrusen in eyes with CSC and PCV and the prevalence was found to be 16.7% and 61.8%, respectively. A previous study has demonstrated an ethnic link in the prevalence of pachydrusen, as pachydrusen were significantly more common in Asian neovascular AMD patients compared with white patients [24]. Our rate of pachydrusen in CSC eyes appeared to be slightly lower compared with most previous studies performed in Asian populations [5–8]. The reported prevalence of pachydrusen in CSC eyes were 27.2% and 40.1% in two studies conducted in Japan [5,7], and 6.8% and 60% in two studies performed in India [6,8]. However, our rate appeared similar to the pachydrusen prevalence of 20% reported by Kim et al. in Korea [25]. The main reason for the lower prevalence of pachydrusen in our CSC patients is likely due to the younger mean age of patients in our study compared with other studies. In our study, the mean age of CSC patients was 46.7 years, whereas studies with higher prevalence of pachydrusen than our study all had a mean age of >50 years [5,7,8]. A study that reported a lower prevalence of pachydrusen in CSC eyes than our study had a mean age of 42.9 years [6], which was younger than our study. The influence of age on the presence of pachydrusen can be demonstrated in our study as well as in previous studies [5,7,8,25], since the mean age of CSC patients with pachydrusen was significantly higher than those without pachydrusen. Takahasi et al. reported the prevalence of pachydrusen in CSC patients was 40.1% and CSC patients with pachydrusen were significantly older than those without, with a mean age of 62.1 years versus 48.8 years, respectively [7]. For PCV, the influence of age on the prevalence of pachydrusen could also be observed, as we also found that patients with pachydrusen were significantly older than those without pachydrusen. Therefore, increasing age appeared to be an important factor for the development of pachydrusen in both CSC and PCV.

FAF is an investigation that can provide in vivo evaluation of RPE function, and abnormalities in FAF are common findings in both CSC and PCV eyes [26–28]. In our study, FAF abnormalities were found in 98.6% of eyes with CSC and in all eyes with PCV. The proportion of eyes with FAF abnormality of $\geq$ 2 disc areas was higher in eyes with PCV than CSC, with 85.3% vs. 47.2%, respectively. We also found that both PCV and CSC eyes with pachydrusen were associated with more extensive RPE dysfunction as demonstrated by FAF abnormalities. The findings suggest pachydrusen might be an indicator of more severe RPE dysfunction and eyes with PCV are associated with more extensive RPE dysfunction compared with CSC. Eyes with PCV generally have larger area of RPE and photoreceptor damage due to macular hemorrhage, exudation, and multiple recurrent pigment epithelial detachments. Therefore, it is likely that PCV eyes will have more extensive RPE dysfunction, resulting in larger area of FAF abnormalities.

There are several limitations associated with our study, including the relatively small sample size and the lack of longitudinal follow-up of the patients. Due to the small sample size, we did not perform multivariate analysis such as regression analysis to evaluate the potential confounding effects on other variables, such as SFCT. In our study, the mean SFCT was found to be similar in eyes with or without pachydrusen in both CSC and PCV eyes. In a large prospective study of over 600 eyes with treatment-naive CSC by Takahasi et al. [7], although the mean SFCT was similar between eyes with or without pachydrusen, SFCT was found to be significantly thicker in eyes with pachydrusen than those without pachydrusen after adjusting for age, gender, and refractive error in multivariate analysis. Notomi et al. also demonstrated that in eyes with pachydrusen and intermediate size drusen, there was a trend of thicker SFCT in these eyes compared with eyes without pachydrusen [29]. However, in the study by Kim et al. [25], pachydrusen was only associated with choroidal thickness in eyes with PCV and not in CSC. Therefore, the interaction between the presence of pachydrusen and choroidal thickness warrants further investigations. In addition, we did not formally evaluate the precise relationship between the location of the pachydrusen and FAF abnormalities. Nonetheless, since the area of FAF abnormality was considerably larger and more widespread than that of pachydrusen, there appeared to be a lack of relationship between the location of the pachydrusen and FAF abnormalities.

Previous follow-up studies have demonstrated that pachydrusen might have important prognostic implications for the progression of PCV [13,14]. In a longitudinal study by Teo et al. [13], the authors evaluated the natural course of 29 eyes with pachydrusen and found that eyes with pachydrusen were significantly more likely to develop into PCV rather than typical neovascular AMD. Similar findings were also observed in a retrospective cohort study by Kim et al. [14], in which 11.5% of 61 eyes with pachydrusen developed into PCV after 5 years, while only 3.3% developed into typical neovascular AMD. In addition to the association with natural history, pachydrusen have also been demonstrated to be a predictor in the treatment response in PCV patients receiving intravitreal anti-VEGF monotherapy [28]. In a retrospective cohort study by Fukuda et al. [30], patients with pachydrusen in the fellow eye had significantly fewer additional intravitreal aflibercept injections following the initial three loading doses for the treatment of PCV. However, similar studies on the influence of pachydrusen on the natural history or treatment outcome have not been performed in CSC. Further longitudinal studies to evaluate the prognostic implications of pachydrusen, especially in eyes with CSC, are therefore warranted. Future studies can also explore the possible association between pachydrusen and persistent subretinal fluid in CSC and PCV eyes following treatment.

5. Conclusions

Pachydrusen are associated with increasing age and have higher prevalence in eyes with PCV than CSC. A more extensive area of FAF abnormality was found in eyes with pachydrusen, suggestive of more widespread RPE dysfunction in eyes with the presence of pachydrusen.

Author Contributions: Conceptualization, T.Y.Y.L.; methodology, T.Y.Y.L., R.Y.K.L., S.K.H.S. and C.Y.C.; formal analysis, T.Y.Y.L. and R.Y.K.L.; investigation, Z.T., A.C.W.L. and R.Y.K.L.; resources, T.Y.Y.L. and C.Y.C.; data curation, T.Y.Y.L., Z.T., A.C.W.L. and R.Y.K.L.; writing—original draft preparation, T.Y.Y.L.; writing—review and editing, T.Y.Y.L., Z.T., A.C.W.L., S.K.H.S., R.Y.K.L. and C.Y.C.; visualization, T.Y.Y.L. and R.Y.K.L. All authors have read and agreed to the published version of the manuscript.

Funding: This research received no external funding.

Institutional Review Board Statement: Patient consent was waived due to the retrospective analysis of anonymized data.

Informed Consent Statement: Ethical review and approval were waived for this study, due to retrospective analysis of anonymized data.

Data Availability Statement: The data presented in this study are available on request from the corresponding author. The data are not publicly available due to privacy.

Conflicts of Interest: The authors declare no conflict of interest.

References

1. Cheung, C.M.G.; Lee, W.K.; Koizumi, H.; Dansingani, K.; Lai, T.Y.Y.; Freund, K.B. Pachychoroid disease. *Eye* **2019**, *33*, 14–33. [CrossRef] [PubMed]
2. Castro-Navarro, V.; Behar-Cohen, F.; Chang, W.; Joussen, A.M.; Lai, T.Y.Y.; Navarro, R.; Pearce, I.; Yanagi, Y.; Okada, A.A. Pachychoroid: Current concepts on clinical features and pathogenesis. *Graefes Arch. Clin. Exp. Ophthalmol.* **2021**, *259*, 1385–1400. [CrossRef] [PubMed]
3. Spaide, R.F. Disease expression in nonexudative age-related macular degeneration varies with choroidal thickness. *Retina* **2018**, *38*, 708–716. [CrossRef] [PubMed]
4. Zhang, X.; Sivaprasad, S. Drusen and pachydrusen: The definition, pathogenesis, and clinical significance. *Eye* **2021**, *35*, 121–133. [CrossRef]
5. Matsumoto, H.; Mukai, R.; Morimoto, M.; Tokui, S.; Kishi, S.; Akiyama, H. Clinical characteristics of pachydrusen in central serous chorioretinopathy. *Graefes Arch. Clin. Exp. Ophthamlol.* **2019**, *257*, 1127–1132. [CrossRef]
6. Singh, S.R.; Chakurkar, R.; Goud, A.; Chhablani, J. Low incidence of pachydrusen in central serous chorioretinopathy in an Indian cohort. *Indian J. Ophthalmol.* **2020**, *68*, 118–122.
7. Takahashi, A.; Hosoda, Y.; Miyake, M.; Miyata, M.; Oishi, A.; Tamura, H.; Ooto, S.; Yamashiro, K.; Tabara, Y.; Matsuda, F.; et al. Clinical and genetic characteristics of pachydrusen in eyes with central serous chorioretinopathy and general Japanese individuals. *Ophthalmol. Retin.* **2021**, *5*, 910–917. [CrossRef]
8. Sheth, J.; Anantharaman, G.; Kumar, N.; Parachuri, N.; Bandello, F.; Kuppermann, B.D.; Loewenstein, A.; Sharma, A. Pachydrusen: The epidemiology of pachydrusen and its relevance to progression of pachychoroid disease spectrum. *Eye* **2020**, *34*, 1501–1503. [CrossRef]
9. Singh, S.R.; Chakurkar, R.; Goud, A.; Rasheed, M.A.; Vupparaboina, K.K.; Chhablani, J. Pachydrusen in polypoidal choroidal vasculopathy in an Indian cohort. *Indian J. Ophthalmol.* **2019**, *67*, 1121–1126.
10. Lee, J.; Byeon, S.H. Prevalence and clinical characteristics of pachydrusen in polypoidal choroidal vasculopathy: Multimodal image study. *Retina* **2019**, *39*, 670–678. [CrossRef]
11. Lee, J.; Kim, M.; Lee, C.S.; Kim, S.S.; Koh, H.J.; Lee, S.C.; Byeon, S.H. Drusen subtypes and choroidal characteristics in Asian eyes with typical neovascular age-related macular degeneration. *Retina* **2020**, *40*, 490–498. [CrossRef] [PubMed]

12. Baek, J.; Lee, J.H.; Chung, B.J.; Lee, K.; Lee, W.K. Choroidal morphology under pachydrusen. *Clin. Exp. Ophthalmol.* **2019**, *47*, 498–504. [CrossRef] [PubMed]
13. Teo, K.; Cheong, K.X.; Ong, R.; Hamzah, H.; Yanagi, Y.; Wong, T.Y.; Chakravarthy, U.; Cheung, C. Macular neovascularization in eyes with pachydrusen. *Sci. Rep.* **2021**, *11*, 7495. [CrossRef] [PubMed]
14. Kim, K.L.; Joo, K.; Park, S.J.; Park, K.H.; Woo, S.J. Progression from intermediate to neovascular age-related macular degeneration according to drusen subtypes: Bundang AMD cohort study report 3. *Acta Ophthalmol.* **2022**, *100*, e710–e718. [CrossRef]
15. Schmitz-Valckenberg, S.; Pfau, M.; Fleckenstein, M.; Staurenghi, G.; Sparrow, J.R.; Bindewald-Wittich, A.; Spaide, R.F.; Wolf, S.; Sadda, S.R.; Holz, F.G. Fundus autofluorescence imaging. *Prog. Retin. Eye Res.* **2021**, *81*, 100893. [CrossRef]
16. Margolis, R.; Mukkamala, S.K.; Jampol, L.M.; Spaide, R.F.; Ober, M.D.; Sorenson, J.A.; Gentile, R.C.; Miller, J.A.; Sherman, J.; Freund, K.B. The expanded spectrum of focal choroidal excavation. *Arch. Ophthalmol.* **2011**, *129*, 1320–1325. [CrossRef]
17. Warrow, D.J.; Hoang, Q.V.; Freund, K.B. Pachychoroid pigment epitheliopathy. *Retina* **2013**, *33*, 1659–1672. [CrossRef]
18. Pang, C.E.; Freund, K.B. Pachychoroid neovasculopathy. *Retina* **2015**, *35*, 1–9. [CrossRef]
19. Zhao, X.; Xia, S.; Chen, Y. Characteristic appearances of fundus autofluorescence in treatment-naive and active polypoidal choroidal vasculopathy: A retrospective study of 170 patients. *Graefes Arch. Clin. Exp. Ophthalmol.* **2018**, *256*, 1101–1110. [CrossRef]
20. van Rijssen, T.J.; van Dijk, E.H.C.; Yzer, S.; Ohno-Matsui, K.; Keunen, J.E.E.; Schlingemann, R.O.; Sivaprasad, S.; Querques, G.; Downes, S.M.; Fauser, S.; et al. Central serous chorioretinopathy: Towards an evidence-based treatment guideline. *Prog. Retin. Eye Res.* **2019**, *73*, 100770. [CrossRef]
21. Han, J.; Cho, N.S.; Kim, K.; Kim, E.S.; Kim, D.G.; Kim, J.M.; Yu, S.Y. Fundus autofluorescence patterns in central serous chorioretinopathy. *Retina* **2020**, *40*, 1387–1394. [CrossRef]
22. Kumar, V.; Azad, S.V.; Verma, S.; Surve, A.; Vohra, R.; Venkatesh, P. Peripapillary pachychoroid syndrome: New insights. *Retina* **2022**, *42*, 80–87. [CrossRef] [PubMed]
23. Schneider, C.A.; Rasband, W.S.; Eliceiri, K.W. NIH Image to ImageJ: 25 years of image analysis. *Nat. Methods* **2012**, *9*, 671–675. [CrossRef] [PubMed]
24. Cheung, C.; Gan, A.; Yanagi, Y.; Wong, T.Y.; Spaide, R. Association between choroidal thickness and drusen subtypes in age-related macular degeneration. *Ophthalmol. Retin.* **2018**, *2*, 1196–1205. [CrossRef] [PubMed]
25. Kim, Y.H.; Chung, Y.R.; Kim, C.; Lee, K.; Lee, W.K. The association of pachydrusen characteristics with choroidal thickness and patient's age in polypoidal choroidal vasculopathy versus central serous chorioretinopathy. *Int. J. Mol. Sci.* **2022**, *23*, 8353. [CrossRef]
26. Govindahari, V.; Singh, S.R.; Rajesh, B.; Gallego-Pinazo, R.; Marco, R.D.; Nair, D.V.; Nair, U.; Chhablani, J. Multicolor imaging in central serous chorioretinopathy—A quantitative and qualitative comparison with fundus autofluorescence. *Sci. Rep.* **2019**, *9*, 11728. [CrossRef]
27. Shinojima, A.; Ozawa, Y.; Uchida, A.; Nagai, N.; Shinoda, H.; Kurihara, T.; Suzuki, M.; Minami, S.; Negishi, K.; Tsubota, K. Assessment of hypofluorescent foci on late-phase indocyanine green angiography in central serous chorioretinopathy. *J. Clin. Med.* **2021**, *10*, 2178. [CrossRef]
28. Yamagishi, T.; Koizumi, H.; Yamazaki, T.; Kinoshita, S. Fundus autofluorescence in polypoidal choroidal vasculopathy. *Ophthalmology* **2012**, *119*, 1650–1657. [CrossRef]
29. Notomi, S.; Shiose, S.; Ishikawa, K.; Fukuda, Y.; Kano, K.; Mori, K.; Wada, I.; Kaizu, Y.; Matsumoto, H.; Akiyama, M.; et al. Drusen and pigment abnormality predict the development of neovascular age-related macular degeneration in Japanese patients. *PLoS ONE* **2021**, *16*, e0255213. [CrossRef]
30. Fukuda, Y.; Sakurada, Y.; Sugiyama, A.; Yoneyama, S.; Matsubara, M.; Kikushima, W.; Tanabe, N.; Parikh, R.; Kashiwagi, K. Pachydrusen in fellow eyes predict response to aflibercept monotherapy in patients with polypoidal choroidal vasculopathy. *J. Clin. Med.* **2020**, *9*, 2459. [CrossRef]

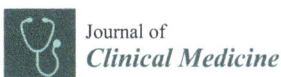

Article

Acute Idiopathic Blind Spot Enlargement Syndrome—New Perspectives in the OCT Era

Julian A. Zimmermann, Nicole Eter and Julia Biermann *

Department of Ophthalmology, University of Muenster Medical Center, Albert-Schweitzer-Campus 1, 48149 Muenster, Germany
* Correspondence: julia.biermann@ukmuenster.de; Tel.: +49-251-83-56001

Abstract: Acute idiopathic blind spot enlargement syndrome (AIBSES) is characterized by unilateral visual field loss in the blind spot area, acute onset photopsia, and funduscopically few or no optic disc changes. AIBSES predominantly affects young adults and is often misdiagnosed as optic neuritis because of low awareness. Optical coherence tomography (OCT) has become the gold standard in diagnosing AIBSES as a disease of the outer retina. In our case series, we present three consecutive patients with AIBSES followed prospectively with and without steroid therapy. The patients, aged 25 to 27 years, presented in our neuroophthalmology department between 2020 and 2021. We report their disease course and management and discuss therapeutic options, as no well-established procedures exist. Common pitfalls and diagnostic errors are analysed. Two women and one man showed unilateral acute-onset photopsia and blind spot enlargement on perimetry without visual acuity reduction. Spectral domain OCT (Heidelberg Engineering, Heidelberg, Germany) revealed marked peripapillary changes in the ellipsoid zone and autofluorescence in all patients, corresponding to faint blurring of the optic disc margin. Characteristically, there was no P100 latency delay in the visual evoked potential in any of the patients. Two patients received weight-adapted oral prednisolone, which was gradually tapered over six to eight weeks. Two patients showed full recovery of their symptoms at six and seven months after onset, while mild defect healing was seen in one treated patient after 12 months. Follow-up OCT showed restoration of the outer retinal layers 6–12 months after disease onset. Careful history taking and an unprejudiced ophthalmological workup helps in diagnosing AIBSES in young adults with unilateral acute visual field defects. While its etiology is still unclear, accurate diagnosis of AIBSES can be made with peripapillary OCT. In our cases, the disease course of AIBSES was much better than its reputation. Early corticosteroid treatment may support outer retinal reorganisation, which can be followed with OCT in accordance with visual field restoration. This should be addressed in a prospective study.

Keywords: blind spot enlargement; optical coherence tomography; retinopathy; optic neuritis; peripapillary; optic disc; visual field defect; young adults

Citation: Zimmermann, J.A.; Eter, N.; Biermann, J. Acute Idiopathic Blind Spot Enlargement Syndrome—New Perspectives in the OCT Era. J. Clin. Med. 2022, 11, 5278. https://doi.org/10.3390/jcm11185278

Academic Editors: Jay Chhablani and Sumit Randhir Singh

Received: 4 August 2022
Accepted: 6 September 2022
Published: 7 September 2022

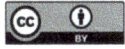

Copyright: © 2022 by the authors. Licensee MDPI, Basel, Switzerland. This article is an open access article distributed under the terms and conditions of the Creative Commons Attribution (CC BY) license (https://creativecommons.org/licenses/by/4.0/).

1. Introduction

In 1988, Fletcher et al., were the first to report acute idiopathic blind spot enlargement syndrome (AIBSES), characterised by acute-onset monocular photopsia and temporal scotoma, corresponding with blind spot enlargement in visual field testing and no or mild funduscopic changes of the retina and the optic nerve head [1]. To our knowledge, fewer than 100 cases have been retrospectively described in the literature, and thus no incidence rates have been reported. However, a higher number of undetected cases must be assumed, especially in the pre–optical coherence tomography (OCT) era.

The etiology of AIBSES as a disease of the outer retina remains unknown. Viral illness and vaccinations have been described as potential triggers [2–6]. An autoimmune cause of the disease has been discussed but is considered unlikely as recurrences are almost non-existent [7]. Furthermore, the idea of choriocapillaris non-perfusion and secondary ischaemia causing dysfunction of the outer retinal layers has been debated [3].

Diagnostic tools used to characterise the features of this disease include fundoscopy, visual field examination, OCT imaging, fluorescein angiography and electrophysiology. However, because OCT can identify AIBSES as a disease of the outer retina surrounding the optic disc, it has become the gold standard. Apart from marked blind spot enlargement, other clinical and diagnostic signs are less obvious (mostly unaffected visual acuity, faint blurring of the optic disc margins, no or mild staining of the optic disc on fluorescein angiography and no P100-delay) [3,7].

The majority of the reported cases of AIBSES have been in young to middle-aged Caucasian females [1,7]. Since unilateral visual field defects and visual phenomena are also found in young adults presenting with optic neuritis, AIBSES is often misdiagnosed, which leads to unnecessary and sometimes invasive diagnostic neurological workup and therapy [8].

Other conditions presenting with blind spot enlargement are papilledema, acute zonal occult outer retinopathy (AZOOR) and multiple evanescent white dot syndrome (MEWDS), the last two of which are also diseases of the outer retina [3,7,9].

No uniform therapy regime has been established so far. The approaches range from observation, in the majority of cases, to the infrequent systemic administration of corticosteroids at different time points. According to the literature, the cure rates have been poor [5,7].

We want to emphasise that AIBSES is an ophthalmic entity that is often missed, with a high estimated number of unreported cases, especially when OCT was not available. The features that distinguish AIBSES from optic neuritis and AZOOR are debated. We present multimodal imaging of three cases, with and without early corticosteroid treatment, which in our experience, supports retinal reorganisation and restoration of the visual field. As papillary OCT is being used increasingly as a diagnostic tool in ophthalmology and neurology, this article aims to increase focus on the outer retinal layers in addition to the well-established retinal nerve fibre layer (RNFL).

2. Case Series

Under the assumption of optic neuritis/papillitis, a serological workup was completed prior to neuroophthalmological assessment. Infectious and autoimmune diseases were ruled out by analysing the following laboratory values: full blood count, urea and electrolytes, thyroid levels, anti-nuclear antibodies (ANAs), anti-neutrophil cytoplasmic antibodies (ANCAs), aquaporin-4 antibodies, anti-glomerular basement membrane antibodies (anti-GBM Ab), viral polymerase chain reaction (PCR) for detection of cytomegalovirus (CMV) and Epstein–Barr virus (EBV), and antibodies against Bartonella henselae, Borrelia burgdorferi, Mycoplasma pneumoniae, and Treponema pallidum. In addition, cases 1 and 2 underwent brain magnetic resonance imaging (MRI) examination and a lumbar puncture, neither of which revealed any pathological findings. In cases 1 and 3, oral azithromycin 500 mg was given preventively for three days as a broad-spectrum therapeutic.

2.1. Case 1

A 26-year-old Caucasian woman consulted the neuroophthalmological department complaining of acute monocular photopsia, more precisely, flickering lights on the temporal half of her left eye, which had started seven days previously. She also reported decreased vision. The referral was made by an ophthalmologist, who suspected papillitis. Apart from flu-like symptoms eight months prior to the visit, the patient's past medical history was unremarkable.

On examination, the patient's best-corrected visual acuity was 20/25 in the right eye (refraction $-0.25/-0.25/\times 118$) and 20/20 in the left eye (refraction $+0.50/-0.50/\times 42$). Pupillary response was normal with no relative afferent pupillary defect (RAPD). Eye motility was normal. The red desaturation test was negative. Intraocular pressure was within the normal range. The findings of an anterior chamber slit lamp examination were physiological in accordance with age. Funduscopically, there was mild left peripapillary blurring with no haemorrhage or shadowing of the retinal vessels and a hypopigmented ring around the disc, which was not seen in the contralateral eye (Figure 1A).

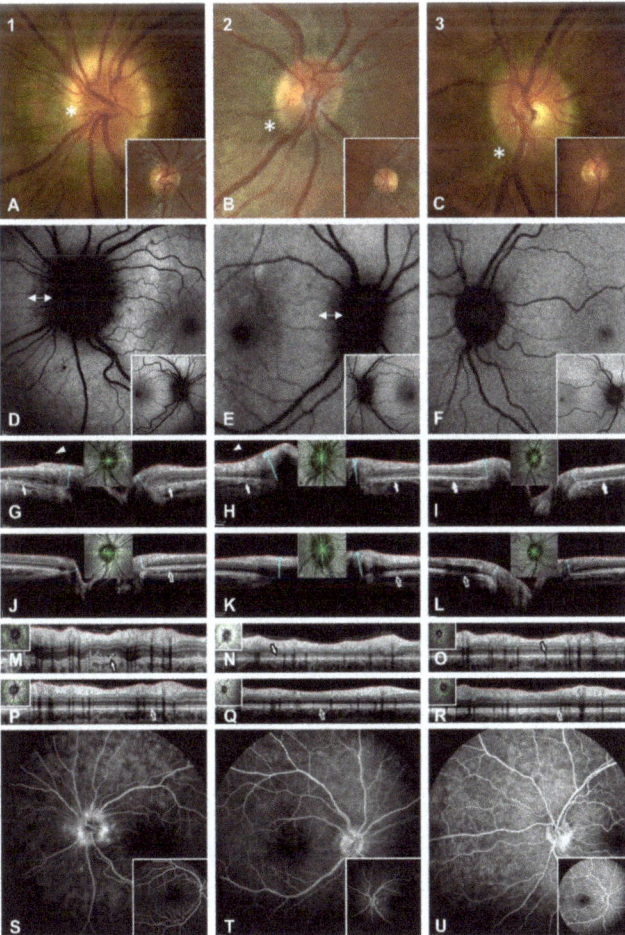

Figure 1. Multimodal imaging of three patients with AIBSES during the first week following the onset of symptoms. Vertical columns show, from left to right, cases 1–3, using SD-OCT (Heidelberg Engineering, Heidelberg, Germany). (**A–C**): Photographs of the optic disc of the affected eye, showing blurred optic disc margins and mild peripapillary colour changes (*), which were most obvious in case 1. Inlets show the contralateral eye. (**D–F**): Fundus autofluorescence imaging discloses circular irregular hypoautofluorescence of the peripapillary retina in cases 1 and 2, marked with arrows. Inlets show the contralateral eye. (**G–L**): Radial OCT cross-sections. Peripapillary irregularity and hyporeflectivity of the retinal pigment epithelium/Bruch's membrane complex, the interdigitation zone, the outer segments of photoreceptors and the ellipsoid zone are present in all affected eyes (arrows in (**G–I**)). The disturbance of retinal layer anatomy is particularly apparent in comparison to the unaffected eyes (empty arrow in (**J–L**)). Furthermore, hyperreflectivity in the preretinal vitreous is seen in (**G,H**) (arrowheads). (**M–R**): Retinal nerve fibre layer (RNFL) analysis. Little RNFL elevation is noticeable in the affected eyes of case 1 and 2 (**M,N**), but not in case 3 (**O**), compared to the unaffected eyes (**P–R**). The impairment of the peripapillary outer retinal layers is also well-displayed

(filled arrows in (**M–O**)). (**S–U**): Intravenous fluorescein angiography (FAG) depicts mild hyperfluorescence/staining of the optic nerve head edges without significant leakage. Speckled hyperfluorescent lesions are depicted in the surrounding disc area in case 1 (**S**), which are also seen in (**D**).

A 30-2 perimetry test (Humphrey visual field analyser 3, Carl Zeiss, Oberkochen, Germany) depicted left blind spot enlargement (Figure 2A). Irregular spotted hypoautofluorescence of the peripapillary retina was found in the left eye with normal appearance in the contralateral eye (Figure 1D). Radial OCT cross-sections revealed peripapillary irregularity and hyporeflectivity of the retinal pigment epithelium/Bruch's membrane complex, the interdigitation zone, the outer segments of photoreceptors and the ellipsoid zone (Figure 1G,J). Furthermore, hyperreflectivity was apparent in the preretinal vitreous, which was not visible by fundoscopy (Figure 1G). RNFL analysis showed very little elevation in comparison to the other eye but distinct irregularity and oedema of the outer retinal layers (Figure 1M,P). Fluorescein angiography (FAG) showed late peripapillary speckled hyperfluorescence but no leakage of the optic disc (Figure 1S). The visual evoked potentials (VEP) showed normal latencies bilaterally but borderline amplitude reduction in the left eye in comparison to the unaffected eye (data not shown).

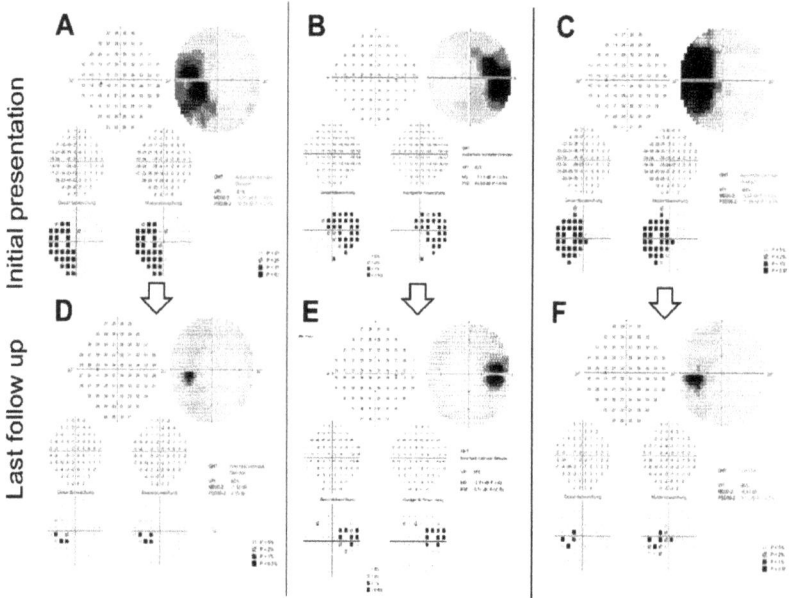

Figure 2. Static perimetry. Results of the 30-2 perimetry examination (Humphrey visual field analyser 3, Zeiss) of the affected eyes of cases 1–3 (from left to right) at first presentation (**A–C**) and at last follow-up, which was after six months in case 1 (**D**), after 12 months in case 2 (**E**) and after seven months in case 3 (**F**). Although all patients reported full recovery of their symptoms, discrete blind spot enlargement persisted in cases 2 and 3 (**E,F**).

As all the findings were highly suggestive of AIBSES, we immediately started treatment with body-weight–based oral prednisolone with an initial dose of 60 mg, which was gradually tapered over six weeks.

Perimetry at the two-month follow-up appointment showed an almost full recovery of the scotoma—the patient no longer complained of visual symptoms. The best-corrected visual acuity remained stable. A fundus examination showed left blurred disc margins and peripapillary retinal pigment epithelium (RPE) irregularity. The OCT scans of the left optic disc showed significant improvement of the outer retinal layer anatomy compared to the initial imaging. The left VEP amplitudes had recovered, and the latencies remained normal. We scheduled several follow-up appointments, which showed further improvement of the visual field and the outer retinal layers on OCT imaging. Full recovery of the blind spot enlargement and almost full restoration of the ellipsoid zone was detectable after six months (Figures 2D and 3A,B).

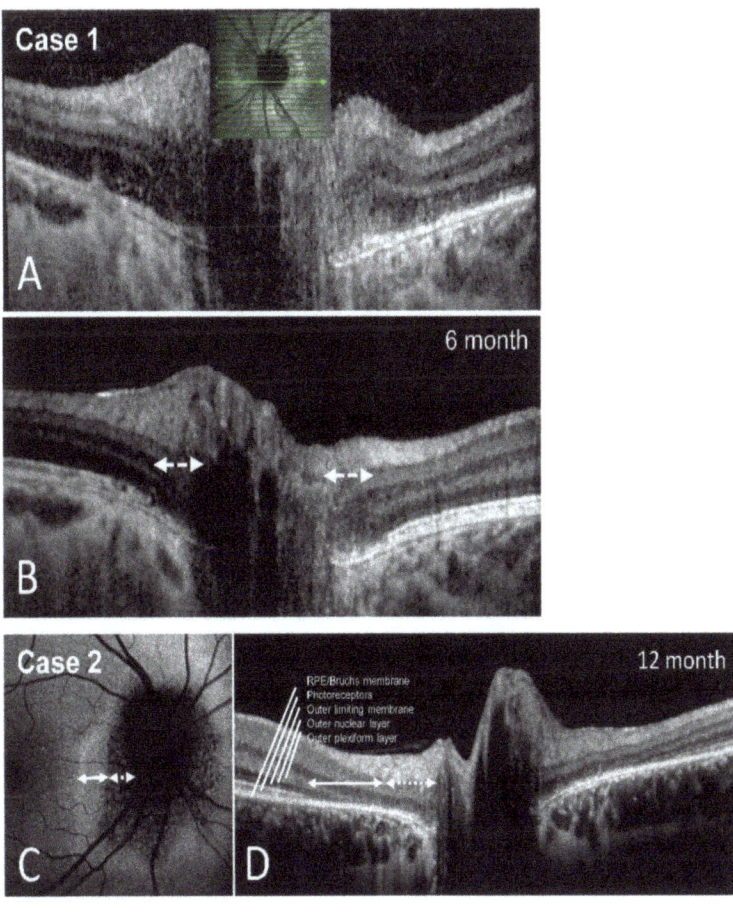

Figure 3. Restoration of outer retinal layer anatomy. SD-OCT scans (Heidelberg Engineering, Heidelberg, Germany). (**A**,**B**): Horizontal OCT cross sections of case 1 at first presentation (**A**) and after six months (**B**), showing restoration of the outer retinal layers in the peripapillary area except of the most proximal disc part, marked with arrows (**B**). (**C**,**D**): Autofluorescence (**C**) and OCT (**D**) of case 2 after 12 months. A hyperfluorescent and hypofluorescent area was apparent over time in the affected zone. Degeneration of the outer plexiform and outer nuclear layers (dotted arrow) represent the difference between both areas, resulting in hypofluorescence.

2.2. Case 2

A 27-year-old female reported a five-day history of gradually worsening photophobia in conjunction with photopsia in the right eye, as well as a mild feeling of ocular pressure. The patient's past medical history included previous episodes of migraine.

On examination, the patient's best-corrected visual acuity was 20/20 in the right eye (refraction +0.00/−0.75/×172) and 20/20 in the left eye (refraction +0.00/−0.50/×45). Pupillary response was normal with no RAPD. Intraocular pressure and examination of the anterior chamber were unremarkable. Funduscopically, there was mild blurring of the right optic disc (Figure 1B). The right anterior vitreous showed no cells. Cells in the posterior vitreous were barely visible funduscopically. OCT, however, clearly showed preretinal hyperreflectivity (Figure 1H). A visual field examination revealed enlargement of the right blind spot (Figure 2B).

Fundus autofluorescence (FAF) showed peripapillary fuzzy hypoautofluorescence (Figure 1E). Fluorescein angiography of the right eye showed no signs of vasculitis but mild staining of the left optic nerve head margin. FAG of the left eye was unremarkable (Figure 1T). When the patient first presented, OCT showed a peripapillary disturbance of the outer retinal layers (Figure 1H,N). VEPs showed normal latencies in both eyes but a check-size dependent decrease of the right amplitudes. Responses in the multifocal electroretinogram (mfERG) were significantly reduced in the affected right eye and normal in the unaffected eye (data not shown).

Based on these findings, we diagnosed the patient with AIBSES and started treating her with oral prednisolone with an initial dose of 60 mg, which was gradually tapered over eight weeks. At the two-month follow-up appointment, the patient reported a subjective reduction of visual impairment with stable visual acuity. Perimetry showed partial but continuing improvement of the scotoma, which continued to improve during one year of follow-up. After one year, a significant but asymptomatic enlargement of the blind spot was still found (Figure 2E). OCT imaging after one year revealed persistent but narrowed peripapillary atrophy of the outer retinal layers (Figure 3C,D) and partial restoration of autofluorescence in the peripheral zone of the defect (Figure 3C).

2.3. Case 3

A 25-year-old Caucasian male was referred by his ophthalmologist with a suspected diagnosis of typical optic neuritis after complaining about a one-week history of flickering monocular sinistral scotoma in the temporal visual field. His past medical history was unremarkable. He had received the diphtheria-tetanus-pertussis vaccination one week prior to the initial presentation.

On examination, the patient's best-corrected visual acuity was 20/20 in both eyes (refraction OD +0.25/−0.75/×138; OS −1.75/−0.50/×36). Red desaturation test, eye motility, intraocular pressure and examination of the anterior chamber were unremarkable in both eyes, with no signs of inflammation. Funduscopically, there was mild blurring of the left optic nerve and peripapillary brightening of the retina (Figure 1C). Perimetry showed enlargement of the left blind spot (Figure 2C). Intravenous FAG depicted mild partial hyperfluorescence of the left optic nerve head without leakage (Figure 1U). OCT imaging depicted peripapillary irregularities of the outer retinal layers, which led to the diagnosis of AIBSES (Figure 1I,O). Visual evoked potentials showed reduced amplitudes and normal latencies in the affected left eye. Responses in the mfERG were significantly reduced in the affected left eye but normal in the unaffected eye (data not shown). Since there was a significant decrease in symptoms and visual field defect size after six days, we decided against applying therapy with systemic corticosteroids.

We scheduled follow-up appointments five and seven months after the initial presentation. Perimetry over the course of seven months showed remarkable improvement without therapy, although a slight blind spot enlargement persisted (Figure 2F). Comparing OCT Bruch's membrane opening (BMO) and RNFL scans over the course of seven months, the most recent multimodal imaging revealed partial recovery of the outer retinal layers (data not shown).

A flowchart of examinations and clinical findings is shown in Figure 4 as a guiding structure in the differential diagnosis.

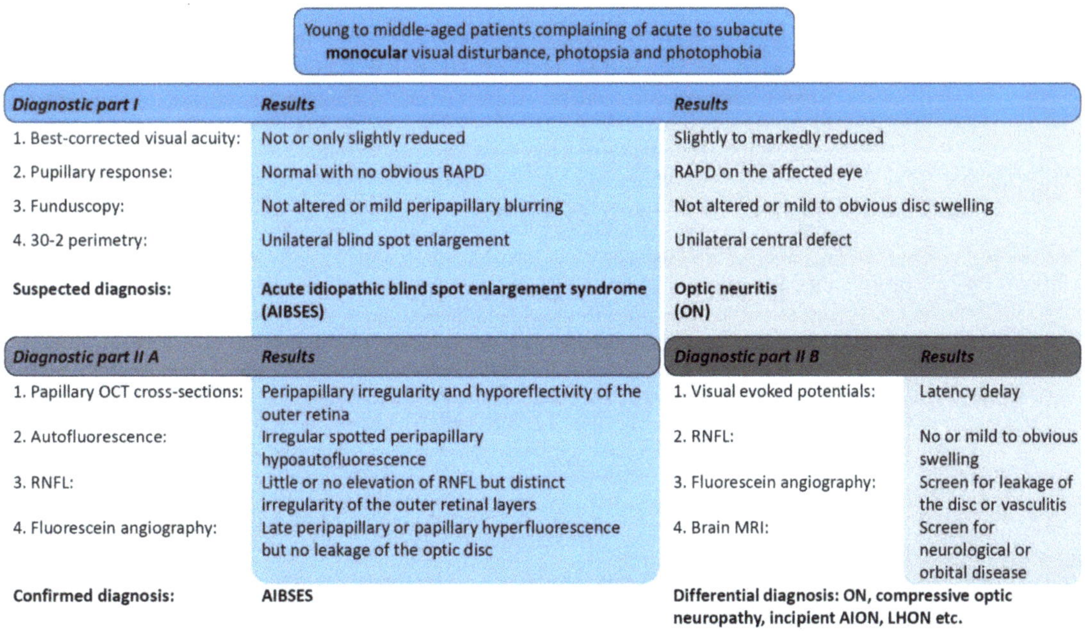

Young to middle-aged patients complaining of acute to subacute monocular visual disturbance, photopsia and photophobia			
Diagnostic part I	*Results*		*Results*
1. Best-corrected visual acuity:	Not or only slightly reduced		Slightly to markedly reduced
2. Pupillary response:	Normal with no obvious RAPD		RAPD on the affected eye
3. Funduscopy:	Not altered or mild peripapillary blurring		Not altered or mild to obvious disc swelling
4. 30-2 perimetry:	Unilateral blind spot enlargement		Unilateral central defect
Suspected diagnosis:	**Acute idiopathic blind spot enlargement syndrome (AIBSES)**		**Optic neuritis (ON)**
Diagnostic part II A	*Results*	*Diagnostic part II B*	*Results*
1. Papillary OCT cross-sections:	Peripapillary irregularity and hyporeflectivity of the outer retina	1. Visual evoked potentials:	Latency delay
2. Autofluorescence:	Irregular spotted peripapillary hypoautofluorescence	2. RNFL:	No or mild to obvious swelling
3. RNFL:	Little or no elevation of RNFL but distinct irregularity of the outer retinal layers	3. Fluorescein angiography:	Screen for leakage of the disc or vasculitis
4. Fluorescein angiography:	Late peripapillary or papillary hyperfluorescence but no leakage of the optic disc	4. Brain MRI:	Screen for neurological or orbital disease
Confirmed diagnosis:	**AIBSES**	**Differential diagnosis:**	ON, compressive optic neuropathy, incipient AION, LHON etc.

Figure 4. Flowchart of diagnostic workup. After the diagnostic part I (**upper part**), a sound clinical suspicion can be made to differentiate AIBSES from optic nerve diseases. The examinations of diagnostic part IIA (**left**) serve to confirm the diagnosis of AIBSES, especially with the use of papillary OCT cross-sections. Fluorescein angiography is not absolutely necessary. The diagnostic part IIB (**right**) can be used to further differentiate between optic neuritis and other retrobulbar diseases, which more often can affect young to middle-aged patients. RAPD: relative afferent pupillary defect; RNFL: retinal nerve fiber layer; MRI: magnetic resonance imaging; AION: anterior ischemic optic neuropathy; LHON: Leber hereditary optic neuropathy.

3. Discussion

The diagnosis of AIBSES must be considered on the basis of the following cardinal findings: acute monocular blind spot enlargement in visual field examination and peripapillary outer retinal abnormalities on OCT imaging in an otherwise unremarkable fundus. The young to middle-aged patients—most of them women—complain of acute to subacute photopsia and photophobia. The condition is unknown to many ophthalmologists and neurologists and therefore is often missed.

Although optic neuritis is a disease of the optic nerve that is often associated with multiple sclerosis, and AIBSES is a disease of the outer retina, the likelihood of confusion between them is present when OCT of the outer retina is not inspected. Two of our patients were initially referred to neurology and given a diagnosis of optic neuritis. This appears reasonable at first, as patients with both diseases are generally (1) young adults, (2) female, (3) with unilateral acute visual symptoms and (4) with no, or very few, funduscopic changes. On a closer look, however, these two disease entities can be distinguished by taking into consideration the hallmarks of typical optic neuritis, which were extensively studied and described in the Optic Neuritis Treatment Trial (ONTT) [10]. The ONTT followed 457 acute optic neuritis patients for eight days following onset between 1988 and 1991 in the United States to investigate treatment with oral or intravenous corticosteroids versus placebo. The clinical profile of typical optic neuritis was summarized as follows: A total of 77.2% of the patients were women. The mean age was 31.8 years. Ocular pain on eye movement was experienced by 92.2% of the patients. The visual loss and visual field defects were severe (only 10.5% showed visual acuity of 20/20 or better in the affected eye) and objectifiable through a relative afferent pupillary defect and latency delay in VEP. The optic disc and fundus appeared normal in 64.7% of the patients or showed only mild optic disc swelling. Atypical optic neuritis must be assumed when the above criteria are not present, and one or both optic discs show significant swelling, haemorrhages or exudates in conjunction with significant and progressive visual loss without pain.

The above findings differ greatly from the clinical presentation of patients with AIBSES, who, in previous studies, did not complain of ocular pain and had normal or only slightly reduced visual acuity in the majority of cases as the central visual field was unaffected, and, therefore, no afferent defect was detectable with VEP or pupil reflex testing [1,7,11]. Instead, OCT reveals that AIBSES patients have outer retinal abnormalities in the peripapillary area, corresponding to the visual field defect, which is a prominent enlarged blind spot. When analysing the patterns of visual field loss in 229 optic neuritis patients, the 1991 Optic Neuritis Study Group found blind spot enlargement in only 2.6% of the patients [10]. Thus, the visual field defect of AIBSES patients must raise concerns about other optic nerve diseases, which typically present with central or nerve fibre bundle visual field defects [12]. None of our patients reported pain, nor was there any reduction in best corrected visual acuity, and the VEP latencies were within normal limits. In a study of 27 patients with AIBSES, 23 complained of positive visual phenomena and 16 patients presented with a visual acuity of 20/20, 10 with a visual acuity between 20/25 and 20/50 and only one with a visual acuity of 20/200 [7].

In the fewer than 100 published cases of AIBSES [1,7,11,13,14], about two-thirds of the patients are women. Although most AIBSES patients are young adults, an age range of 16 to 63 years has been reported [1,7,11,13–15]. Unilateral courses are the rule. Recurrence of the disease cannot be ruled out but is highly uncommon. Six of the 27 cases described by Volpe suffered a recurrence between one and 15 years after the first occurrence. In two cases, the contralateral eye was affected [7].

Although no optic disc swelling was found in our patients, blurring of the optic disc margins was seen, and discrimination between possible diagnoses by fundoscopy alone was unfeasible. Blurred margins of the optic disc have been previously described as a common funduscopic finding representing peripapillary retinal damage [7], although other authors have reported no abnormalities of the optic disc [7,16]. Vitritis was present in only three of the 27 cases in Volpe et al.'s study, the largest AIBSES cohort collected to date. Vitreal hyperreflectivity was found adjacent to the inner retinal layers in two out of the three cases presented here, depicted in OCT images (Figure 1G,H). Due to this location, there was no funduscopic evidence of cells in the anterior vitreous, which is accessible by indirect fundoscopy. Fluorescein angiography revealed late staining of the optic nerve head edges in our three patients and mild peripapillary leakage in one case (Figure 1S,U). This finding was present in almost 50% of the 27 patients described previously [7].

The gold standard for diagnosing AIBSES nowadays, however, is a papillary SD-OCT. Common findings include microstructural irregularities and loss of the ellipsoid zone and outer nuclear layers of the retina [4,17,18]. Some authors have described cases in which recovery of the ellipsoid zone on OCT imaging, formerly known as the inner and outer segments of retinal photoreceptors, corresponded with visual improvement, which is consistent with our findings [17,18]. Over the observation period of our cases, recovery of the irregular outer retina was found (Figure 3). Therefore, we highlight the importance of SD-OCT for the diagnosis of AIBSES and for follow-up.

In the pre-OCT era, the use of ERG to detect abnormalities of the retinal photoreceptors was suggested for diagnosing patients with AIBSES [1,5,7,19]. Multifocal electroretinogram amplitudes were abnormally reduced in both of our patients who had ERG, consistent with the results of previous studies, in which eight of nine patients showed abnormal nasal parafoveal focal ERG results [7]. In their retrospective analysis of 22 patients, Watzke et al. showed that multifocal ERG results revealed more extensive and even bilateral retinal damage than perimetric results and clinical examination would have suggested [13].

Interestingly, Piri et al. also describe a case with reduced perifoveal mfERG responses in the asymptomatic contralateral eye [17]. This was not a finding in our patients, where we found changes only in the symptomatic eye without evidence of changes to the unaffected eye. In summary, multifocal ERG can be considered a supporting diagnostic tool for characterising outer retinal function in AIBSE patients but is dispensable in cases with an unambiguous OCT finding.

No general agreement has been reached regarding the exact classification of AIBSES in relation to other disease entities affecting the outer retina or choriocapillaris, especially AZOOR and MEWDS [4]. Whether AIBSES is an independent disease or just a facet of AZOOR [7,20] is still being debated. This is reasonable, as AIBSES and AZOOR show some similarities. In both disease entities, changes at the level of the outer retinal bands on OCT seem to lead to photopsia and visual field loss on perimetry, but, interestingly, without decreasing visual acuity significantly [2]. On SD-OCT, AZOOR patients show changes at the photoreceptor level—mainly irregularities of the ellipsoidal zone, drusenoid deposits and atrophy of the photoreceptors and retinal pigment epithelium (Mrejen et al., 2014). Young women are particularly affected—the average age of AZOOR patients is 30 years [2]. Further similarities include the mostly inconspicuous funduscopic findings at the beginning of the disease and the occasional finding of cells in the vitreous body. However, after reviewing the literature and based on our findings, we argue in favour of classifying AZOOR and AIBSES as different entities. AZOOR is often described as bilateral (in nine of 13 patients described by Gass [2]), and ERG changes were measureable in both eyes in 50% of patients, some of whom were clinically asymptomatic [2]. AIBSES however, is a unilateral disease. While in AIBSES the enlargement of the blind spot is the pathological hallmark resulting from the one peripapillary focus, an exclusive enlargement of the blind spot is rarely found in AZOOR patients—only in 19% of the published cases, which mostly show multifocal visual field defects [19]. Of the 51 patients reported in the largest published AZOOR cohort to date, recurrence of the disease with at least one episode occurred in 16 cases. The median time to recurrence was 39 months [19]. Documented recurrences of AIBSES are rare, as reported above. Finally, another distinctive feature seems to be the poor recovery of photopsias and visual field defects in AZOOR patients, in whom depigmentation and atrophic changes of the retinal pigment epithelium developed and correlated with the persisting visual field defects [19]. In contrast, our AIBSES patients showed a good regression of their symptoms, with and without corticosteroids, as well as a significant improvement of the visual field defect over time.

While the clinical symptoms of MEWDS and AIBSES are often similar (unilaterality; spontaneous occurrence of photopsia; visual field defects), diagnostic differences can help to distinguish the two entities. The funduscopically faint white dots in the mid-periphery, which give MEWDS its name, were not present in our patients, nor have they been described for AIBSES patients. The fluorescence angiography of our patients showed hyperfluorescence exclusively around or on the optic disc. Patchy areas of late hyperfluorescence in the periphery, as described for MEWDS, were not found, nor were peripheral changes in fundus autofluorescence. MEWDS is known to be a self-limiting disease while spontaneous recovery in AIBSES has not yet been reported in the majority of cases.

The etiology of AIBSES remains unclear. For both AIBSES and AZOOR, viral infections, autoimmune diseases and vaccinations have been found to be potential triggers [2–5,21]. Genetic and hormonal factors are also possible, with the clear predominance of female patients [7]. Cimino et al. suggest that choriocapillaris non-perfusion and secondary ischemia may cause dysfunction of the outer retinal layers, and this may be the mechanism behind primary inflammatory choriocapillaropathies (PICCP), including AIBSES and MEWDS [3]. However, none of our patients reported a recent history of a viral infection or disease, while only one patient (case 3) reported recent vaccination. However, a careful history of COVID-19 disease and vaccination showed no causal relationship with the beginning of visual symptoms in this patient. In our opinion, an autoimmune/parainfectious inflammatory etiology can be hypothesised, as vitreous cellular hyperreflectivity is often present preretinally but is visible only in the OCT. We can only speculate about the potential impact of steroid treatment on recovery to support this idea.

Currently, no established therapeutic regime exists to treat AIBSES. The use of systemic steroids has been reported in single case descriptions. The reported results vary from spontaneous improvement of signs and symptoms without intervention within six to 10 weeks to the use of systemic immunosuppressive drugs [3–5]. There are no references to potential therapies in either the earliest description of AIBSES [1] or in the largest collection of 27 patients [7]. The majority of individual case descriptions and small case series, however, report no or only partial regression of the visual field defect [1,5,7,18]. We saw visual field improvement in all our prospectively followed patients, two of whom received treatment with systemic steroids and one of whom received no treatment but recovered spontaneously very quickly. With a relatively low spectrum of side-effects and an impressive reduction in visual field defects and irregularities of the outer retina on OCT in both of our patients treated with systemic steroids, we currently consider the administration of weight-adapted corticosteroids for some weeks to be advisable for the treatment of AIBSES. Further controlled studies are needed to draw stronger conclusions about the impact of timing and dosing.

4. Conclusions

To the best of our best knowledge, fewer than 100 cases of AIBSES have been published, and the accurate classification of disease entities affecting the outer retina continues to pose difficulties. However, a higher number of undetected cases must be assumed, especially in the pre-OCT era. A careful history taking, and unprejudiced ophthalmological workup, helps in diagnosing AIBSES in young adults in whom unilateral acute blind spot enlargement is identified in visual field examination. Although the etiology is still unclear, AIBSES can be accurately diagnosed with peripapillary OCT, perimetry and a lack of a distinct relative afferent pupillary defect. An autoimmune/parainfectious inflammatory etiology seems possible as preretinal vitreous cellular hyperreflectivity is often present. Early treatment with corticosteroids may support outer retinal reorganisation and restoration of the visual field; precise dosage, administration and duration of treatment should be addressed in detail in a prospective study. The course of our prospectively followed patients raises doubts about the often-stated view that AIBSES is a disease with a poor prognosis. AIBSES is a noteworthy ophthalmologic condition that can be clearly distinguished from optic neuritis. Neurologists should be suspicious if referred patients show unilateral blind spot enlargement, which is a very rare finding in optic neuritis. As there is an increasing use of papillary OCT diagnostic in ophthalmology and neurology, this article aims to increase focus on the outer retinal layers in addition to the familiar RNFL.

Author Contributions: Conceptualization, J.B.; methodology, J.B. and J.A.Z.; investigation, J.B. and J.A.Z.; resources, N.E.; data curation, J.B. and J.A.Z.; writing—original draft preparation, J.B. and J.A.Z.; writing—review and editing, all authors; supervision, J.B. and N.E. All authors have read and agreed to the published version of the manuscript.

Funding: This research received no external funding.

Informed Consent Statement: Patient consent was waived due to local regulations of the Ethics Committee of the University of Muenster, Germany, as this study meets the criteria of § 6 health data protection law NRW.

Data Availability Statement: Not applicable.

Acknowledgments: We acknowledge support from the Open Access Publication Fund of the University of Muenster.

Conflicts of Interest: The authors declare no conflict of interest.

References

1. Fletcher, W.A.; Imes, R.K.; Goodman, D.; Hoyt, W.F. Acute idiopathic blind spot enlargement. A big blind spot syndrome without optic disc edema. *Arch. Ophthalmol.* **1988**, *106*, 44–49. [CrossRef] [PubMed]
2. Gass, J.D. Acute zonal occult outer retinopathy. Donders Lecture: The Netherlands Ophthalmological Society, Maastricht, Holland, June 19, 1992. *J. Clin. Neuroophthalmol.* **1993**, *13*, 79–97. [PubMed]
3. Cimino, L.; Mantovani, A.; Herbort, C.P. Primary Inflammatory Choriocapillaropathies. In *Uveitis and Immunological Disorders*; Krieglstein, G.K., Weinreb, R.N., Pleyer, U., Mondino, B., Eds.; Springer: Berlin/Heidelberg, Germany, 2005; pp. 209–231. ISBN 3-540-20045-2.
4. Jampol, L.M.; Wiredu, A. MEWDS, MFC, PIC, AMN, AIBSE, and AZOOR: One disease or many? *Retina* **1995**, *15*, 373–378. [PubMed]
5. Quinones, X.; Ortiz, J.; Santos, C.; Oliver, A.L.; Rodríguez, J. Acute idiopathic blind spot enlargement syndrome following influenza vaccination. *Am. J. Ophthalmol. Case Rep.* **2020**, *20*, 100949. [CrossRef] [PubMed]
6. Wong, M.; Campos-Baniak, M.G.; Colleaux, K. Acute idiopathic blind spot enlargement syndrome following measles, mumps and rubella vaccination. *Can. J. Ophthalmol.* **2019**, *54*, e199–e203. [CrossRef] [PubMed]
7. Volpe, N.J.; Rizzo, J.F.; Lessell, S. Acute idiopathic blind spot enlargement syndrome: A review of 27 new cases. *Arch. Ophthalmol.* **2001**, *119*, 59–63. [PubMed]
8. Stunkel, L.; Kung, N.H.; Wilson, B.; McClelland, C.M.; van Stavern, G.P. Incidence and Causes of Overdiagnosis of Optic Neuritis. *JAMA Ophthalmol.* **2017**, *136*, 76–81. [CrossRef] [PubMed]
9. Fisayo, A.; Bruce, B.B.; Newman, N.J.; Biousse, V. Overdiagnosis of idiopathic intracranial hypertension. *Neurology* **2016**, *86*, 341–350. [CrossRef] [PubMed]
10. Beck, R.W. The Optic Neuritis Treatment Trial. *Arch. Ophthalmol.* **1988**, *106*, 1051–1053. [CrossRef] [PubMed]
11. Singh, K.; Frank, M.P.; de Shults, W.T.; Watzke, R.C. Acute Idiopathic Blind Spot Enlargement. *Ophthalmology* **1991**, *98*, 497–502. [CrossRef]
12. Rizzo, J.F.; Lessell, S. Optic neuritis and ischemic optic neuropathy. Overlapping clinical profiles. *Arch. Ophthalmol.* **1991**, *109*, 1668–1672. [CrossRef] [PubMed]
13. Watzke, R.C.; Shults, W.T. Clinical features and natural history of the acute idiopathic enlarged blind spot syndrome. *Ophthalmology* **2002**, *109*, 1326–1335. [CrossRef]
14. Sugahara, M.; Shinoda, K.; Matsumoto, S.C.; Satofuka, S.; Hanazono, G.; Imamura, Y.; Mizota, A. Outer retinal microstructure in a case of acute idiopathic blind spot enlargement syndrome. *Case Rep. Ophthalmol.* **2011**, *2*, 116–122. [CrossRef] [PubMed]
15. Makino, S. Acute Idiopathic Blind Spot Enlargement Syndrome in A 63-Year-Old Man. *Internet J. Ophthalmol. Vis. Sci.* **2014**, *11*, 1.
16. Liu, X.; Chen, B.; Zhang, M.; Huang, H. Clinical features and differential diagnosis of acute idiopathic blind spot enlargement syndrome. *Eye Sci.* **2014**, *29*, 143–150. [PubMed]
17. Piri, N.; Kaplan, H.J.; Sigford, D.K.; Tezel, T.H. High-definition optical coherence tomography findings in acute idiopathic blind spot enlargement (AIBSE) syndrome. *Ocul. Immunol. Inflamm.* **2014**, *22*, 494–496. [CrossRef] [PubMed]
18. Trese, M.G.J.; Cohen, S.R.; Besirli, C.G. Recovery of outer retina in acute idiopathic blind spot enlargement (AIBSE). *Am. J. Ophthalmol. Case Rep.* **2016**, *1*, 13–15. [CrossRef] [PubMed]
19. Gass, J.D.; Agarwal, A.; Scott, I.U. Acute zonal occult outer retinopathy: A long-term follow-up study. *Am. J. Ophthalmol.* **2002**, *134*, 329–339. [CrossRef]
20. Wang, M.; Sadaka, A.; Prager, T.; Lee, A.G.; Pellegrini, F.; Cirone, D.; Simone, L.; de Cimino, L. From A ... to ... Z(OOR): The Clinical Spectrum of Acute Zonal Occult Outer Retinopathy. *Neuro Ophthalmol.* **2018**, *42*, 215–221. [CrossRef] [PubMed]
21. Wang, Q.; Jiang, L.; Yan, W.; Wei, W.; Lai, T.Y.Y. Fundus Autofluorescence Imaging in the Assessment of Acute Zonal Occult Outer Retinopathy. *Ophthalmologica* **2017**, *237*, 153–158. [CrossRef] [PubMed]

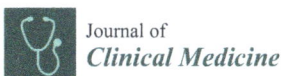

Article

Risk Factors for Progression of Age-Related Macular Degeneration: Population-Based Amish Eye Study

Muneeswar G. Nittala [1,†], Federico Corvi [1,†], Jyotsna Maram [1], Swetha B. Velaga [1], Jonathan Haines [2], Margaret A. Pericak-Vance [3], Dwight Stambolian [4] and SriniVas R. Sadda [1,5,*]

1. Doheny Image Reading Center, Doheny Eye Institute, Los Angeles, CA 90033, USA
2. Department of Epidemiology & Biostatistics, Case Western Reserve University, Cleveland, OH 44106, USA
3. John P. Hussman Institute for Human Genomics, University of Miami Miller School of Medicine, Miami, FL 33136, USA
4. Department of Ophthalmology, Perelman School of Medicine, University of Pennsylvania, Philadelphia, PA 19104, USA
5. Department of Ophthalmology, David Geffen School of Medicine at UCLA, Los Angeles, CA 90095, USA
* Correspondence: ssadda@doheny.org
† These authors contributed equally to this work.

Abstract: Objective: To evaluate the optical coherence tomography (OCT)-based risk factors for progression to late age-related macular degeneration (AMD) in a population-based study of elderly Amish. Methods: A total of 1332 eyes of 666 consecutive subjects who completed a 2-year follow-up visit were included in this multicenter, prospective, longitudinal, observational study. Imaging features were correlated with 2-year incidence of late AMD development. Odds ratios for imaging features were estimated from logistic regression. Baseline OCT images were reviewed for the presence of drusen volume ≥ 0.03 mm^3 in the central 3 mm ring, intraretinal hyperreflective foci (IHRF), hyporeflective drusen cores (hDC), subretinal drusenoid deposits (SDD), and drusenoid pigment epithelium detachment (PED). Subfoveal choroidal thickness, drusen area, and drusen volume within 3 and 5 mm circles centered on the fovea were also assessed. Results: Twenty-one (1.5%) of 1332 eyes progressed to late AMD by 2 years. The mean age of the study subjects was 65 ± 10.17 ($\pm$SD) years and 410 subjects were female. Univariate logistic regression showed that drusen area and volume in both 3 mm and 5 mm circles, subfoveal choroidal thickness, drusen volume ≥ 0.03 mm^3 in the 3 mm ring, SDD, IHRF, and hDC were all associated with an increased risk for development of late AMD. The multivariate regression model identified that drusen volume in the 3 mm ring (OR: 2.59, $p = 0.049$) and presence of IHRF (OR: 57.06, $p < 0.001$) remained as independent and significant risk factors for progression to late AMD. Conclusions: This population-based study confirms previous findings from clinic-based studies that high central drusen volume and IHRF are associated with an increased risk of progression to late AMD. These findings may be of value in risk-stratifying patients in clinical practice or identifying subjects for early intervention clinical trials.

Keywords: age-related macular degeneration; Amish eye study; complete retinal pigment epithelial and outer retina atrophy; geographic atrophy; optical coherence tomography

1. Introduction

Age-related macular degeneration (AMD) affects almost 200 million people worldwide in 2020, which will increase to 288 million by 2040 [1]. AMD is a complex disease in which demographic and environmental factors—including age, gender, smoking, and diet—contribute to the risk of developing disease [2,3]. Despite the complexity of the phenotype, eyes with AMD are classified in different stages of severity in which late stages are defined by the presence of macular neovascularization (MNV) and/or geographic atrophy (GA).

Considering the GA progression, several trials are ongoing to test different agents to determine whether they can slow the progression of the atrophic changes. However, progression of AMD is not fully understood and is highly variable [4]. Increasingly, there has been a desire to intervene at an earlier stage in these AMD patients before irreversible atrophic lesions appear [5]. In order to design such studies, however, it essential to identify biomarkers and patients who are at greatest risk for progression to late AMD.

Recently, OCT has been introduced as an essential tool for identifying atrophy. The Classification of Atrophy Meetings (CAM) group defined the terms complete retinal pigment epithelial (RPE) and outer retinal atrophy (cRORA) using specific OCT criteria [6].

In addition, a number of OCT risk factors for progression to atrophy have been defined in retinal clinic studies and post-hoc analysis of retina clinical trials. These risk factors include central drusen volume ≥ 0.03 mm^3, intraretinal hyperreflective foci (IHRF), hyporeflective drusen cores (hDC), and subretinal drusenoid deposits (SDD) [7–12]. A retina clinic population, however, may be confounded by selection bias and may not reflect the diversity of AMD in the general population.

The Amish migrated from eastern Europe to the U.S. in the early 18th century to escape religious persecution. Due to the founder effect, genetic changes within the Amish population have increased in frequency making it possible to identify genetic anomalies with a much smaller sample size than would be needed from the general population. Therefore, genetic studies on the Amish afford researchers the opportunity to identify variants of European origin without the burden of recruiting a much larger number of subjects. As the Amish population is a founder population which is genetically and culturally isolated, it features a uniform environment and reduced genetic diversity. Moreover, the Amish do not indulge in smoking, reducing the amount of AMD risk attributable to smoking. The possibility to study this population represents a unique opportunity to evaluate in a clear view the impact of different risk factors in the progression of late AMD. Thus, the purpose of this study is to evaluate the suggested OCT risk factors for atrophy in the context of a longitudinal prospective study from the patients enrolled in the AMISH eye study.

2. Methods

The Amish eye study is a multicenter, prospective, longitudinal, observational study with NEI-supported clinical research investigation aimed at understanding genetic associations with AMD progression. Of the 1339 subjects (2668 eyes) who were initially enrolled in the Amish eye study, the first 666 consecutive subjects (49.7%; 1332 eyes or roughly half the cohort) returned for their 2-year follow up visit and were thus included in this analysis. Patients were identified from three settlements in Ohio, Indiana, and Pennsylvania. The human subject protocols have been approved by the Institutional Review Boards of the University of Pennsylvania, University of Miami, Case Western Reserve University, and University of California Los Angeles. All study procedures followed the tenets of the Declaration of Helsinki. Written informed consent was obtained from all subjects after explaining the nature and possible consequences of the study. Inclusion criteria were: (1) age $\geq$ 50 years; (2) self-identification as Amish; (3) membership in a sibship with at least 1 individual reported to have AMD; (4) follow-up data for at least 2 years. Exclusion criteria included inadequate image quality, any previous or concomitant ophthalmological condition that could confound the interpretation of AMD features on imaging, and presence of late AMD in the study eye at baseline.

2.1. Study Design

The data collection and imaging protocols were detailed in previous Amish eye study reports [13]. Data collection was standardized and included measurements taken by clinical research coordinators, ophthalmic technicians, and board-certified ophthalmologists in respective study sites. Patients were evaluated after a 2-year follow-up to assess which cases progressed and which cases did not progress to late AMD.

2.2. Study Procedures

Demographic information collected at baseline and at the 2-year follow-up visit included age, sex, family history of AMD, and the presence of any other eye diseases. All individuals received a comprehensive eye exam, including visual acuity measured using a Snellen chart at 20 feet, and a panel of multimodal imaging studies consisting of stereo color fundus photographs (CFPs), blue light fundus autofluorescence (FAF; Spectralis), infrared reflectance (IR; Spectralis), and dense-volume OCT (Cirrus and Spectralis).

2.2.1. OCT Image Acquisition

All structural OCT images were acquired by both the Cirrus HD-OCT (Carl Zeiss Meditec, Dublin, CA, USA), using a macular cube protocol of 128 horizontal B-scans and 512 A-scans per line (6 × 6 mm, foveal centered), and the Spectralis OCT (Spectralis; Heidelberg Engineering, Heidelberg, Germany), using a macular cube protocol of 97 horizontal B-scans and 512 A-scans per line and automatic real-time tracking (ART) of 9 (6 × 6 mm, foveal centered and EDI mode off). In addition to the fovea-centered scan, an additional OCT volume was captured centered on the optic disk. Two devices were originally incorporated in the study to take advantage of the unique capabilities of each instrument, such as the automated drusen quantification by the Cirrus and the better visualization of the outer retinal substructures and choroid by the averaged scans of the Spectralis. Scans were repeated in the case of motion artifacts and/or low signal strength (SS). In accordance with the manufacturer's recommendations and the reading center's guidelines, to be acceptable for inclusion, an OCT volume had to have SS > 30 on Spectralis and SS ≥ 7 on the Cirrus.

2.2.2. Structural OCT Image Analysis

All images were reviewed by two independent and masked graders (MGN and SBV) at baseline and after 2 years for the presence of cRORA, drusenoid pigment epithelium detachment (PED), IHRF, hDC, SDD, and drusen volume ≥0.03 mm^3 within 3 mm circle (Figure 1), as well as to measure drusen volume and area as continuous metrics within the central 3 mm and central 5 mm circles and subfoveal choroidal thickness.

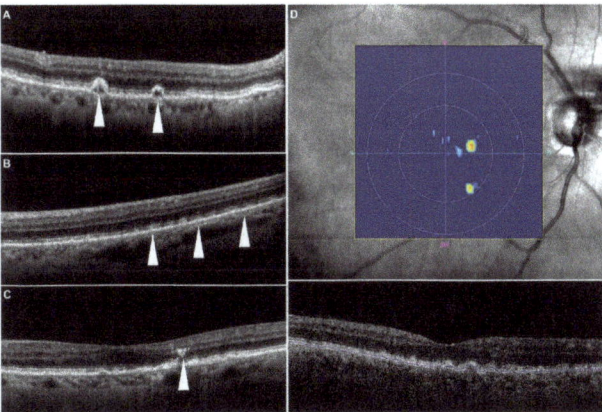

Figure 1. Representative examples of structural optical coherence tomography risk factors. (**A**) Drusenoid lesions with a hyporeflective core (white arrowheads)—note there is no evidence of any shadow artifact to explain the hyporeflectivity; (**B**) subretinal drusenoid deposits (white arrowheads); (**C**) intraretinal hyperreflective focus (white arrowhead)—here seen above the apex of the drusen; (**D**) drusen volume map from the Cirrus Advanced RPE analysis software—the algorithm segments the RPE band following the RPE contour and also estimates the original RPE position (termed the RPE fit) in the absence of an RPE elevation. The region between the RPE band and the RPE fit is then quantified as the drusen volume.

A cRORA lesion was identified according to the CAM criteria as containing a region of hypertransmission of at least 250 μm in diameter, a zone of attenuation or disruption of the RPE of at least 250 μm in diameter, evidence of overlying photoreceptor degeneration, and the absence of scrolled RPE or other signs of an RPE tear [6].

Drusen volume and drusen area were analyzed using the manufacturer's FDA-cleared Cirrus Advanced RPE Analysis software (version 6.0) as previously described [14]. The accuracy and reproducibility of automated drusen segmentation in eyes with non-neovascular age-related macular degeneration has been reported in previous publications [15].

IHRF were identified as well-circumscribed hyperreflective lesions within the neurosensory retina, with a minimum size of 3 pixels and a reflectivity equal to or more than that of the RPE band [16]. hDC lesions were identified based on the presence of hyporeflective spaces within drusen with a minimum height of at least 40 μm as previously reported [17]. SDD were identified as medium-reflective to hyperreflective mounds or cones, either at the level of the ellipsoid zone or between the ellipsoid zone and the RPE surface [9]. Subfoveal choroidal thickness was measured using the caliper tool on the central B-scan in the Spectralis device. Calipers were set at the Bruch's membrane line and the inner surface of the sclera to obtain thickness measurements.

2.3. Statistical Analysis

The primary objective of the study was to evaluate structural OCT biomarkers for their ability to predict progression from intermediate AMD to late AMD, defined as the appearance of cRORA (based on Beckman AMD classification scale, Figure 2). Data analyses were conducted with IBM SPSS (version 26.0; IBM Corporation, Armonk, NY, USA). The normality of sample distribution was evaluated by Kolmogorov–Smirnov and Shapiro–Wilk tests. The χ^2 test and Student's t-test for independent samples were used to evaluate differences in proportions and means among categorical and continuous variables, respectively. Logistic regression (univariate followed by multivariate) was also performed, using baseline drusen area in the 3 mm and 5 mm circles, drusen volume ≥ 0.03 mm^3 in the 3 mm and 5 mm rings, drusenoid PED, SDD, subfoveal choroidal thickness, IHRF, and hDC as independent variables and the progression to cRORA as the dependent variable. Intraclass correlation coefficient (ICCs) and Cohen's kappa (κ) were computed to measure the intergrader repeatability for quantitative and qualitative assessments. A p value < 0.05 was considered to be statistically significant.

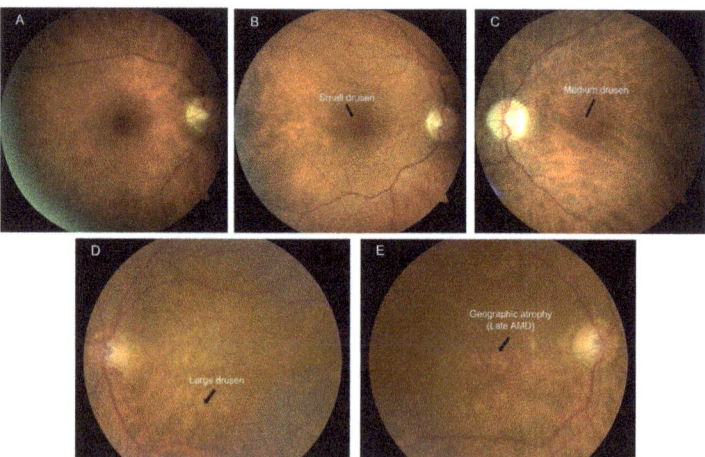

Figure 2. Illustration of the Beckman's clinical classification of AMD based on color fundus photos. (**A**) No apparent aging changes; (**B**) Normal aging changes; (**C**) Early AMD; (**D**) Intermediate AMD; (**E**) Late AMD evidenced by geographic atrophy.

3. Results

A total of 1332 eyes of 666 consecutive subjects with a two-year follow-up were included in this analysis. Of these 1332 eyes, twenty-one eyes (1.58%) progressed to late AMD at 2 years.

The mean age of the cohort in this analysis was 65.43 ± 10.17 years and 410 were females (61.56%). Patients who progressed to cRORA within 2 years were older (76.30 ± 6.01 years compared to 65.19 ± 10.14 years for those who did not progress; $p < 0.001$) and more likely to be male (52.9% male among those progressing to cRORA vs. 38.1% among those who did not progress; $p < 0.001$).

The univariate logistic regression comparing eyes which progressed to cRORA and those which did not progress demonstrated that drusen area in the 3 mm and 5 mm ring, drusen volume ≥ 0.03 mm^3 in the 3 mm and 5 mm ring, subfoveal choroidal thickness, SDD, IHRF, and hDC were all associated with an increased probability of cRORA development (OR = 2.31, 95% CI 1.65–3.23, $p < 0.001$), (OR = 1.65 95% CI 1.33–2.05, $p < 0.001$), (OR = 153.12, 95% CI 8.98–2610; $p = 0.001$), (OR = 78.03, 95% CI 7.49–813, $p < 0.001$) (OR = 1.01, 95% CI 1.00–1.01, $p = 0.002$), (OR = 8.65, 95% CI 3.49–21.46, $p < 0.001$) (OR = 40.23, 95% CI 14.41–112.37, $p < 0.001$), (OR = 4.1, 95% CI 2.77–6.07, $p < 0.001$) (Table 1 and Figure 3). The multivariate regression model confirmed the association between drusen volume ≥ 0.03 mm^3 in the 3 mm ring and IHRF (Table 1).

Table 1. Regression Analysis to Study the Effect of Various Biomarkers on GA incidence.

	Univariate Analysis			Multivariate Analysis		
	Odds Ratio	95% CI	p	Odds Ratio	95% CI	p
Drusen volume ≥ 0.03 mm^3 in the center 3 mm ring *						
No	1			1		
Yes	10.53	4.09–27.09	<0.001	3.47	0.42–28.34	0.25
Intraretinal hyperreflective foci (IHRF) *						
No	1			1		
Yes	40.23	14.41–112.37	<0.001	57.06	10.02–324.87	<0.001
Hyporeflective drusen core (hDC) *						
No	1			1		
Yes	6.32	2.53–15.77	<0.001	1.94	0.53–7.03	0.32
Presence of subretinal drusenoid deposits (SDD)/Reticular Pseudodrusen (RPD) *						
No	1			1		
Yes	8.65	3.49–21.46	<0.001	0.66	0.17–2.67	0.56
Drusenoid PED *						
No	1			1		
Yes	11.42	4.55–28.69	<0.001	1.17	0.23–5.91	0.85
Drusen Area in 3 mm ring #	2.31	1.65–3.23	<0.001	0.03	0.001–1.12	0.06
Drusen Area in 5 mm ring #	1.65	1.33–2.05	<0.001	24.06	0.89–652.73	0.06
Drusen Volume in 3 mm ring #	153.12	8.98–2610	0.001	2.59	1.46–6.54	**0.049**
Drusen Volume in 5 mm ring #	78.03	7.49–813	<0.001	1.49	5.76–38.71	0.06
Subfoveal choroidal thickness (microns) #	0.99	0.985–0.997	**0.002**	1	0.99–1.01	0.65

* Qualitative and categorical parameters; # Quantitative and continuous parameters; PED—Pigment epithelium detachment.

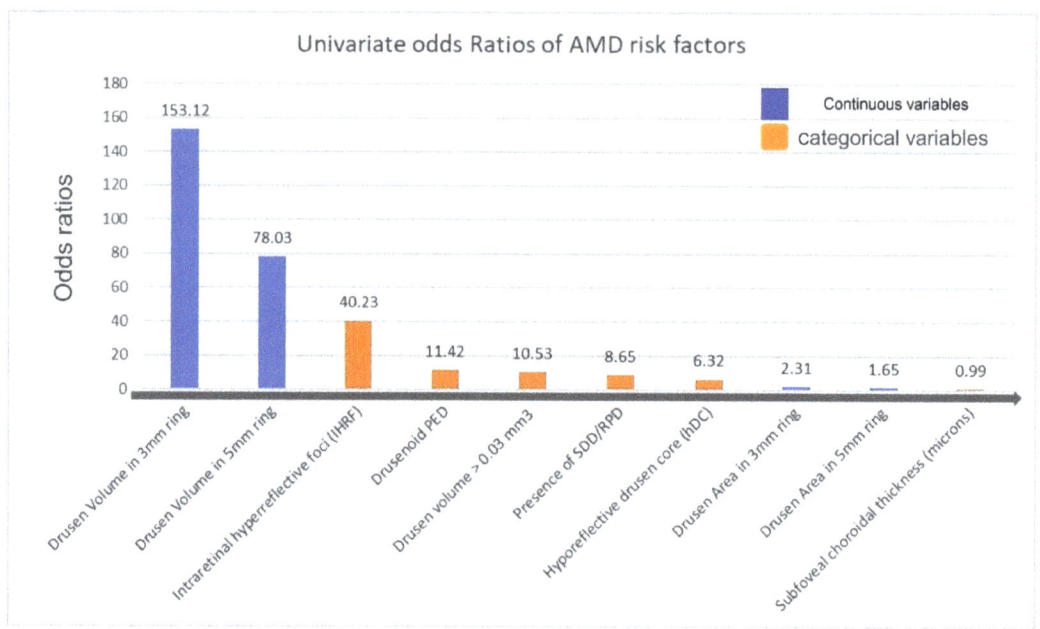

Figure 3. Bar plot showing the odds ratios from the univariate regression analysis (gray arrow indicates the direction of higher to lower risk for late AMD development).

Following a multivariate regression analysis performed by removing collinear variables like drusen area and drusen volume in 5 mm circles, results showed IHRF (OR: 37.66, (95% CI 10.75–131.98, $p < 0.001$) is still an independent and significant risk factor for late AMD progression.

4. Discussion

In this study, we evaluated structural OCT biomarkers for their ability to predict progression from intermediate AMD to cRORA in the prospective Amish eye study. The univariate analysis revealed that previously identified OCT risk factors appeared to predict progression to late AMD in this cohort. Importantly, IHRF and drusen volume in the 3 mm circle remained independent predictors of progression even when other structural OCT biomarkers were considered.

A few studies have evaluated the relationship between specific AMD biomarkers and AMD progression. Recently, Lei et al., proposed an OCT-based scoring system for the progression of AMD which included the presence of IHRF, SDD, hDC, and drusen volume within a central 3 mm circle ≥ 0.03 mm^3 [12].

Consistently, across multiple studies, IHRF have been identified as one of the strongest risk factors for atrophy and late AMD [7,16,18–20]. Histopathologic, laboratory, and OCT studies have suggested that IHRF represent the migration of activated RPE cells into the inner retinal layers which may be the result of an inflammatory response due to the oxidative damage and complement-activation processes in the pathophysiology of AMD [16]. Christenbury and colleagues observed that an increasing number of IHRF was associated with a greater incidence of geographic atrophy at 2 years [19]. Nassisi et al., observed a correlation between the quantity of IHRF in the eyes with intermediate AMD and the 1-year risk of progression to late AMD [21]. Recently, the presence of IHRF was also highlighted as an important risk factor by Schmidt-Erfurth et al., using an artificial intelligence model [18]. In our study, IHRF was confirmed to be a strong and independent predictor of late AMD.

Drusen volume ≥ 0.03 mm^3 within the central 3 mm of the macula has also been noted be an important risk factor for progression. Abdelfattah and colleagues were able to demonstrate that a drusen volume ≥ 0.03 mm^3 was associated with a higher risk of progression to late-stage AMD, and in particular to GA [10]. In this study, we confirmed the importance of drusen volume as both a categorical and a quantitative and continuous parameter.

Numerous studies have identified hDC as risk factors for progression to atrophy in several studies [7,12,18,20]. In particular, it was hypothesized that increasing heterogeneity within the drusen (which initially have a homogenous medium-reflective appearance) may reflect progressive impairment of RPE function and impending collapse of the drusen leading to atrophy. Recently, Tan and colleagues were able to show that these hyporeflective cores corresponded histologically to multi-lobular calcific hydroxyapatite nodules that seemed to gradually lead to the complete loss of overlying RPE [22].

SDD are considered another important risk factor in the progression of AMD [9]. In particular, the presence of SDD strongly correlate with the progression from intermediate AMD to late AMD. Marsiglia and colleagues evaluated GA progression in eyes with dry AMD, finding a high correlation between the presence of SDD and the presence and expansion of GA [23]. It has been observed that SDD eyes are generally characterized by a progressive reduction in choroidal and choriocapillaris blood flow during the progression of AMD [24,25]. Interestingly, in this study, SDD and a thin choroid were found to be associated with development of late AMD. In fact, eyes with GA and SDD generally manifest a thinner choroid compared to normal eyes of similar age [26].

Our univariate analysis confirmed that hDC and SDD were significant risk factors for progression from iAMD to cRORA. However, they did not remain significant in the multivariate model when including an IHRF and a high central drusen volume. It is possible that with a longer time frame and larger sample they may have remained significant.

Our study is not without limitations which must be considered when assessing our findings. First, the follow-up evaluation occurred at 2 years which may be a short time in the context of AMD. As a result, there were relatively few progression events in this cohort. Other risk factors may have been identified with a longer follow-up. Second, we used only structural OCT to identify both risk factors and progression to the late AMD end point. Other imaging modalities such as fundus autofluorescence, fluorescein angiography, and OCT angiography were not included in this analysis. On the other hand, structural OCT is widely available, and OCT-based biomarkers may be of the greatest clinical value. Despite these limitations, our study does have several strengths including the use of two masked, independent, experienced reading-center graders for each image and the use of standardized protocols and data collection in the context of a large prospective observational study.

In summary, we observed that the presence of IHRF and a high drusen volume in the central 3 mm ring were independently and significantly associated with development of late AMD. Other previously described AMD biomarkers such as hyporeflective drusen cores and subretinal drusenoid deposits did not remain as independent predictors in the multivariable model, highlighting their collinearity with other factors. This population-based study confirms the findings from previous clinic-based studies regarding the importance of IHRF and high central drusen volume as risk factors for progression to late AMD. These findings may of value in risk-stratifying patients in clinical practice, establishing follow-up intervals for re-assessment, and for identifying subjects for early-intervention clinical trials.

Author Contributions: Data curation, M.G.N., J.M. and S.B.V.; Formal analysis, M.G.N., J.M. and S.B.V.; Funding acquisition, J.H., M.A.P.-V., D.S. and S.R.S.; Resources, M.G.N., M.A.P.-V. and D.S.; Writing—original draft, M.G.N. and F.C.; Writing—review & editing, S.R.S. All authors have read and agreed to the published version of the manuscript.

Funding: Supported by the National Eye Institute, Bethesda, Maryland (grant #RO1 EY023164), the Department of Ophthalmology at the Perelman School of Medicine, Univ. of Pennsylvania, Philadelphia, Pennsylvania, John P. Hussman Institute of Human Genomics at the University of Miami Miller School of Medicine, Miami, Florida and the Institute for Computational Biology, Case Western Reserve University, Cleveland, Ohio. Funds also were received from the F.M. Kirby Foundation and Research to Prevent Blindness.

Institutional Review Board Statement: The study is approved by IRB protocol number 14-001476.

Informed Consent Statement: Informed consent was obtained from all subjects involved in the study.

Data Availability Statement: Not applicable.

Conflicts of Interest: M.G. Nittala, F. Corvi, J. Maram, S.B. Velaga, J.L. Haines, M.A. Pericak-Vance, D. Stambolian declare no conflicts of interest. S.R. Sadda reports consulting fees from Amgen, Allergan, Regeneron, Roche/Genentech, Novartis, Merck, 4DMT, Optos, Heidelberg, and Centervue. He also receives research instruments from Topcon, Nidek, Heidelberg, Centervue, Optos, and Carl Zeiss Meditec, outside the submitted work.

Abbreviations

AMD	Age-related Macular Degeneration
iAMD	intermediate age-related Macular Degeneration
cRORA	Complete Retinal Pigment Epithelial and Outer Retina Atrophy
iRORA	Incomplete Retinal Pigment Epithelial and Outer Retina Atrophy
OCT	Optical Coherence Tomography
IHRF	Intraretinal Hyperreflective Foci
SDD	Subretinal Drusenoid Deposits
hDC	Hyporeflective drusen cores
RPE	Retinal Pigment Epithelium
MNV	Macular Neovascularization
GA	Geographic Atrophy
OR	odds ratio

References

1. Wong, W.L.; Su, X.; Li, X.; Cheung, C.M.G.; Klein, R.; Cheng, C.-Y.; Wong, T.Y. Global Prevalence of Age-Related Macular Degeneration and Disease Burden Projection for 2020 and 2040: A Systematic Review and Meta-Analysis. *Lancet Glob. Health* **2014**, *2*, e106–e116. [CrossRef]
2. Age-Related Eye Disease Study Research Group. Risk Factors Associated with Age-Related Macular Degeneration: A Case-Control Study in the Age-Related Eye Disease Study: Age-Related Eye Disease Study Report Number 3. *Ophthalmology* **2000**, *107*, 2224–2232. [CrossRef]
3. Naj, A.C.; Scott, W.K.; Courtenay, M.D.; Cade, W.H.; Schwartz, S.G.; Kovach, J.L.; Agarwal, A.; Wang, G.; Haines, J.L.; Pericak-Vance, M.A. Genetic Factors in Nonsmokers with Age-Related Macular Degeneration Revealed through Genome-Wide Gene-Environment Interaction Analysis. *Ann. Hum. Genet.* **2013**, *77*, 215–231. [CrossRef]
4. Tikellis, G.; Robman, L.D.; Dimitrov, P.; Nicolas, C.; McCarty, C.A.; Guymer, R.H. Characteristics of Progression of Early Age-Related Macular Degeneration: The Cardiovascular Health and Age-Related Maculopathy Study. *Eye* **2007**, *21*, 169–176. [CrossRef]
5. Holz, F.G.; Sadda, S.R.; Busbee, B.; Chew, E.Y.; Mitchell, P.; Tufail, A.; Brittain, C.; Ferrara, D.; Gray, S.; Honigberg, L.; et al. Efficacy and Safety of Lampalizumab for Geographic Atrophy Due to Age-Related Macular Degeneration: Chroma and Spectri Phase 3 Randomized Clinical Trials. *JAMA Ophthalmol.* **2018**, *136*, 666–677. [CrossRef]
6. Sadda, S.R.; Guymer, R.; Holz, F.G.; Schmitz-Valckenberg, S.; Curcio, C.A.; Bird, A.C.; Blodi, B.A.; Bottoni, F.; Chakravarthy, U.; Chew, E.Y.; et al. Consensus Definition for Atrophy Associated with Age-Related Macular Degeneration on OCT: Classification of Atrophy Report 3. *Ophthalmology* **2018**, *125*, 537–548. [CrossRef]
7. Ouyang, Y.; Heussen, F.M.; Hariri, A.; Keane, P.A.; Sadda, S.R. Optical Coherence Tomography-Based Observation of the Natural History of Drusenoid Lesion in Eyes with Dry Age-Related Macular Degeneration. *Ophthalmology* **2013**, *120*, 2656–2665. [CrossRef]
8. Finger, R.P.; Chong, E.; McGuinness, M.B.; Robman, L.D.; Aung, K.Z.; Giles, G.; Baird, P.N.; Guymer, R.H. Reticular Pseudodrusen and Their Association with Age-Related Macular Degeneration: The Melbourne Collaborative Cohort Study. *Ophthalmology* **2016**, *123*, 599–608. [CrossRef]
9. Spaide, R.F.; Ooto, S.; Curcio, C.A. Subretinal Drusenoid Deposits AKA Pseudodrusen. *Surv. Ophthalmol.* **2018**, *63*, 782–815. [CrossRef]

10. Abdelfattah, N.S.; Zhang, H.; Boyer, D.S.; Rosenfeld, P.J.; Feuer, W.J.; Gregori, G.; Sadda, S.R. Drusen Volume as a Predictor of Disease Progression in Patients With Late Age-Related Macular Degeneration in the Fellow Eye. *Investig. Ophthalmol. Vis. Sci.* **2016**, *57*, 1839–1846. [CrossRef]
11. Nassisi, M.; Lei, J.; Abdelfattah, N.S.; Karamat, A.; Balasubramanian, S.; Fan, W.; Uji, A.; Marion, K.M.; Baker, K.; Huang, X.; et al. OCT Risk Factors for Development of Late Age-Related Macular Degeneration in the Fellow Eyes of Patients Enrolled in the HARBOR Study. *Ophthalmology* **2019**, *126*, 1667–1674. [CrossRef] [PubMed]
12. Lei, J.; Balasubramanian, S.; Abdelfattah, N.S.; Nittala, M.G.; Sadda, S.R. Proposal of a Simple Optical Coherence Tomography-Based Scoring System for Progression of Age-Related Macular Degeneration. *Graefe's Arch. Clin. Exp. Ophthalmol.* **2017**, *255*, 1551–1558. [CrossRef] [PubMed]
13. Nittala, M.G.; Song, Y.E.; Sardell, R.; Adams, L.D.; Pan, S.; Velaga, S.B.; Horst, V.; Dana, D.; Caywood, L.; Laux, R.; et al. AMISH EYE STUDY: Baseline Spectral Domain Optical Coherence Tomography Characteristics of Age-Related Macular Degeneration. *Retina* **2019**, *39*, 1540–1550. [CrossRef]
14. Gregori, G.; Wang, F.; Rosenfeld, P.J.; Yehoshua, Z.; Gregori, N.Z.; Lujan, B.J.; Puliafito, C.A.; Feuer, W.J. Spectral Domain Optical Coherence Tomography Imaging of Drusen in Nonexudative Age-Related Macular Degeneration. *Ophthalmology* **2011**, *118*, 1373–1379. [CrossRef]
15. Nittala, M.G.; Ruiz-Garcia, H.; Sadda, S.R. Accuracy and Reproducibility of Automated Drusen Segmentation in Eyes with Non-Neovascular Age-Related Macular Degeneration. *Investig. Ophthalmol. Vis. Sci.* **2012**, *53*, 8319–8324. [CrossRef]
16. Ho, J.; Witkin, A.J.; Liu, J.; Chen, Y.; Fujimoto, J.G.; Schuman, J.S.; Duker, J.S. Documentation of Intraretinal Retinal Pigment Epithelium Migration via High-Speed Ultrahigh-Resolution Optical Coherence Tomography. *Ophthalmology* **2011**, *118*, 687–693. [CrossRef]
17. Lee, S.Y.; Stetson, P.F.; Ruiz-Garcia, H.; Heussen, F.M.; Sadda, S.R. Automated Characterization of Pigment Epithelial Detachment by Optical Coherence Tomography. *Investig. Ophthalmol. Vis. Sci.* **2012**, *53*, 164–170. [CrossRef]
18. Schmidt-Erfurth, U.; Waldstein, S.M.; Klimscha, S.; Sadeghipour, A.; Hu, X.; Gerendas, B.S.; Osborne, A.; Bogunovic, H. Prediction of Individual Disease Conversion in Early AMD Using Artificial Intelligence. *Investig. Ophthalmol. Vis. Sci.* **2018**, *59*, 3199–3208. [CrossRef]
19. Christenbury, J.G.; Folgar, F.A.; O'Connell, R.V.; Chiu, S.J.; Farsiu, S.; Toth, C.A. Progression of Intermediate Age-Related Macular Degeneration with Proliferation and Inner Retinal Migration of Hyperreflective Foci. *Ophthalmology* **2013**, *120*, 1038–1045. [CrossRef]
20. Corvi, F.; Tiosano, L.; Corradetti, G.; Nittala, M.G.; Lindenberg, S.; Alagorie, A.R.; McLaughlin, J.A.; Lee, T.K.; Sadda, S.R. Choriocapillaris Flow Deficit as a Risk Factor for Progression of Age-Related Macular Degeneration. *Retina* **2021**, *41*, 686–693. [CrossRef]
21. Nassisi, M.; Fan, W.; Shi, Y.; Lei, J.; Borrelli, E.; Ip, M.; Sadda, S.R. Quantity of Intraretinal Hyperreflective Foci in Patients With Intermediate Age-Related Macular Degeneration Correlates With 1-Year Progression. *Investig. Ophthalmol. Vis. Sci.* **2018**, *59*, 3431–3439. [CrossRef] [PubMed]
22. Tan, A.C.S.; Pilgrim, M.G.; Fearn, S.; Bertazzo, S.; Tsolaki, E.; Morrell, A.P.; Li, M.; Messinger, J.D.; Dolz-Marco, R.; Lei, J.; et al. Calcified Nodules in Retinal Drusen Are Associated with Disease Progression in Age-Related Macular Degeneration. *Sci. Transl. Med.* **2018**, *10*, eaat4544. [CrossRef]
23. Marsiglia, M.; Boddu, S.; Bearelly, S.; Xu, L.; Breaux, B.E.; Freund, K.B.; Yannuzzi, L.A.; Smith, R.T. Association between Geographic Atrophy Progression and Reticular Pseudodrusen in Eyes with Dry Age-Related Macular Degeneration. *Investig. Ophthalmol. Vis. Sci.* **2013**, *54*, 7362–7369. [CrossRef]
24. Querques, G.; Querques, L.; Forte, R.; Massamba, N.; Coscas, F.; Souied, E.H. Choroidal Changes Associated with Reticular Pseudodrusen. *Investig. Ophthalmol. Vis. Sci.* **2012**, *53*, 1258–1263. [CrossRef]
25. Corvi, F.; Souied, E.H.; Capuano, V.; Costanzo, E.; Benatti, L.; Querques, L.; Bandello, F.; Querques, G. Choroidal Structure in Eyes with Drusen and Reticular Pseudodrusen Determined by Binarisation of Optical Coherence Tomographic Images. *Br. J. Ophthalmol.* **2017**, *101*, 348–352. [CrossRef]
26. Lindner, M.; Bezatis, A.; Czauderna, J.; Becker, E.; Brinkmann, C.K.; Schmitz-Valckenberg, S.; Fimmers, R.; Holz, F.G.; Fleckenstein, M. Choroidal Thickness in Geographic Atrophy Secondary to Age-Related Macular Degeneration. *Investig. Ophthalmol. Vis. Sci.* **2015**, *56*, 875–882. [CrossRef]

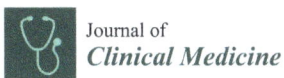

Article

Optical Coherence Tomography as a Biomarker for Differential Diagnostics in Nystagmus: Ganglion Cell Layer Thickness Ratio

Khaldoon O. Al-Nosairy [1], Elisabeth V. Quanz [1], Julia Biermann [2,†] and Michael B. Hoffmann [1,3,*,†]

1. Department of Ophthalmology, Faculty of Medicine, Otto-von-Guericke University, 39120 Magdeburg, Germany
2. Department of Ophthalmology, University of Muenster Medical Centre, 48149 Muenster, Germany
3. Center for Behavioral Brain Sciences, 39118 Magdeburg, Germany
* Correspondence: michael.hoffmann@med.ovgu.de
† These authors contributed equally to this work.

Abstract: In albinism, with the use of optical coherence tomography (OCT), a thinning of the macular ganglion cell layer was recently reported. As a consequence, the relevant OCT measure, i.e., a reduction of the temporal/nasal ganglion cell layer thickness quotient (GCLTQ), is a strong candidate for a novel biomarker of albinism. However, nystagmus is a common trait in albinism and is known as a potential confound of imaging techniques. Therefore, there is a need to determine the impact of nystagmus without albinism on the GCLTQ. In this bi-center study, the retinal GCLTQ was determined (OCT Spectralis, Heidelberg Engineering, Heidelberg, Germany) for healthy controls ($n = 5$, 10 eyes) vs. participants with nystagmus and albinism ($N_{albinism}$, $n = 8$, 15 eyes), and with nystagmus of other origins (N_{other}, $n = 11$, 17 eyes). Macular OCT with 25 horizontal B scans 20 × 20° with 9 automated real time tracking (ART) frames centered on the retina was obtained for each group. From the sectoral GCLTs of the early treatment diabetic retinopathy study (ETDRS) circular thickness maps, i.e., 3 mm and 6 mm ETDRS rings, GCLTQ I and GCLTQ II were determined. Both GCLTQs were reduced in $N_{albinism}$ (GCLTQ I and II: 0.78 and 0.77, $p < 0.001$) compared to N_{other} (0.91 and 0.93) and healthy controls (0.89 and 0.95). The discrimination of $N_{albinism}$ from N_{other} via GCLTQ I and II had an area under the curve of 80 and 82% with an optimal cutoff point of 0.86 and 0.88, respectively. In conclusion, lower GCLTQ in $N_{albinism}$ appears as a distinguished feature in albinism-related nystagmus as opposed to other causes of nystagmus.

Keywords: nystagmus; GCLT quotient; OCT; macular thickness asymmetry; misrouting; albinism; foveal hypoplasia; retina

1. Introduction

Optical coherence tomography (OCT) provides non-invasive surrogate structural biomarkers that aid diagnosis and/or further understanding of various ophthalmological diseases. Albinism, for example, demonstrates characteristic structural retinal abnormalities, i.e., foveal hypoplasia (FH), where OCT holds promising potentials as a defining biomarker [1].

Albinism, a rare inherited disorder, affects hair, skin, and eyes, i.e., oculocutaneous albinism, or eyes only, i.e., ocular albinism [2]. In fact, albinism demonstrates several ophthalmic characteristics including nystagmus, iris translucency, and optic nerve fibers' misrouting at the optic chiasm [3]. Further, albinism shows inter-subject variability in the typical ocular features and this variability can overlap with other diagnoses associated with the infantile nystagmus syndrome (INS) [3]. Actually, there is no single defining feature in albinism, as highlighted in a recent investigation of more than 500 participants with albinism [3], where no single diagnostic test had 100% penetrance. Even misrouting, determined by visual evoked potential (VEP), was not detected in 16% of the above

patient cohort [3]. In the present study, OCT was additionally employed to address this heterogeneity and the limited availability of molecular diagnosis in albinism.

The use of OCT has been suggested for the identification of FH in albinism [4–6]. However, this is not straightforward, as FH may be absent in albinism and present in other diseases than albinism [3] or may occur without any disease status [7]. In fact, more detailed quantitative OCT assessments might offer better insights into retinal characterizations in these disease entities. A stimulating macular OCT finding in this respect was the report of the thinning of the temporal ganglion cell layer thickness (GCLT), and hence a reduction of the temporal/nasal GCLT quotient (GCLTQ) in albinism-related FH compared to other causes of FH and to healthy controls [1]. In fact, this OCT approach of macular GCLT assessment might be of assistance to establish a novel diagnostic biomarker in albinism [1].

Importantly, nystagmus is a common trait of albinism. Nystagmus is known, however, to have the potential to interfere with imaging measures. It is therefore critical to assess whether the above GCLTQ reduction is exclusive to albinism-related nystagmus or whether it might be more generally associated with nystagmus, especially in the absence of FH. In this study, we therefore aimed to (i) investigate and compare GCLTQ in nystagmus participants driven by albinism vs. other etiologies and (ii) to estimate the area under the curve (AUC) of GCLTQ as a diagnostic biomarker in albinism vs. nystagmus of other origins. In the present study, we propose that the GCLTQ reduction, previously observed in albinism, is a novel OCT biomarker specific to albinism as opposed to other causes of nystagmus.

2. Materials and Methods

This bi-center study adhered to the tenets of the Declaration of Helsinki and the Ethical Committee of the Otto-von-Guericke University of Magdeburg and Muenster approved the study protocol. The consents of two participants from the Magdeburg cohort were utilized with the standard diagnostic procedure performed in the clinic.

2.1. Participants

In this bi-centric study, participants were recruited from the university eye hospitals in Magdeburg and Münster into three groups: (a) healthy controls (HC; $n = 5$; mean age (range) [y]: 37 (21–56)), i.e., logMAR ≤ 0 best corrected visual acuity; (b) participants with nystagmus and without misrouting of the optic nerves (N_{other}; $n = 11$; 7 acquired, 4 with infantile nystagmus syndrome (INS); (mean age range) [y]: 27 (8–56)); and (c) participants with nystagmus and misrouting of the optic nerves ($N_{albinism}$; $n = 8$; (mean age range) [y]: 19 (5–52)) diagnosed as albinism after Kruijt et al. [3], i.e., each of 3 major criteria: (I) FH $\geq$ grade 2, (II) negative VEP correlations, and (III) ocular hypopigmentation, i.e., iris translucency or fundus hypopigmentation, or 2 major and 2 minor criteria, i.e., minor criteria are: (i) nystagmus, (ii) FH grade 1, (iii) fundus hypopigmentation grade 1, and (iv) skin and hair hypopigmentation, i.e., lighter than that of their siblings and parents.

FH was classified after Thomas et al. [8] into grades: G1, absence of plexiform layers' extrusion; G2, G1 plus absence of the foveal pit; G3, G2 plus the absence of outer segment lengthening; and G4, G3 plus absence of outer nuclear layer lengthening.

Fundus hypopigmentation was graded after Schmitz et al. [9] as follows into grades: G1, peripheral retinal hypopigmentation; G2, distinct G1 plus central hypopigmentation; G3, strongly pronounced G2 (macular and foveal hypoplasia); and G4, G3 plus atypical choroideremia. The included participants of the present study are detailed in Table 1.

Table 1. Participants' grouping and key features.

Center-ID	Eye	Group	Nystagmus Type	BCVA OD/OS	Fundus Hypopigmentation OD/OS	Misrouting VEP	Foveal Hypoplasia OD/OS
MD-BWZ133	Both	HC	None	−0.1/−0.2	0/0	−	0/0
MD-KZJ780	Both	HC	None	−0.1/−0.1	0/0	−	0/0
MD-LHP483	Both	HC	None	0/0	0/0	−	0/0
MD-RKM968	Both	HC	None	−0.2/−0.2	0/0	−	0/0
MD-YHW227	Both	HC	None	−0.2/−0.2	0/0	−	0/0
MD-BJA815	OS	INS	J/H	0.2/0.2	0/0	−	n.a./0
MD-ENH995	Both	INS	J/H	0.6/0.49	0/0	−	0/0
MD-JDG458	Both	INS	P/H	0.3/0.3	0/0	−	0/0
MD-MFY773	OD	INS	J/H	0.1/0.3	0/0	−	0/n.a.
MD-PEP763	Both	INS	J/H	0/0.4	0/0	−	0/0
MD-SUQ660	Both	INS	J/H	−0.1/−0.1	0/0	−	0/0
MD-WQE170	OD	INS	P/H	0.2/0.2	0/0	−	1/n.a.
MS-MS01	OS	INS	J/H	0.1/0.3	0/0	n.a.	n.a./0
MS-MS02	OD	INS	J/H	0.4/0.4	0/0	n.a.	4/n.a.
MD-TGY248	Both	AN	J/V	0/0	0/0	−	0/0
MD-TIO945	Both	AN	J/H	0/−0.1	0/0	−	0/0
MD-HAA059	Both	Albinism *	n.a. ‡	0.6/0.7	3/3	+	3/4
MD-JTE807	Both	Albinism	J/H	0.4/0.8	0/0	+	4/4
MD-NLE254	Both	Albinism *	n.a. ‡	0.4/0.4	2/2	+	3/3
MD-PYV946	OS	Albinism	J/H	0.4/0.4	2/2	+	n.a./1
MD-TCU787	Both	Albinism *	n.a. ‡	0.8/0.6	2/2	+	3/3
MS-MS03	Both	Albinism	J/H	0.5/0.4	2/2	n.a.	3/3
MS-MS04	Both	Albinism	P/H	0.4/0.4	3/3	+	3/3
MS-MS05	Both	Albinism *	J/H	0.5/0.4	3/3	n.a.	3/4

MD/MS: Magdeburg/Muenster cohort; OD: right eye; OS: left eye; BCVA [logMAR]: best corrected visual acuity; VEP: misrouting visual evoked potential; "+"/"−" indicates presence/absence of optic nerve (negative/positive correlation coefficient between both eyes' inter-hemispherical activation difference); INS: idiopathic infantile syndrome (excluding albinism); HC: healthy control; AN: acquired nystagmus (causes: Arnold-Chiari syndrome, pons bleeding, hydrocephalus shunt operation); J/H: jerk horizontal nystagmus; P/H: pendular horizontal nystagmus; J/V: jerk vertical nystagmus; "n.a.": was not assessed; ‡ nystagmus diagnosis was made by qualified ophthalmologist. Albinism diagnosis: according to Kruijt et al.'s criteria [3], as detailed in Materials and Methods together with the grading schemes. * Indicates the presence of iris translucency.

Exclusion criteria were epilepsy, dizziness, diabetic retinopathy, and neurological diseases unrelated to nystagmus. There were no significant differences of the mean age between groups (healthy vs. N_{other} vs. $N_{albinism}$ group (mean age): 37 vs. 27 vs. 19; $p = 0.12$). The BCVA was significantly lowest in the latter group, i.e., 0.4 logMAR, while it was the highest for the healthy group, i.e., −0.15 logMAR; see Table 2.

Table 2. Studied groups' characteristics.

	HC	N_{other}	$N_{albinism}$	p	HC vs. N_{other}	HC vs. $N_{albinism}$	N_{other} vs. $N_{albinism}$
n (f)	5 (3)	11 (6)	8 (5)				
Age [y]	37 (21–56)	27 (8–56)	19 (5–52)	0.12			
Eyes (OD)	10 (5)	17 (9)	15 (7)	1.0§			
SE [Diopters] ‡	[−0.25 (−2−+3.4)]	[−1.0 (−7−+3.5)]	[1.5 (−4.4−+6.3)]	0.005 ‡	0.16	0.07	0.001
BCVA [LogMAR] ‡	[−0.15 (0−−0.20)]	[0.20 (+1−−0.1)]	[0.4 (+0.8−+0.4)]	<0.001 ‡	<0.001	<0.001	<0.001
(n of Eyes) Ophthalmological examination	10	17	15				
Strabismus	0	2	4	0.16 §			
Iris translucency	0	0	8	<0.001 §			

Table 2. Cont.

	HC	N$_{other}$	N$_{albinism}$	p	HC vs. N$_{other}$	HC vs. N$_{albinism}$	N$_{other}$ vs. N$_{albinism}$
Fundus hypopigmentation				<0.001 §			
0	10	17	2				
1	0	0	0				
2	0	0	7				
3	0	0	6				
OCT							
FH				<0.001 §			
0	10	15	0				
1	0	1	1				
2	0	0	0				
3	0	0	10				
4	0	1	4				
Retinal GCLT [µm]							
Nasal II	37 ± 3	37 ± 4	35 ± 5	0.31			
Nasal I ‡	[55 (52–58)]	[51 (46–60)]	[47 (17–56)]	<0.001 ‡	>0.05	<0.001	0.004
Central ‡	[19 (10–23)]	[16 (11–42)]	[37 (17–57)]	<0.001 ‡	>0.05	<0.001	<0.001
Temporal I	49 ± 2	48 ± 5	35 ± 10	<0.001	>0.05	<0.001	<0.001
Temporal II	35 ± 4	35 ± 3	27 ± 6	<0.001	>0.05	<0.001	<0.001
GCLTQ I [ratio]	0.89 ± 0.04	0.91 ± 0.07	0.78 ± 0.14	**0.001**	0.60	**0.025**	**0.002**
GCLTQ II [ratio]	0.95 ± 0.08	0.93 ± 0.09	0.77 ± 0.17	**<0.001**	0.99	**0.003**	**0.002**

n: number; f: female; OD: right eye; SE: spherical equivalent; GCLT: ganglion cell layer thickness; GCLTQ I and II: GCLT quotient of temporal and nasal quadrants within the 3 mm and 6 mm ETDRS rings. Comparisons: healthy (HC) vs. (i) nystagmus without albinism (N$_{other}$) and (ii) nystagmus with albinism (N$_{albinism}$) groups and (iii) N$_{other}$ vs. MSR N$_{albinism}$. ± standard deviation; § Fisher's exact test; ‡ nonparametric tests: Kruskal Wallis test and data in [median (range)]. Significant p values are given in bold.

2.2. Procedure and Measurements

All participants underwent complete ophthalmic examinations. Visual fields were tested where necessary utilizing a Humphrey Field Analyzer 3 (Carl Zeiss Meditec AG, Jena, Germany; Swedish Interactive Threshold Algorithm 24–2 protocol (SITA Faster)).

2.2.1. Visual Evoked Potentials

Three scalp electrodes (Oz, O1, O2) were placed and referenced to the Fz (according to the international 10–20 System) [10]. Following the International Society for Clinical Electrophysiology of Vision (ISCEV) standards for VEP recordings [11], the EP2000 evoked potential system was used for stimulation, recording, and analysis of pattern onset–offset VEP in all but four participants of the Magdeburg cohort [12] and in one participant of the Münster cohort. The stimuli were presented on a monochrome CRT monitor (MDG403, Philips; P45 phosphor; 75 Hz) in a dimly lit room. The stimulation and recording were set up according to the EP2000 testing paradigm which included a pattern onset epoch of 40 ms and 468 ms offset presenting 3 check sizes, i.e., 0.5°, 1°, and 2° with a spaced-averaged mean luminance of 50 cd/m^2 and contrast of 100% at a viewing distance of 114 cm. The VEP signals were connected to an amplifier (Grass Model 15, Astro-Med Inc., West Warwick, RI, USA), 100,000 times amplified, and band pass filtered (0.3, 70 Hz). VEP trials with a threshold of 90 µV were online rejected. Two VEP blocks were monocularly recorded and later averaged using IGOR (IGOR Pro, WaveMetrics, Portland, OR, USA). VEPs were digitally filtered (high-pass and low-pass cutoff: 0 and 40 Hz) and averaged using IGOR. To determine the presence of misrouting, the difference of the averaged VEP over the opposing hemisphere were calculated for each eye's recording. Subsequently, the correlation of the interhemispheric difference traces for the two eyes was determined via the correlation coefficient [13]. Albinotic misrouting of the optic nerves typically results in negative correlation coefficients in albinism between right and left eyes difference traces [12].

2.2.2. Optical Coherence Tomography (OCT)

The OCT for the macula was performed with 25 horizontal B scans 20° × 20° volume scans centered on the retina with 9 automated real time tracking (ART) frames with the Spectral domain OCT (OCT Spectralis, Heidelberg Engineering, Heidelberg, Germany). FH as well as GCLTQ were graded and calculated after Thomas et al. as detailed above [8]. Based on the macular scan, GCLT was computed using the inbuilt multilayer segmentation algorithm of the Heidelberg OCT device. GCLTs within the two nasal and two temporal quadrants of the ETDRS areas established by the Early Treatment Diabetic Retinopathy study were exported to calculate temporal/nasal GCLTQ [1]. GCLTQ I and II are the ratios within the 3 mm and 6 mm ETDRS rings, respectively.

2.3. Statistics

Further analysis for VEP and OCT was conducted using the programs IGOR and R [14]. The Shapiro–Wilk test was used to check the normality of the data and parametric or nonparametric tests were applied accordingly. p values were adjusted with the Sidak correction for multiple testing. The area under the curve (AUC) of the receiver operating characteristics was also calculated for GCLTQ I and II to differentiate between eyes with albinism and other eyes. Sample size was calculated based on Brücher et al. [1] where an area under the curve of 89% of ganglion cell thickness ratio II between the albinism and non-albinism groups with a power of 95% and p value < 0.05 mandated the inclusion of 10 eyes per group.

3. Results

3.1. Overview of Ophthalmological Characteristics

As expected, the presence of iris transillumination defects, fundus hypopigmentation, and FH were significantly prevalent in $N_{albinism}$ compared to the other two groups (Fisher's exact tests $p \leq 0.001$). $N_{albinism}$ displayed the only eyes with iris translucency ($n = 8/15$) and fundus hypopigmentation ($n = 13$) (Grade 3 ($n = 7$), Grade 4 ($n = 6$)). Further, FH was more likely associated with $N_{albinism}$ ($n = 15/15$) (Grade 1 ($n = 1$), Grade 3 ($n = 10$), Grade 4 ($n = 4$)) while only two eyes ($n = 2/17$) (Grade 1 ($n = 1$) and Grade 4 ($n = 1$) from two separate individuals) were affected in N_{other}.

3.2. OCT Analysis: GCLTQ

The GCLT was significantly different between the albinism and the reference groups for the N1, T1, central, and T2 quadrants; see Figure 1a. The central GCLT was, in accordance with the prevalence of FH, significantly thicker in the $N_{albinism}$ group than the other two groups ($p < 0.001$). In contrast, the paracentral GCTL was significantly reduced in $N_{albinism}$ for the quadrants N1, T1, and T2 compared to healthy and N_{other}. There is, in accordance with previous records [1,15], an asymmetry of the pericentral thinning of the GCLT in albinism, which is reflected by the GCLTQ as reported previously. The GCLTQ I was statistically lower ($p = 0.001$) in the $N_{albinism}$ group, i.e., a mean of 0.78, vs. healthy and N_{other}, i.e., 0.89 and 0.91, respectively. Likewise, GCLTQ II showed the same trend ($p < 0.001$), i.e., 0.77 vs. 0.95 and 0.93, respectively; see Figure 1b.

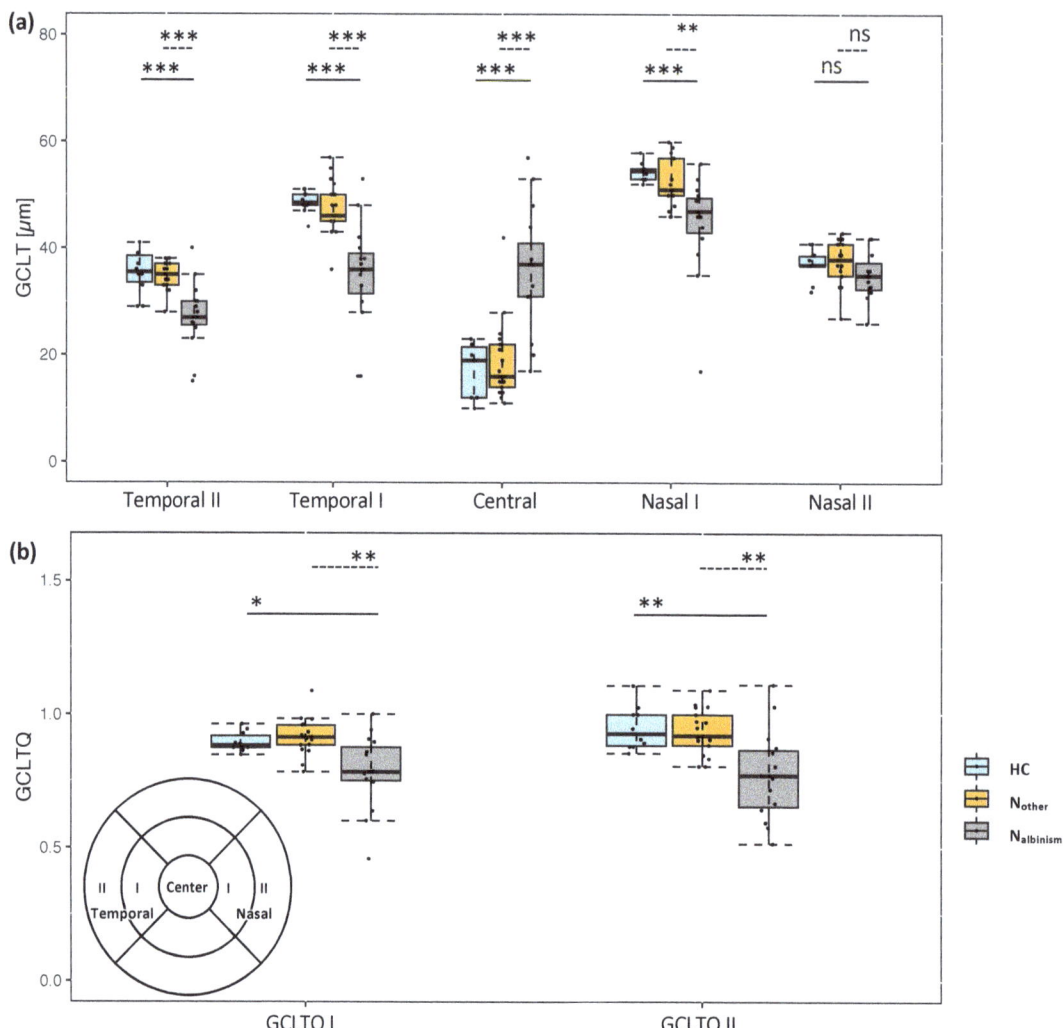

Figure 1. Paracentral ganglion cell layer thickness (GCLT) and quotient (GCLTQ) analysis. (**a**) Comparison of the GCLT in the 5 relevant sectors within the ETDRS macular OCT scan for healthy (HC) vs. albinism ($N_{albinism}$) and other causes of nystagmus (N_{other}). (**b**) Group comparisons of the GCLT quotients (GCLTQs) of temporal to nasal quadrants within the 3 mm macular ETDRS ring, i.e., GCLTQ I, and the outer 6 mm ring, i.e., GCLTQ II. Lower left panel is the ETDRS scan layout with areas of interest. p values were corrected after Sidak. * $p < 0.05$; ** $p < 0.01$; *** $p < 0.0001$. ns = non-significant p value.

3.3. GCLTQ Diagnostic Performance

In order to establish the sensitivity of this OCT metric to detect albinism-related macular changes from other groups, we determined the cut-off points for GCLT I and II ratios and their respective AUC. The calculated optimal cutoff points were 0.857 and 0.875, respectively. The GCLT I ratio had an AUC of 80% with a sensitivity and specificity of 73% and 89% at the determined cutoff point, respectively, and the GCLT II ratio showed a comparable performance, i.e., 82% AUC with 80% and 81% at the optimal cutoff point, respectively.

4. Discussion

We tested whether the OCT finding of decreased GCLTQ, which was previously reported for albinism, is independent of the presence of nystagmus, a condition that is common to albinism. Here, we confirmed previous findings of decreased GCLTQ in albinism and extended this finding by demonstrating normal GCLTQ for a critical control group, i.e., patients with nystagmus in the absence of albinism and (except for two of the patients) without FH. This strongly suggests that GCLTQ reduction is indeed specific to albinism and that it might be employed as a diagnostic metric in albinism independent from the presence of nystagmus.

Stimulated by a previous incidental finding in a Japanese family [16], Brücher et al. and Woertz et al. [1,15] reported a thinning of temporal paracentral GCLT in albinism with FH vs. other causes of FH. Brücher et al. [1] set a cut-off of the temporal/nasal GCLTQ to identify FH with albinism where GCLTQ II is more sensitive than GCLTQ I, 0.72 vs. 0.80, respectively. In the present study, we observed a similar trend, but with slightly higher optimal cut-off points, i.e., of 0.88 vs. 0.86 for GCLTQ II and I, respectively, in albinism with nystagmus vs. other groups. Further, Brücher et al. [1] reported somewhat higher AUCs (89% and 91%) than our present study (80% and 82%) for GCLTQ I and II, respectively. Both studies have in common that the sensitivity was highest for GCLTQ II than I (Brücher et al. [1]: 100% vs. 90%; present study: 80% vs. 73%). Taken together, the discrimination performance in the present study appears slightly inferior to the preceding study, which is likely associated with the different non-albinotic reference group in the present study, i.e., N_{other}.

Beyond its clinical relevance, the finding of temporal thinning of macular GCLT raises the question of the (i) underlying mechanisms and (ii) its relevance to the post-retinal visual pathway architecture in albinism [17–20]. (i) The origin of the GCLT thinning in albinism might be related to the severity of retinal changes in albinism, especially FH, a typical trait of albinism. For this purpose, future studies on datasets with greater sample sizes are needed to perform meaningful correlation analyses of the relationship of temporal GCLT thinning and the grade of FH. (ii) Normally the line of decussation, which separates the retinal ganglion cells that project to the opposite hemisphere from those that remain ipsilateral, coincides with the fovea. In albinism, the misrouting of the optic nerves at the optic chiasm leads to a shift of the line of decussation into the temporal retina [21], and thus substantially more axons cross the midline. The size of this lateral shift affects on average 8 degrees in the visual field, but has been reported to vary between 2 and 15 degrees of visual angle, underlining a large interindividual variability in albinism [13,21]. This variability is to some degree related to the severity of the pigmentation deficit of the affected individuals [22]. It is generally assumed and supported by experimental evidence [2] that the projection error of part of the temporal retinal ganglion cells is related to changes in the retinal physiology and development and its inter-individual variability. It is currently unclear whether there is a link between the GCLTQ reduction in albinism and the degree of optic nerve misrouting. This prompts the question of whether the severity of retinal changes, as reflected by the GCLTQ reduction in albinism, is related to changes in the post-retinal pathways, e.g., the degree of misrouting of the optic nerves. Uncovering these relations is likely to assist uncovering the nature and origin of the changes of the visual pathway architecture in albinism. Datasets with greater sample sizes are needed to perform the necessary correlation analyses. Therefore, the publication of datasets from these rare patients [23] is highly desirable, as these can be merged subsequently for the required analyses.

Although the present study is unique by its investigation of GCLTQ in groups with nystagmus with and without albinism, the following limitations deserve attention: (i) There was a comparatively small sample size; however, the rarity of patients with albinism or nystagmus made it difficult to include more. (ii) The long scanning time required to acquire meaningful OCT data led to the exclusion of a number of patients as they had fixation that was too unstable. As the technical evolution of retinal OCT is proceeding rapidly, faster scanning times and optimized eye tracking will hopefully lead to an extension of explorable patients in future.

In conclusion, the present study lends further support of selective thinning of the paracentral temporal retina specifically in albinism. While this might serve as a biomarker to aid in the identification of albinism, it might also help to uncover the impact of these retinal changes on the post-retinal visual pathways in albinism.

Author Contributions: M.B.H.: funding and supervision, study concept and design. K.O.A.-N.: investigation and data analysis, manuscript draft. E.V.Q.: investigation, data analysis. J.B.: funding, study concept and design, investigation. All authors: comments on results, comments and revision of the manuscript. All authors have read and agreed to the published version of the manuscript.

Funding: This work was supported by funding of the German Research Foundation (DFG, HO2002/10-3, Project number 149341228) to M.B.H. and of the Bielschowsky Society to J.B. and M.B.H.

Institutional Review Board Statement: The study was conducted according to the guidelines of the Declaration of Helsinki, and approved by Ethics Committee of Faculty of Medicine, Otto-von-Guericke University, Magdeburg (153/18) and Faculty of Medicine, Muenster (2019-002-f-S).

Informed Consent Statement: Informed consent was obtained from all subjects involved in the study.

Data Availability Statement: Data are available upon request.

Acknowledgments: Thanks are given to Francie H. Kramer and Juliane Reupsch for their assistance with the study. We thank the study participants and the German nystagmus network (Nystagmus Netzwerk e.V.) for their support.

Conflicts of Interest: The authors declare no conflict of interest.

References

1. Brücher, V.C.; Heiduschka, P.; Grenzebach, U.; Eter, N.; Biermann, J. Distribution of macular ganglion cell layer thickness in foveal hypoplasia: A new diagnostic criterion for ocular albinism. *PLoS ONE* **2019**, *14*, e0224410. [CrossRef] [PubMed]
2. Bakker, R.; Wagstaff, P.E.; Kruijt, C.C.; Emri, E.; van Karnebeek, C.D.M.; Hoffmann, M.B.; Brooks, B.P.; Boon, C.J.F.; Montoliu, L.; van Genderen, M.M.; et al. The retinal pigmentation pathway in human albinism: Not so black and white. *Prog. Retin. Eye Res.* **2022**, 101091, in press. [CrossRef] [PubMed]
3. Kruijt, C.C.; de Wit, G.C.; Bergen, A.A.; Florijn, R.J.; Schalij-Delfos, N.E.; van Genderen, M.M. The Phenotypic Spectrum of Albinism. *Ophthalmology* **2018**, *125*, 1953–1960. [CrossRef] [PubMed]
4. Cronin, T.H.; Hertle, R.W.; Ishikawa, H.; Schuman, J.S. Spectral domain optical coherence tomography for detection of foveal morphology in patients with nystagmus. *J. AAPOS* **2009**, *13*, 563–566. [CrossRef]
5. Kuht, H.J.; Maconachie, G.D.E.; Han, J.; Kessel, L.; van Genderen, M.M.; McLean, R.J.; Hisaund, M.; Tu, Z.; Hertle, R.W.; Gronskov, K.; et al. Genotypic and Phenotypic Spectrum of Foveal Hypoplasia: A Multicenter Study. *Ophthalmology* **2022**, *129*, 708–718. [CrossRef]
6. Kuht, H.J.; Thomas, M.G.; McLean, R.J.; Sheth, V.; Proudlock, F.A.; Gottlob, I. Abnormal foveal morphology in carriers of oculocutaneous albinism. *Br. J. Ophthalmol.* **2022**. [CrossRef]
7. Noval, S.; Freedman, S.F.; Asrani, S.; El-Dairi, M.A. Incidence of fovea plana in normal children. *J. Am. Assoc. Pediatric Ophthalmol. Strabismus* **2014**, *18*, 471–475. [CrossRef]
8. Thomas, M.G.; Kumar, A.; Mohammad, S.; Proudlock, F.A.; Engle, E.C.; Andrews, C.; Chan, W.-M.; Thomas, S.; Gottlob, I. Structural Grading of Foveal Hypoplasia Using Spectral-Domain Optical Coherence Tomography: A Predictor of Visual Acuity? *Ophthalmology* **2011**, *118*, 1653–1660. [CrossRef]
9. Schmitz, B.; Schaefer, T.; Krick, C.M.; Reith, W.; Backens, M.; Käsmann-Kellner, B. Configuration of the Optic Chiasm in Humans with Albinism as Revealed by Magnetic Resonance Imaging. *Investig. Ophthalmol. Vis. Sci.* **2003**, *44*, 16–21. [CrossRef]
10. American Electroencephalographic Society. Guideline thirteen: Guidelines for standard electrode position nomenclature. *J. Clin. Neurophysiol.* **1994**, *11*, 111–113. [CrossRef]
11. Odom, J.V.; Bach, M.; Brigell, M.; Holder, G.E.; McCulloch, D.L.; Mizota, A.; Tormene, A.P. ISCEV standard for clinical visual evoked potentials: (2016 update). *Doc. Ophthalmol.* **2016**, *133*, 1–9. [CrossRef]
12. Hoffmann, M.B.; Wolynski, B.; Bach, M.; Meltendorf, S.; Behrens-Baumann, W.; Golla, F. Optic Nerve Projections in Patients with Primary Ciliary Dyskinesia. *Investig. Ophthalmol. Vis. Sci.* **2011**, *52*, 4617–4625. [CrossRef]
13. Hoffmann, M.B.; Lorenz, B.; Morland, A.B.; Schmidtborn, L.C. Misrouting of the Optic Nerves in Albinism: Estimation of the Extent with Visual Evoked Potentials. *Investig. Ophthalmol. Vis. Sci.* **2005**, *46*, 3892–3898. [CrossRef]
14. R Core Team. *R: The R Project for Statistical Computing*; R Foundation for Statistical Computing: Vienna, Austria, 2013; Available online: https://www.r-project.org/ (accessed on 1 January 2020).

15. Woertz, E.N.; Omoba, B.S.; Dunn, T.M.; Chiu, S.J.; Farsiu, S.; Strul, S.; Summers, C.G.; Drack, A.V.; Carroll, J. Assessing Ganglion Cell Layer Topography in Human Albinism Using Optical Coherence Tomography. *Investig. Ophthalmol. Vis. Sci.* **2020**, *61*, 36. [CrossRef]
16. Oki, R.; Yamada, K.; Nakano, S.; Kimoto, K.; Yamamoto, K.; Kondo, H.; Kubota, T. A Japanese Family with Autosomal Dominant Oculocutaneous Albinism Type 4. *Investig. Ophthalmol. Vis. Sci.* **2017**, *58*, 1008–1016. [CrossRef]
17. Bridge, H.; von dem Hagen, E.A.H.; Davies, G.; Chambers, C.; Gouws, A.; Hoffmann, M.; Morland, A.B. Changes in brain morphology in albinism reflect reduced visual acuity. *Cortex* **2014**, *56*, 64–72. [CrossRef]
18. Hoffmann, M.B.; Dumoulin, S.O. Congenital visual pathway abnormalities: A window onto cortical stability and plasticity. *Trends Neurosci.* **2015**, *38*, 55–65. [CrossRef]
19. Puzniak, R.J.; Prabhakaran, G.T.; Hoffmann, M.B. Deep Learning-Based Detection of Malformed Optic Chiasms From MRI Images. *Front. Neurosci.* **2021**, *15*, 755785. [CrossRef]
20. Puzniak, R.J.; Ahmadi, K.; Kaufmann, J.; Gouws, A.; Morland, A.B.; Pestilli, F.; Hoffmann, M.B. Quantifying nerve decussation abnormalities in the optic chiasm. *NeuroImage Clin.* **2019**, *24*, 102055. [CrossRef]
21. Hoffmann, M.B.; Tolhurst, D.J.; Moore, A.T.; Morland, A.B. Organization of the Visual Cortex in Human Albinism. *J. Neurosci.* **2003**, *23*, 8921–8930. [CrossRef]
22. Von Dem Hagen, E.A.H.; Houston, G.C.; Hoffmann, M.B.; Morland, A.B. Pigmentation predicts the shift in the line of decussation in humans with albinism. *Eur. J. Neurosci.* **2007**, *25*, 503–511. [CrossRef]
23. Puzniak, R.J.; McPherson, B.; Ahmadi, K.; Herbik, A.; Kaufmann, J.; Liebe, T.; Gouws, A.; Morland, A.B.; Gottlob, I.; Hoffmann, M.B.; et al. CHIASM, the human brain albinism and achiasma MRI dataset. *Sci. Data* **2021**, *8*, 308. [CrossRef]

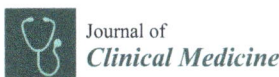

Article

Choroidal Vascularity Index in Central and Branch Retinal Vein Occlusion

Pasquale Loiudice [1,2,*], Giuseppe Covello [1], Michele Figus [1], Chiara Posarelli [1], Maria Sole Sartini [1] and Giamberto Casini [1]

1 Department of Surgical, Medical and Molecular Pathology and Critical Care Medicine, University of Pisa, 56124 Pisa, Italy
2 Complex Operative Ophthalmology Unit, "F. Lotti" Hospital, 56025 Pontedera, Italy
* Correspondence: pasquale.loiudice@phd.unipi.it

Abstract: (1) Background: we aimed to evaluate choroidal vascularity change in eyes with central and branch retinal vein occlusion (RVO). (2) Methods: in this retrospective cross-sectional study, we reviewed the records of 47 patients with recent-onset, naïve, unilateral retinal vein occlusion. Enhanced-depth imaging optical coherence tomography scans were binarized using the ImageJ software; luminal area (LA) and total choroidal area (TCA) were measured. The choroidal vascularity index (CVI) was calculated as the proportion of LA to TCA. Depending on the pattern of macular oedema, eyes were classified as having no macular oedema (nME), cystoid macular oedema (CME), cystoid macular oedema with serous retinal detachment (mixed). (3) Results: CVI, TCA and LA were greater in eyes with RVO than in fellow, unaffected eyes. No difference was found between central and branch RVO except for central macular thickness (CMT). When compared with controls, eyes with CME presented a significant increase in subfoveal choroidal thickness, CMT, TCA, LA and CVI; eyes with mixed macular oedema had greater CMT and CVI than contralateral eyes; no significant differences in any of the considered parameters were observed in eyes with nME. (4) Conclusions: The results suggest that RVO alters the vascularity of the choroid that varies according to the type of macular oedema.

Keywords: branch vein occlusion; central vein occlusion; choroid; choroidal vascularity index; image binarization; macular oedema; optical coherence tomography; retinal vein occlusion

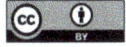

1. Introduction

Retinal vein occlusion (RVO) is an expression used to cover a spectrum of conditions characterized by impaired retinal venous flow. RVOs can be classified as central retinal vein occlusion (CRVO), hemi-retinal vein occlusion (HRVO) and branch retinal vein occlusion (BRVO), depending on the location of the obstruction. Taken together, they represent the second leading cause of blindness due to retinal vascular disorders after diabetic retinopathy [1]. Symptomatology can range from nearly asymptomatic to impaired light perception due to macular edema and ischemia, optic neuropathy, vitreous hemorrhage, neovascular glaucoma, proliferative retinopathy, tractional or combined tractional/rhegmatogenous retinal detachment [2,3].

Since the use of enhanced deep image optical coherence tomography (EDI-OCT) has allowed better visualization of the choroid [4], several authors have studied choroidal change in eyes with CRVO or BRVO leading to discordant results. On the one hand, an increase in subfoveal choroidal thickness was found (SFCT) in patients with RVO if compared with unaffected fellow eyes [5–7]; on the other hand, other authors did not find any significant difference in SFCT between eyes with RVO and contralateral ones [8,9].

Derived from the research of Sonoda and colleagues [10] and further developed by Agrawal and co-workers [11], the choroidal vascularity index (CVI) has been considered a promising tool to evaluate choroidal vascular change since it is not influenced by age, gender, refractive error, axial length or intraocular pressure. Defined as the proportion of luminal area (LA) to total choroidal area (TCA), it has been employed in several ocular diseases such as central serous chorioretinopathy, age-related macular degeneration, type-2 diabetes and Vogt–Koyanagi–Harada Disease [12–15].

The present study aimed to evaluate if, in eyes with recent-onset, naïve, unilateral retinal vein occlusion, (1) CRVO and BRVO induce modification in choroidal vascularity assessed by the CVI, (2) there is any difference in CVI between central and branch RVO, (3) there is a relationship between the type of macular edema and choroidal response to retinal vein occlusion.

2. Materials and Methods

This retrospective cross-sectional study was approved by the local Institutional Review Board (Comitato Etico Area Vasta Nord-Ovest, Prot. n. 17441) of Pisa University Hospital, Pisa, Italy. The study was conducted in adherence with the tenets of the current version of the Declaration of Helsinki (64th WMA General Assembly, Fortaleza, Brazil, October 2013). All patients signed an informed consent form.

We reviewed the medical records of patients with recent-onset, naïve, unilateral retinal vein occlusion who were referred to Pisa University Hospital between September 2020 and March 2021. All patients underwent fluorescein angiography and spectral-domain optical coherence tomography (SD-OCT) using the Heidelberg Spectralis (Heidelberg Retinal Angiography; Heidelberg Engineering, Heidelberg, Germany, Software version 6.9) platform. These exams were performed between five and fifteen days from the clinical diagnosis. Data regarding best-corrected visual acuity (BCVA), refraction, age, sex, medical history, and slit-lamp examination were also recorded. Visual acuity was converted in the logarithm of the minimal angle of resolution (logMAR) for statistical purposes. We excluded cases with spherical equivalent greater than ±6 diopters and cylinder greater than ±2 diopters, previous laser photocoagulation or anti-vascular endothelial growth factor therapy in any eye, history of trauma or intraocular surgery except for cataract extraction at least 180 days before enrollment, other retinal disorders that could interfere with the measurement including age-related macular degeneration, diabetic retinopathy, central serous chorioretinopathy, any history of uveitis.

OCT images were obtained with the enhanced deep image (EDI) protocol acquiring 20 equally spaced OCT B-scan sections in a 20° × 20° horizontal raster pattern. Choroidal thickness (CT) was measured in the subfoveal region using the built-in caliper of the software of the instrument at a single point below the fovea extending from the bottom of the hyperreflective layer corresponding to Bruch's membrane to the hyperreflective layer at the sclerochoroidal border. Central macular thickness (CMT) was recorded for all patients using the embedded tool.

We classified the images into 3 categories, depending on the pattern of macular edema: no macular edema (nME), cystoid macular edema (CME), cystoid macular edema with serous retinal detachment (mixed).

2.1. Image Binarization

The same full-length scan used for CT measurement was utilized for binarization employing the open-source software ImageJ (version 1.52; National Institutes of Health, USA, http://imagej.nih.gov/ij, accessed on 9 June 2022). The polygon tool was used to select the TCA. The selection was added to the region of interest (ROI) manager. The image was then downgraded to 8-bit and adjusted with Niblack auto local threshold. Color threshold was used to select the LA which was added to the ROI manager. CVI was calculated as the proportion of LA to TCA. Stromal area (SA) was calculated by subtracting LA from TCA (Figure 1).

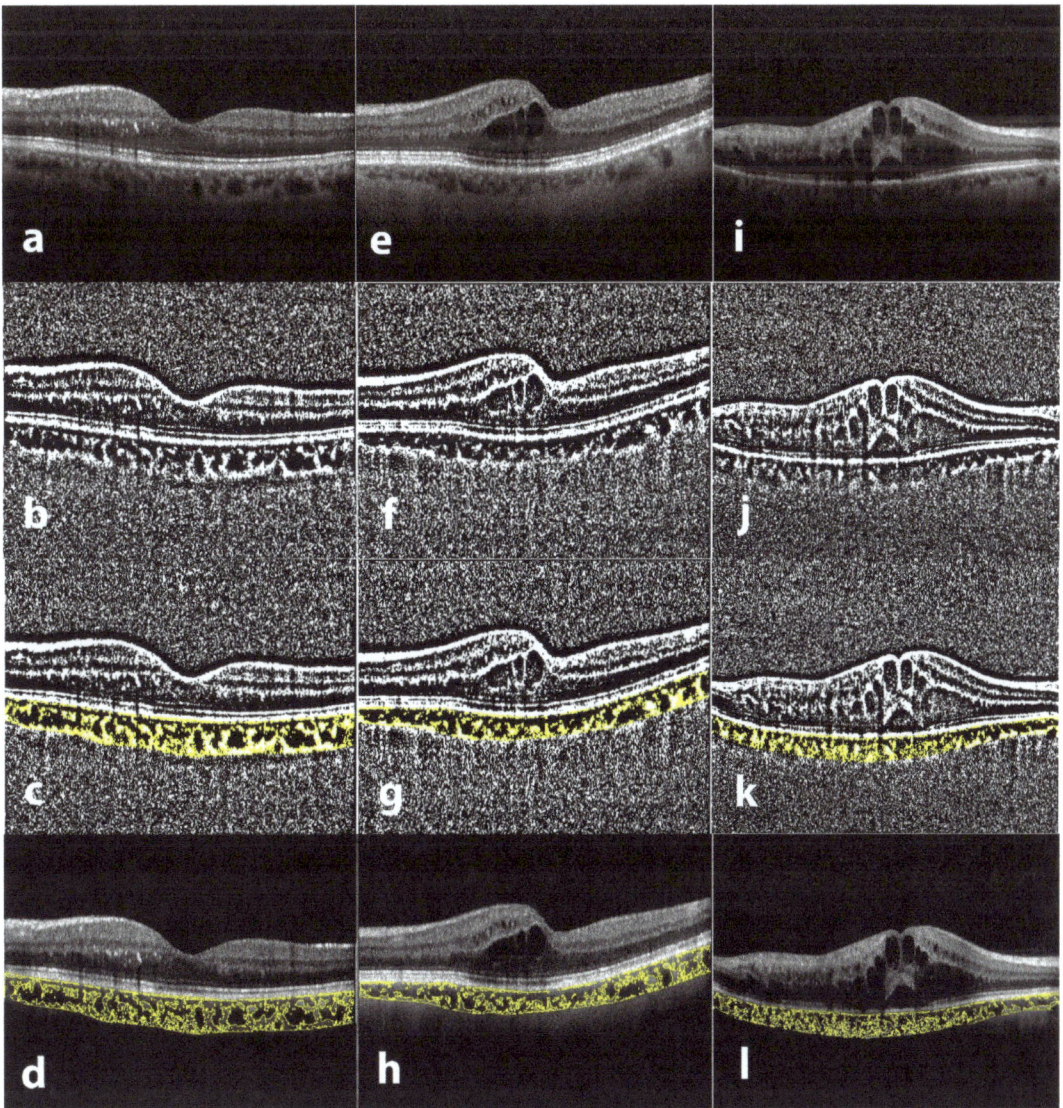

Figure 1. Binarization and identification of the luminal and stromal areas of the choroid. Spectral-domain optical coherence tomography (SD-OCT) acquired using enhanced deep image (EDI) mode. (**a,e,i**) Original subfoveal scan; (**b,f,j**) The image was downgraded to 8-bit and Niblack auto local threshold was applied; (**c,g,k**) Color threshold was used to select luminal area; (**d,h,l**) Overlay of region of interest on the original image. Depending on the pattern of macular edema, eyes were classified into 3 categories: no macular edema (**a**), cystoid macular edema (**e**), cystoid macular edema with serous retinal detachment (**i**).

2.2. Statistical Analysis

Statistical analysis was performed using the SPSS software version 20.0 for Windows (SPSS Inc., Chicago, IL, USA). The normality of distribution of data was assessed using Kolmogorov–Smirnov and Shapiro–Wilk tests. Differences in SFCT, CMT, TCA, SA, LA and CVI were assessed with a two-side independent sample t-test. Fisher's exact test was applied for categorical variables. Analysis of variance test and Pearson χ^2 test were used comparing demographics and clinical features between different types of macular edema. p values < 0.05 were considered statistically significant.

3. Results

Seventy-six consecutive patients affected by BRVO or CRVO were screened. Among these, 29 were excluded due to poor image quality, concomitant retinal diseases, or recent surgery; the remaining 47 subjects were included in the study. Patient demographics and clinical characteristics are displayed in Table 1.

Table 1. Patient demographics and clinical characteristics in subjects with recent-onset retinal vein occlusion.

	RVO	BRVO	CRVO	p Value
No. of eyes	47	36	11	
Gender (male/female)	26/21	20/16	6/5	0.610 [†]
Eye (right/left)	28/19	23/13	5/6	0.312 [†]
Age (years, mean ± SD)	72.40 ± 11.64	73.03 ± 14.45	64.57 ± 8.61	0.431 [*]
Systemic disease				
Hypertension	28	22	6	0.697 [†]
Diabetes mellitus	6	4	2	0.538 [†]
Glaucoma	9	7	2	0.925 [†]
Ischemic/non ischemic	21/26	14/22	7/4	0.181 [†]
Type of macular oedema				
nME	9	9	0	n/a
CME	23	18	5	0.791 [†]
Mixed	15	9	6	0.065 [†]
BCVA	0.623 ± 0.38	0.565 ± 0.39	0.811 ± 0.30	0.041 [*]

RVO = retinal vein occlusion; BRVO = branch retinal vein occlusion; CRVO = central retinal vein occlusion; nME = no macular oedema; CME = cystoid macular oedema; Mixed = cystoid macular oedema + serous retinal detachment; BCVA = best corrected visual acuity. [*] BRVO compared to CRVO, independent-sample t-test. [†] Fisher's exact test.

The eyes of subjects with BRVO or CRVO did not significantly differ regardless of gender and laterality distribution, mean age, concomitant systemic diseases, ischemic pattern, and type of macular edema. BCVA was significantly lower in patients with CRVO than in those with BRVO (0.811 ± 0.30 (20/126) and 0.565 ± 0.39 (20/73), respectively, p = 0.041, independent sample t-test). The type of macular edema was nME in 9 cases, CME in 23 cases and mixed in 15 cases (Table 2).

Table 2. Demographics and clinical features according to type of macular oedema in subjects with recent-onset central or branch retinal vein occlusion.

	Macular Oedema Group				
	nME Group (n = 9)	CME Group (n = 23)	Mixed Group (n = 15)	Control Group (n = 47)	p Value
Age (mean ± SD)	63.11 ± 14.61	74.74 ± 11.45	74.40 ± 6.96	72.40 ± 11.64	0.025 [*]
Gender(male/female)	5/4	14/9	7/8	26/21	0.690 [†]
Eye (right/left)	5/4	16/7	7/8	28/19	0.359 [†]
BCVA (logMAR)	0.2 ± 0.16	0.63 ± 0.32	0.87 ± 0.35	0.62 ± 0.38	0.142 [*]
Type (CRVO/BRVO)	0/9	3/20	8/7	11/36	0.003 [†]

BCVA = best-corrected visual acuity; nME = no macular oedema; CME = cystoid macular oedema; Mixed = cystoid macular oedema + serous retinal detachment; CRVO = central retinal vain occlusion; BRVO = branch retinal vein occlusion. [*] Analysis of variance test. [†] Pearson χ^2 test.

Mean age was significantly lower in eyes with nME (p = 0.025, analysis of variance test). No difference was observed between groups in gender, laterality distribution and BCVA.

Comparing eyes with RVO with their unaffected fellow eyes, we observed no significant difference in subfoveal choroidal thickness and SA. In contrast, eyes with RVO had greater values of CMT, TCA, LA and CVI (Table 3).

Table 3. Optical coherence tomography parameters in patients with recent-onset retinal vein occlusion.

Parameter	Study Eye	Fellow Eye	p *
Subfoveal choroidal thickness (μm)	200.87 ± 56.24	176.83 ± 44.89	0.24
Central macular thickness (μm)	505.49 ± 218.28	276.93 ± 28.45	**<0.001**
Total choroidal area (mm²)	0.44 ± 0.13	0.39 ± 0.11	**0.046**
Luminal area (mm²)	0.17 ± 0.05	0.13 ± 0.04	**0.002**
Stromal area (mm²)	0.27 ± 0.08	0.25 ± 0.07	0.218
Choroidal vascularity index (%)	38.46 ± 3.89	35.64 ± 3.24	**<0.001**

* Independent-sample t-test. Significant p values are in bold.

Table 4 displays OCT parameters according to the type of macular edema. When compared with controls, eyes with nME had no significant differences in SFCT, CMT, TCA, LA, SA and CVI. Eyes with CME presented a significant increase in SFCT, CMT, TCA, LA and CVI. Finally, eyes with mixed macular edema had greater CMT and CVI than contralateral eyes.

Table 4. Optical coherence tomography parameters according to type of macular oedema secondary to retinal vein occlusion.

Parameter/Group	nME	Control	p Value *	CME	Control	p Value †	Mixed	Control	p Value ‡
SFCT (μm)	216.22 ± 80.63	205.89 ± 44.19	0.740	208.91 ± 51.61	174.39 ± 43.94	**0.019**	179.33 ± 163.13	163.13 ± 41.45	0.295
CMT (μm)	332.44 ± 87.44	290.66 ± 38.09	0.207	464.82 ± 166.19	270.39 ± 24.98	**<0.001**	671.66 ± 239.22	278.73 ± 25.59	**<0.001**
TCA (mm²)	0.51 ± 0.17	0.47 ± 0.14	0.634	0.44 ± 0.13	0.37 ± 0.10	**0.039**	0.39 ± 0.92	0.37 ± 0.89	0.426
LA (mm²)	0.19 ± 0.06	0.16 ± 0.05	0.380	0.17 ± 0.05	0.13 ± 0.03	**0.006**	0.15 ± 0.04	0.13 ± 0.04	0.111
SA (mm²)	0.32 ± 0.11	0.30 ± 0.10	0.802	0.27 ± 0.08	0.23 ± 0.06	0.115	0.24 ± 0.05	0.23 ± 0.05	0.981
CVI (%)	37.53 ± 3.33	35.50 ± 3.55	0.230	38.28 ± 3.55	36.10 ± 3.12	**0.032**	39.29 ± 4.72	35.01 ± 3.35	**0.008**

SFCT = subfoveal choroidal thickness; CMT = central macular thickness; TCA = total choroidal area; LA = luminal area; SA = stromal area; CVI = choroidal vascularity index; nME = no macular oedema; CME = cystoid macular oedema; Mixed = cystoid macular oedema + serous retinal detachment. * nME group compared to control group, independent-sample t test. † CME group compared to control group, independent-sample t test. ‡ Mixed group compared to control group, independent-sample t test. Significant p values are in bold.

Considering OCT parameters according to the type of retinal occlusion, eyes with CRVO and BRVO did not significantly differ except for CMT (Table 5).

Table 5. Optical coherence tomography parameters according to type of retinal vein occlusion.

Parameter/Group	BRVO	CRVO	p Value *
SFCT (μm)	199.08 ± 58.68	206.76 ± 49.46	0.673
CMT (μm)	443.28 ± 167.59	709.09 ± 247.66	**0.005**
TCA (mm²)	0.45 ± 0.14	0.39 ± 0.09	0.090
LA (mm²)	0.17 ± 0.05	0.14 ± 0.04	0.091
SA (mm²)	0.28 ± 0.09	0.24 ± 0.05	0.115
CVI (%)	38.83 ± 3.87	37.22 ± 3.88	0.245

CRVO = central retinal vein occlusion; BRVO = branch retinal vein occlusion; SFCT = subfoveal choroidal thickness; CMT = central macular thickness; TCA = total choroidal area; LA = luminal area; SA = stromal area; CVI = choroidal vascularity index. * Independent-sample t test. Significant p values are in bold.

We also compared OCT parameters in eyes with CRVO; no significant difference was found between eyes with ischemic and non-ischemic subtype.

4. Discussion

In this cross-sectional study, we evaluated choroidal vascularity changes in patients affected by retinal vein occlusion, both central and branch, using their unaffected fellow eyes as control. We further aimed to investigate if there was any difference in choroidal response among central and branch RVO and if there was a relationship between choroidal vascularity and the type of macular edema.

Taken together, we observed an increase in CVI as well as TCA and LA in affected eyes compared to controls. Comparing eyes with central and branch RVO, there was no difference in any of the considered OCT parameters except for CMT. Similar findings were reported by Tang and colleagues [16] meaning that the vascularity choroidal changes may be equal regardless of the type of occlusion. A recent study found that CVI was significantly lower in patients with RVO than in fellow eyes. However, the measurements were performed at least 1 month after an anti-vascular endothelial growth factor (VEGF) injection or steroid (dexamethasone) implant [17]. Consequently, the lower values of CVI could have been influenced by the effect of the drugs and the reduction of macular edema, although the effect of steroids on choroid is still controversial. Similarly, it has been reported that choroidal thickness reduced after anti-VEGF or intravitreal steroid therapy [8,18,19].

In our study, no differences in subfoveal choroidal thickness arose between the study and contralateral eyes. Recent research evaluating choroidal thickness change in patients with RVO reported discordant results. Some authors demonstrated a greater choroidal thickness in eyes with RVO if compared with the unaffected fellow eyes [7,16,20]. In contrast, others [8,9] showed no differences in choroidal thickness between the affected and contralateral eyes. Even after treatment, changes in choroidal thickness were different [8]. Some studies reported a significant SFCT change after intravitreal injections [7], whereas other studies reported that SFCT did not decrease after treatment [21].

Furthermore, SFCT did not change in functional non-responders after 3 monthly anti-VEGF therapy [5,22]. Although the reasons for this difference were not completely understood, a possible explanation may be attributed to several factors such as type of RVO, central or branch, RVO phase (acute or longstanding), type of macular edema, age, axial length, gender, anterior chamber depth, and lens thickness. The CVI has the advantage of overlooking the limitations related to the use of CT since it is not influenced by the aforementioned variables.

Comparing eyes with CRVO and BRVO, we found that CMT was greater in eyes with CRVO. Previous studies [23,24] demonstrated that SFCT was thicker in eyes with CRVO than in those with BRVO. It had been observed that CRVO eyes had a higher ischemic index and VEGF level compared with BRVO eyes [25]. Increased VEGF may be the main cause of increased choroidal thickness inducing vascular hyperpermeability and dilated vessels in the choroidal layer [26,27]. It may also explain the increased CMT observed in eyes with CRVO.

We stratified our results according to the type of macular edema. There was no difference between subtypes of macular oedema regardless of age, gender, laterality and BCVA. If compared with controls, eyes with CME had higher values of SFCT, CMT, TCA, LA and CVI. Increased CMT and CVI have been observed also in eyes with a mixed pattern of macular edema (intraretinal and subfoveal). In contrast, we noticed no difference in SFCT, CMT, TCA, LA, SA and CVI in the nME group.

We hypothesize that eyes with CME and mixed macular edema could have a greater inflammatory response secondary to RVO comparing with nME eyes. It is known that, when RVO occurs, the choriocapillaris increases its permeability under the influence of soluble VEGF and other inflammatory mediators [28]. VEGF induces choroidal vascular hyperpermeability and, subsequently, choroidal thickening [7]. Moreover, choroidal thickening is also due to nitric oxide production, triggered by VEGF expression [28]. It is possible that in eyes with nME, this inflammatory response was absent or reduced so even choroidal thickening does not occur. To confirm this theory, our results showed an increased CVI only in eyes in which macular edema had developed.

Although CVI has been extensively discussed and globally recognized as a reliable and promising tool for the study of choroidal vascularity, there are some limitations in its routine use by regular ophthalmologists in their daily activity. The EDI-OCT images should be binarized which requires a certain familiarity with the software. However, CVI could provide interesting information as it could be used as a prognostic parameter to be taken into consideration in the proper management of eyes with RVO.

This study suffers from certain limitations including the retrospective design and the small sample sizes in the subgroups. Additionally, we measured only a single scan going through the fovea; a volume scan over the macular area could provide more comprehensive information.

5. Conclusions

In conclusion, our results support a dilatation of the choroidal vessels in eyes with RVO. Choroidal vascularity, assessed by the CVI, varied according to the pattern of macular edema (nME, CME, mixed) and was independent of the type of RVO (branch or central).

Supplementary Materials: The following supporting information can be downloaded at: https://www.mdpi.com/article/10.3390/jcm11164756/s1, Table S1: data set.

Author Contributions: Conceptualization, P.L.; formal analysis, P.L.; investigation, C.P.; data curation, G.C. (Giuseppe Covello) and M.S.S.; writing—original draft preparation, P.L. and G.C. (Giuseppe Covello); writing—review and editing, P.L. and M.F.; supervision, M.F. and G.C. (Giamberto Casini) All authors have read and agreed to the published version of the manuscript.

Funding: This research received no external funding.

Institutional Review Board Statement: The study was conducted in accordance with the Declaration of Helsinki and approved by the Institutional Review Board (Comitato Etico Area Vasta Nord-Ovest) of Pisa University Hospital, Pisa, Italy (protocol code 17441).

Informed Consent Statement: Informed consent was obtained from all subjects involved in the study.

Data Availability Statement: Data supporting reported results can be found in Supplementary Materials, Table S1.

Conflicts of Interest: The authors declare no conflict of interest.

References

1. Klein, R.; Klein, B.E.; Moss, S.E.; Meuer, S.M. The epidemiology of retinal vein occlusion: The Beaver Dam Eye Study. *Trans. Am. Ophthalmol. Soc.* **2000**, *98*, 133–141, discussion 141–143. [PubMed]
2. Rehak, J.; Rehak, M. Branch retinal vein occlusion: Pathogenesis, visual prognosis, and treatment modalities. *Curr. Eye Res.* **2008**, *33*, 111–131. [CrossRef]
3. Patel, A.; Nguyen, C.; Lu, S. Central Retinal Vein Occlusion: A Review of Current Evidence-based Treatment Options. *Middle East Afr. J. Ophthalmol.* **2016**, *23*, 44–48. [CrossRef]
4. Spaide, R.F.; Koizumi, H.; Pozzoni, M.C. Enhanced depth imaging spectral-domain optical coherence tomography. *Am. J. Ophthalmol.* **2008**, *146*, 496–500. [CrossRef]
5. Rayess, N.; Rahimy, E.; Ying, G.S.; Pefkianaki, M.; Franklin, J.; Regillo, C.D.; Ho, A.C.; Hsu, J. Baseline choroidal thickness as a short-term predictor of visual acuity improvement following antivascular endothelial growth factor therapy in branch retinal vein occlusion. *Br. J. Ophthalmol.* **2019**, *103*, 55–59. [CrossRef]
6. Kim, K.H.; Lee, D.H.; Lee, J.J.; Park, S.W.; Byon, I.S.; Lee, J.E. Regional Choroidal Thickness Changes in Branch Retinal Vein Occlusion with Macular Edema. *Ophthalmologica* **2015**, *234*, 109–118. [CrossRef] [PubMed]
7. Tsuiki, E.; Suzuma, K.; Ueki, R.; Maekawa, Y.; Kitaoka, T. Enhanced depth imaging optical coherence tomography of the choroid in central retinal vein occlusion. *Am. J. Ophthalmol.* **2013**, *156*, 543–547.e541. [CrossRef] [PubMed]
8. Lee, E.K.; Han, J.M.; Hyon, J.Y.; Yu, H.G. Changes in choroidal thickness after intravitreal dexamethasone implant injection in retinal vein occlusion. *Br. J. Ophthalmol.* **2015**, *99*, 1543–1549. [CrossRef] [PubMed]
9. Du, K.F.; Xu, L.; Shao, L.; Chen, C.X.; Zhou, J.Q.; Wang, Y.X.; You, Q.S.; Jonas, J.B.; Wei, W.B. Subfoveal choroidal thickness in retinal vein occlusion. *Ophthalmology* **2013**, *120*, 2749–2750. [CrossRef] [PubMed]
10. Sonoda, S.; Sakamoto, T.; Yamashita, T.; Uchino, E.; Kawano, H.; Yoshihara, N.; Terasaki, H.; Shirasawa, M.; Tomita, M.; Ishibashi, T. Luminal and stromal areas of choroid determined by binarization method of optical coherence tomographic images. *Am. J. Ophthalmol.* **2015**, *159*, 1123–1131.e1121. [CrossRef] [PubMed]
11. Agrawal, R.; Gupta, P.; Tan, K.A.; Cheung, C.M.; Wong, T.Y.; Cheng, C.Y. Choroidal vascularity index as a measure of vascular status of the choroid: Measurements in healthy eyes from a population-based study. *Sci. Rep.* **2016**, *6*, 21090. [CrossRef] [PubMed]
12. Agrawal, R.; Li, L.K.; Nakhate, V.; Khandelwal, N.; Mahendradas, P. Choroidal Vascularity Index in Vogt-Koyanagi-Harada Disease: An EDI-OCT Derived Tool for Monitoring Disease Progression. *Transl. Vis. Sci. Technol.* **2016**, *5*, 7. [CrossRef]
13. Agrawal, R.; Chhablani, J.; Tan, K.A.; Shah, S.; Sarvaiya, C.; Banker, A. Choroidal vascularity index in central serous chorioretinopathy. *Retina* **2016**, *36*, 1646–1651. [CrossRef] [PubMed]
14. Kim, M.; Ha, M.J.; Choi, S.Y.; Park, Y.H. Choroidal vascularity index in type-2 diabetes analyzed by swept-source optical coherence tomography. *Sci. Rep.* **2018**, *8*, 70. [CrossRef] [PubMed]

15. Koh, L.H.L.; Agrawal, R.; Khandelwal, N.; Sai Charan, L.; Chhablani, J. Choroidal vascular changes in age-related macular degeneration. *Acta Ophthalmol.* **2017**, *95*, e597–e601. [CrossRef] [PubMed]
16. Tang, F.; Xu, F.; Zhong, H.; Zhao, X.; Lv, M.; Yang, K.; Shen, C.; Huang, H.; Lv, J.; Zeng, S.; et al. Comparison of subfoveal choroidal thickness in eyes with CRVO and BRVO. *BMC Ophthalmol.* **2019**, *19*, 133. [CrossRef] [PubMed]
17. Aribas, Y.K.; Hondur, A.M.; Tezel, T.H. Choroidal vascularity index and choriocapillaris changes in retinal vein occlusions. *Graefes Arch. Clin. Exp. Ophthalmol.* **2020**, *258*, 2389–2397. [CrossRef] [PubMed]
18. Okamoto, M.; Yamashita, M.; Sakamoto, T.; Ogata, N. Choroidal blood flow and thickness as predictors for response to anti-vascular endothelial growth factor therapy in macular edema secondary to branch retinal vein occlusion. *Retina* **2018**, *38*, 550–558. [CrossRef] [PubMed]
19. Esen, E.; Sizmaz, S.; Demircan, N. Choroidal thickness changes after intravitreal dexamethasone implant injection for the treatment of macular edema due to retinal vein occlusion. *Retina* **2016**, *36*, 2297–2303. [CrossRef] [PubMed]
20. Coban-Karatas, M.; Altan-Yaycioglu, R.; Ulas, B.; Sizmaz, S.; Canan, H.; Sariturk, C. Choroidal thickness measurements with optical coherence tomography in branch retinal vein occlusion. *Int. J. Ophthalmol.* **2016**, *9*, 725–729. [CrossRef] [PubMed]
21. Park, J.; Lee, S.; Son, Y. Effects of two different doses of intravitreal bevacizumab on subfoveal choroidal thickness and retinal vessel diameter in branch retinal vein occlusion. *Int. J. Ophthalmol.* **2016**, *9*, 999–1005. [CrossRef] [PubMed]
22. Rayess, N.; Rahimy, E.; Ying, G.S.; Pefkianaki, M.; Franklin, J.; Regillo, C.D.; Ho, A.C.; Hsu, J. Baseline Choroidal Thickness as a Predictor for Treatment Outcomes in Central Retinal Vein Occlusion. *Am. J. Ophthalmol.* **2016**, *171*, 47–52. [CrossRef] [PubMed]
23. Quinlan, P.M.; Elman, M.J.; Bhatt, A.K.; Mardesich, P.; Enger, C. The natural course of central retinal vein occlusion. *Am. J. Ophthalmol.* **1990**, *110*, 118–123. [CrossRef]
24. Minturn, J.; Brown, G.C. Progression of nonischemic central retinal vein obstruction to the ischemic variant. *Ophthalmology* **1986**, *93*, 1158–1162. [CrossRef]
25. Pe'er, J.; Shweiki, D.; Itin, A.; Hemo, I.; Gnessin, H.; Keshet, E. Hypoxia-induced expression of vascular endothelial growth factor by retinal cells is a common factor in neovascularizing ocular diseases. *Lab. Investig.* **1995**, *72*, 638–645. [PubMed]
26. Maruko, I.; Iida, T.; Sugano, Y.; Ojima, A.; Sekiryu, T. Subfoveal choroidal thickness in fellow eyes of patients with central serous chorioretinopathy. *Retina* **2011**, *31*, 1603–1608. [CrossRef] [PubMed]
27. Maruko, I.; Iida, T.; Sugano, Y.; Furuta, M.; Sekiryu, T. One-year choroidal thickness results after photodynamic therapy for central serous chorioretinopathy. *Retina* **2011**, *31*, 1921–1927. [CrossRef] [PubMed]
28. Mrejen, S.; Spaide, R.F. Optical coherence tomography: Imaging of the choroid and beyond. *Surv. Ophthalmol.* **2013**, *58*, 387–429. [CrossRef] [PubMed]

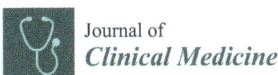

Article

Large Amplitude Iris Fluttering Detected by Consecutive Anterior Segment Optical Coherence Tomography Images in Eyes with Intrascleral Fixation of an Intraocular Lens

Makoto Inoue *, Takashi Koto and Akito Hirakata

Kyorin Eye Center, Kyorin University School of Medicine, 6-20-2 Shinkawa, Mitaka 186-8611, Tokyo, Japan
* Correspondence: inoue@eye-center.org; Tel.: +81-422475511

Abstract: Saccadic eye movements induce movements of the aqueous and vitreous humor and iris fluttering. To evaluate iris fluttering during eye movements, anterior segment optical coherence tomography (AS-OCT) was used in 29 eyes with pars plana vitrectomy (PPV) and intrascleral fixation of an intraocular lens (ISF group) and 15 eyes with PPV and an IOL implantation into lens capsular bag (control group). The height of the iris from the iris plane (the line between the anterior chamber angles) was compared every 0.2 s after the eye had moved from a temporal to the primary position (time 0). The height of the nasal iris in the ISF group decreased to -0.68 ± 0.43 mm at 0 s ($p < 0.001$) and returned to -0.06 ± 0.23 mm at 0.2 s. The height of the temporal iris increased to 0.45 ± 0.31 mm at 0 s ($p < 0.001$) and returned to -0.06 ± 0.18 mm at 0.2 s. The height of the nasal iris at 0 s in the ISF group was significantly lower, and that of the temporal iris was significantly higher than the control (-0.05 ± 0.09 mm, 0.03 ± 0.06 mm, $p < 0.001$, respectively). Iris fluttering can act as a check valve for aqueous and vitreous humor movements and can be quantified by consecutive AS-OCT images. Large amplitude iris fluttering in eyes with intrascleral fixation is important because it can lead to a reverse pupillary block.

Keywords: intrascleral fixation; intraocular lens; anterior segment optical coherence tomography; iris capture; reverse pupillary block; peripheral iridectomy

Citation: Inoue, M.; Koto, T.; Hirakata, A. Large Amplitude Iris Fluttering Detected by Consecutive Anterior Segment Optical Coherence Tomography Images in Eyes with Intrascleral Fixation of an Intraocular Lens. *J. Clin. Med.* **2022**, *11*, 4596. https://doi.org/10.3390/jcm11154596

Academic Editors: Sumit Randhir Singh and Jay Chhablani

Received: 29 June 2022
Accepted: 4 August 2022
Published: 6 August 2022

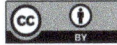

Copyright: © 2022 by the authors. Licensee MDPI, Basel, Switzerland. This article is an open access article distributed under the terms and conditions of the Creative Commons Attribution (CC BY) license (https://creativecommons.org/licenses/by/4.0/).

1. Introduction

Intrascleral fixation or ciliary suturing of an intraocular lens (IOLs) has been used on eyes without adequate support by the lens capsule [1–8]. A fluttering of the iris can be seen more frequently in eyes without a lens capsule behind the iris through the slit-lamp microscope when the patient blinks. The flow of the aqueous and vitreous humor through the gap around the optics of the IOL during eye movements causes the iris to oscillate back and forth, i.e., flutter. This is important because excessive iris movements can lead to a pupillary capture by the intraocular lens, causing a reverse pupillary block, one of the major complications after intrascleral fixation and ciliary sulcus fixation of an IOL [9–12]. Pupillary capture by the IOL can cause an increase in intraocular pressure and mild eye pain and discomfort, called Uveitis-Glaucoma-Hyphema (UGH) syndrome. In addition, the capture by the IOL can deform the pupil, which can reduce visual acuity by decreasing the depth of focus and increasing ocular aberrations.

The eye is filled with fluid, and saccadic eye movements and body motions cause movement of the intraocular fluids, which generates shear stress on the ocular tissues in contact with the fluids [13]. The movement of the aqueous humor and vitreous humor during eye movements have been analyzed with a computational model because it is difficult to observe and measure them in situ in live human eyes [13–17].

The anterior segment optical coherence tomographic (AS-OCT) devices were designed to record cross-sectional images of the anterior segment of the eye [18,19]. The smoothness of the anterior surface of the iris in Fuchs uveitis [20,21], morphological change after laser peripheral iridectomy in eyes with primary angle closure glaucoma and uveitic secondary glaucoma have been evaluated by AS-OCT [22,23]. Swept-source AS-OCT uses a longer wavelength light source of 1310 nm, which enables the scanning of the anterior and posterior surface of an IOL. It also enables high-speed scanning leading to images of the entire anterior chamber angle, and the repetitive imaging of the same section of the anterior chamber will appear similar to a continuous movie scan [18,19]. With the dynamic scanning ability of swept-source AS-OCT, evaluation of iris movement during pupil constriction with light revealed that the iris stiffness was higher in patients with primary angle-closure glaucoma than in healthy controls [24]. Detection of peripheral anterior synechia has been described by corneal deformation using an air-puff dynamic AS-OCT system [25].

We present a dynamic analysis with swept-source AS-OCT, which allowed us to evaluate and quantify the degree of iris fluttering produced by eye movements in eyes with an intrasclerally fixed IOL. The purpose of this study was to determine whether iris flutter immediately after a saccadic eye movement can be detected and quantified. Another purpose was to determine whether the movement of the iris can lead to a pupillary capture by the IOL after intrascleral fixation.

2. Materials and Methods

This single-center, observational study was approved by the Institutional Review Committee of the Kyorin University School of Medicine (1507). It adheres to the tenets of the Declaration of Helsinki. All of the patients received a detailed explanation of the surgical and ophthalmic procedures, and all signed an informed consent form. All of the patients consented to our review of their medical records and their anonymized use in medical publications.

2.1. Subjects

The findings in 29 eyes of 29 patients after pars plana vitrectomy (PPV) and intrascleral fixation of an IOL (ISF group) were compared to that in 15 eyes of 15 patients after PPV combined with cataract surgery with implantation of an IOL in the lens capsular bag (control group). In the ISF group, the surgery was performed on 21 eyes with IOL dislocation, 4 eyes with lens dislocation, and 4 eyes with aphakia. In the control group, there were 6 eyes with an epiretinal membrane, 6 eyes with a macular hole, 1 eye each with a lamellar macular hole, proliferative diabetic retinopathy, and rhegmatogenous retinal detachment. The eyes with a posterior synechia, impending reverse pupillary block, and intraoperative complications, including posterior capsule rupture during cataract surgery in the control group, were excluded. The age, sex, laterality, axial length, and anterior chamber depth (ACD) were compared between the ISF and the control groups and with and without peripheral iridectomy (PI) in the ISF group.

The axial length was measured with the OA2000 Optical Biometer (TOMEY Corp, Nagoya, Japan). Swept-source AS-OCT (CASIA2, TOMEY Corp, Nagoya, Japan) with a scan rate of 50,000 A-scan per second was used. The ACD was measured from the corneal endothelium to the anterior surface of the IOL along the visual axis with caliper software integrated into the AS-OCT device.

2.2. Measurement of Iris Flutter by Anterior Segment Optical Coherence Tomography (AS-OCT)

Cross-sectional images of the anterior segment, including the iris, were obtained by swept-source AS-OCT (CASIA2). Consecutive images were recorded with the movie mode from both groups one month after the surgery. For this, the patient's head was fixed to the head holders of the AS-OCT device, and the patient was instructed to fixate a target located 30 degrees laterally from the primary visual axis for 1 s and then move the eye back to the primary position and to hold this eye position for 3 s (Figure 1a,b). This sequence was repeated several times, and the sequences with blinking were excluded from the analyses. The timing of the eye movements was controlled by the sound of a metronome with a repetition rate of one second. Video images were recorded with the AS-OCT device at

5 frames/sec. In each sequence, the time when the eye stopped at the primary position was set to 0.

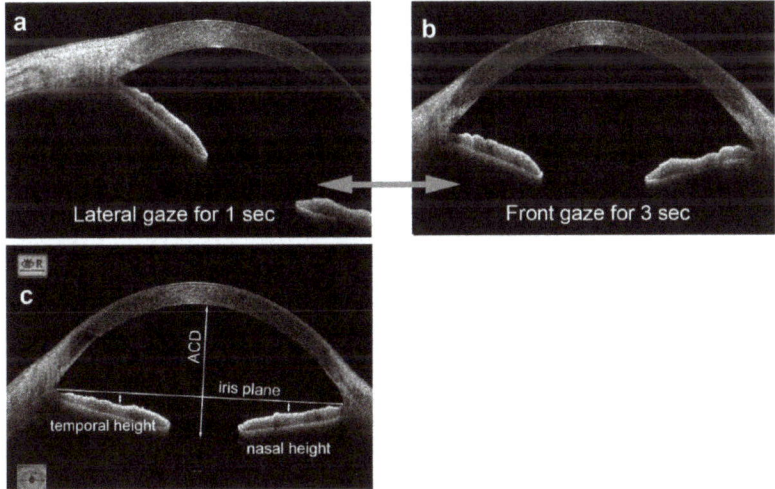

Figure 1. Anterior segment optical coherence tomographic (AS-OCT) images are taken when the eye is fixed on a temporal target and then moves to the primary position. Also shown are images that show the parameters of the AS-OCT images that are measured. (**a**). AS-OCT image when the patient is looking at a point located 30 degrees temporal from the visual axis. (**b**). AS-OCT image taken immediately after the patient has moved the eye to the primary position and holds this position for 3 s. (**c**). The heights of the temporal and nasal sectors of the iris are defined as the distance from the iris plane (the line between anterior chamber angles) to the anterior surface of the nasal and temporal sectors of the mid-iris.

The iris height was defined as the distance to the anterior surface of the middle sector of the iris from the iris plane, which is a reference line connecting the anterior chamber angles (Figure 1c) and measured at the primary position for the temporal and nasal sectors with the caliper function of the ImageJ software (National Institute of Health, Bethesda, MD, USA). The baseline values were measured at the primary position without an eye movement. The iris height was compared between the eyes in the ISF group and the control group. The iris height was also compared with or without PI in the ISF group.

2.3. Surgical Procedures

The PPV and all other surgical procedures were performed by two surgeons (TK and MI) with 27-gauge instruments of the Constellation® Vision System (Alcon Laboratories, Fort Worth, TX, USA) under local anesthesia. The surgery of the ISF group was for a dislocated or subluxated crystalline lens or an IOL, or aphakia. For these eyes, the dislocated lens was lifted by suction of a vitreous cutter and then phacoemulsified or extracted. A dislocated acrylic or silicone IOL was cut into 2 or 3 pieces by scissors and then extracted through a transconjunctival single plane corneoscleral incision. A residual posterior hyaloid cortex was made more visible by intravitreal injection of triamcinolone acetonide (MaQaid®, Wakamoto Pharmaceutical Co., Ltd., Tokyo, Japan), and the residual posterior hyaloid cortex was removed by suction with a vitreous cutter if it was present.

The intrascleral fixation was performed as described by Yamane et al. [7,8]. The limbal positions where the haptics of the IOL were extracted were at approximately 2 and 8 o'clock, which were marked with a toric marker. Two angled parallel incisions were made at 2 mm posterior to the limbus at the marked positions by 30-gauge thin-walled needles. A 3-piece IOL with 7 mm diameter optics (NX-70, Santen Pharma, Osaka, Japan) was implanted in the anterior chamber, and both haptics of the IOL were inserted into 30-gauge needles and extracted with the needles. The excess lengths of the haptics were cut, and the ends were flanged with a coagulator (Accu-Temp®, Alcon Laboratories, Fort Worth, TX, USA).

The control group underwent PPV combined with cataract surgery and implantation of an IOL in the lens capsular bag before the PPV. Posterior vitreous detachment, membrane peeling, internal limiting peeling with the aid of brilliant blue G, endo-photocoagulation, tamponade by air, or 20% sulfur hexafluoride (SF6) were performed as needed.

2.4. Statistical Analyses

The significance of the differences in the baseline characteristics and the degree and time course of the iris fluttering between the 2 groups was determined by the Wilcoxon signed rank tests, Mann–Whitney U tests, or Fisher's exact probability tests. All statistical analyses were performed using SPSS (version 28.0; IBM, Armonk, New York, NY, USA).

3. Results

The differences in age, sex distribution, and axial length between the ISF and the control groups were not significant (Table 1). However, the ACD of the eyes at the baseline in the ISF group was significantly deeper, and the heights of the iris in the temporal and nasal sectors were significantly lower than that of the control group when the eye was in the primary position.

Table 1. Baseline characteristics between the eyes after intrascleral fixation and vitrectomy combined with cataract surgery.

	ISF	Control	p-Value
Eyes	29	15	
Age	66.2 ± 17.7	65.1 ± 8.0	0.435 *
Sex (M/W)	22/7	7/8	0.056 **
Laterality (R/L)	14/15	9/6	0.338 **
Axial length (mm)	25.32 ± 1.73	24.75 ± 2.05	0.202 *
Nasal height of iris (mm)	−0.20 ± 0.16	−0.06 ± 0.17	0.007 *
Temporal height of iris (mm)	−0.23 ± 0.13	−0.08 ± 0.16	0.006 *
ACD (mm)	5.82 ± 0.58	5.25 ± 0.31	<0.001 *
Peripheral iridectomy	20	0	

ISF = intrascleral fixation, M = man, W = woman, R = right, L = left, ACD = anterior chamber depth, * = Mann–Whitney U test, ** = Fisher's exact probability test.

3.1. Time Course of Changes in Height of Temporal and Nasal Sectors of Iris after an Eye Movement

At the time when the AS-OCT was used to evaluate iris fluttering, one month after the implantation of the IOL, no intravitreal gas bubbles were seen in any of the eyes that had undergone a gas tamponade in both groups.

After the eye moved from the lateral to the primary position, the height of the nasal sector of the iris in the ISF group decreased significantly from the baseline at −0.20 ± 0.16 mm to −0.88 ± 0.40 mm at 0 s ($p < 0.001$, Wilcoxon signed-rank test, $p < 0.01$ was taken to be significant with Bonferroni correction, Figures 2 and 3, Video S1). The height of the nasal iris returned to −0.27 ± 0.29 mm at 0.2 s ($p = 0.207$), to −0.24 ± 0.22 mm at 0.4 s ($p = 0.163$), to −0.22 ± 0.17 mm at 0.6 s ($p = 0.396$), and to −0.21 ± 0.17 mm at 0.8 s ($p = 0.977$) while the eye remained in the primary position. The height of the nasal iris in the control group decreased from the baseline at −0.06 ± 0.17 mm to −0.11 ± 0.19 mm at 0 s ($p = 0.058$) and returned to −0.05 ± 0.16 mm at 0.2 s ($p = 0.813$), to -0.08 ± 0.17 mm at 0.4 s ($p = 0.041$), to −0.06 ± 0.17 mm at 0.6 s ($p = 0.475$), and to −0.06 ± 0.16 mm at 0.8 s ($p = 0.762$) but were not significant ($p < 0.01$ was taken to be significant with Bonferroni correction).

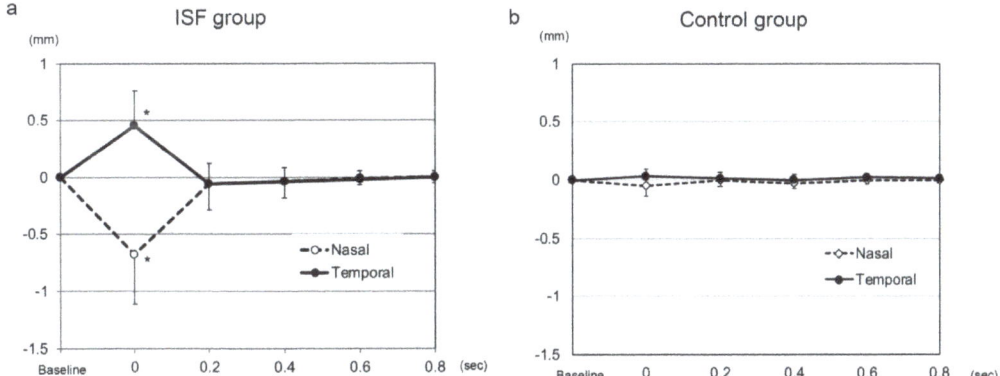

Figure 2. A plot of changes in the height of the temporal and nasal sectors of the iris immediately after a movement of the eye from a 30° temporal position to the primary position in an eye with an intrascleral fixation (ISF) of an intraocular lens (IOL). Also plotted are the values of an eye in which the IOL was implanted in the lens capsule, the control group. (**a**). The height of the nasal sector of the iris of eyes in the ISF group decreases significantly from the baseline at 0 s ($p < 0.001$) and returns at 0.2 s. The height of the temporal sector in eyes of the ISF group increases significantly from the baseline at 0 s and returns to the baseline at 0.2 s. (**b**). The height of the nasal sector of the iris in the ISF group at 0 s was significantly smaller than that of the control group ($p < 0.001$). The temporal height of the ISF group at 0 s was greater than that of the control ($p < 0.001$). The nasal height of the ISF group at 0 s was smaller than that of the control ($p < 0.001$). (* $p < 0.01$).

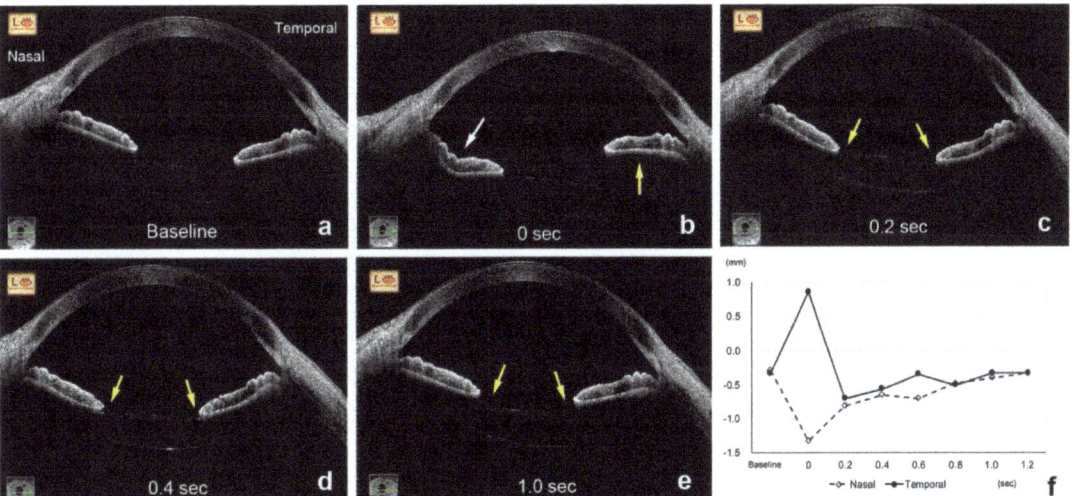

Figure 3. AS-OCT images of a 72-year-old woman in the ISF group. The nasal height of the iris (white arrow) decreases, and the temporal height (yellow arrow) increases at 0 s (**b**) from the baseline (**a**). The height of the nasal and temporal iris (yellow arrows) remains at the lower level at 0.2 s (**c**) and 0.4 s (**d**) and returns to the baseline level at 1.0 s (**e**,**f**).

The amount of height change of the nasal iris from the baseline was significantly greater at 0 s in the ISF group (-0.68 ± 0.43 mm) than in the control group (-0.05 ± 0.09 mm, $p < 0.001$, Figures 2 and 4, Video S2). However, the amount of height change of the nasal iris was not significantly different between these 2 groups at 0.2 s ($p = 0.154$), 0.4 s ($p = 0.931$),

0.6 s ($p = 0.832$), and 0.8 s ($p = 0.89$). The amount of height change of the nasal iris from the baseline was only significant at 0 s in the ISF group, and this amount of height change of the nasal iris at 0 s was not significant group with age ($p = 0.321$, Spearman partial correlation coefficient), ACD ($p = 0.446$), and axial length ($p = 0.365$). The amount of height change of the nasal iris from the baseline was not significant at 0 s in the control group, and this height change at 0 s was also not significant with age ($p = 0.745$), ACD ($p = 0.788$), and axial length ($p = 0.176$).

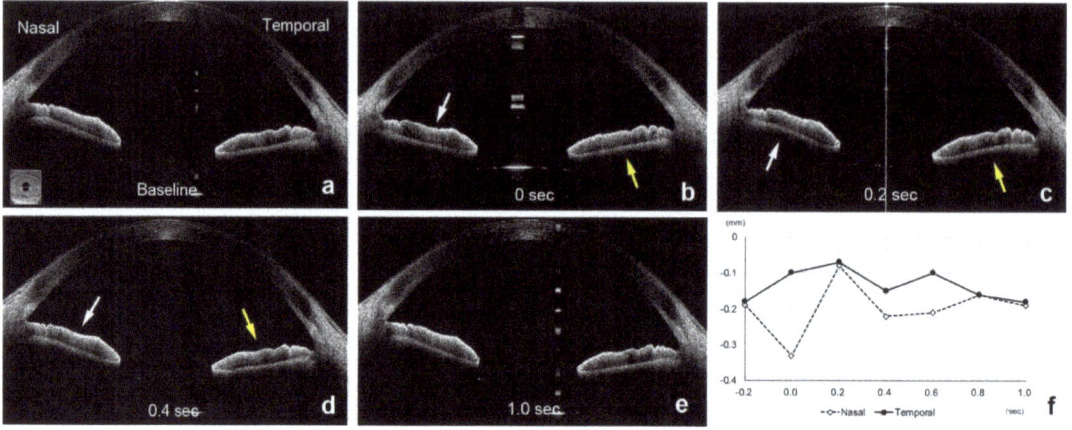

Figure 4. AS-OCT images of a 67-year-old man in the control group who had undergone vitrectomy combined with cataract surgery for an idiopathic macular hole and had the IOL implanted in the capsular bag. The nasal height of the iris (white arrow) decreases at time 0 s (**b**) immediately after the eye stops at the primary position from the baseline (**a**). The nasal height (white arrows) increases at 0.2 s (**c**) and decreases (white arrows) at 0.4 s (**d**). The nasal height returns at 1.0 s (**e**) to the baseline position (**f**). The temporal height of the iris (yellow arrow) increases at 0 s and remains higher at 0.2 s (yellow arrow, **c**) and then returns to the baseline position at 0.4 s (**d**–**f**).

The direction of the changes in the height of the temporal sector of the iris was in the opposite direction from that of the nasal sector. Thus, the height of the temporal iris in the eyes of the ISF group increased significantly from the baseline (-0.23 ± 0.13 mm) to 0.22 ± 0.32 mm at 0 s ($p < 0.001$, Wilcoxon signed-rank test, $p < 0.01$ was taken to be significant with Bonferroni correction), and then returned to -0.29 ± 0.22 mm at 0.2 s ($p = 0.071$), to -0.26 ± 0.18 mm at 0.4 s ($p = 0.124$), to -0.25 ± 0.15 mm at 0.6 s ($p = 0.008$), and to -0.23 ± 0.14 mm at 0.8 s ($p = 0.483$). The height of the temporal iris in the control group decreased from the baseline at -0.08 ± 0.16 mm to -0.05 ± 0.19 mm at 0 s ($p = 0.091$) and returned to -0.07 ± 0.16 mm at 0.2 s ($p = 0.682$), to -0.08 ± 0.14 mm at 0.4 s ($p = 0.694$), to -0.07 ± 0.15 mm at 0.6 s ($p = 0.027$), and to -0.08 ± 0.15 mm at 0.8 s ($p = 0.079$) but were not significant ($p < 0.01$ was taken to be significant with Bonferroni correction).

The amount of change in the height of the temporal iris from the baseline was significantly greater (0.45 ± 0.31 mm, $p < 0.001$) in the ISF group at 0 s than that in the control group (0.03 ± 0.06 mm). However, the amount of height change of the temporal iris was not significantly different between these 2 groups at 0.2 s ($p = 0.084$), 0.4 s ($p = 0.244$), 0.6 s ($p = 0.019$), and 0.8 s ($p = 0.089$). The amount of height change of the temporal iris from the baseline was only significant at 0 s in the ISF group, and this amount of height change of the temporal iris at 0 s was not significant with age ($p = 0.386$, Spearman partial correlation coefficient), ACD ($p = 0.482$), and axial length ($p = 0.082$). The amount of height change of the temporal iris from the baseline was not significant at 0 s in the control group, and this change at 0 s was significant with axial length ($p = 0.009$) but not with age ($p = 0.086$), and ACD ($p = 0.889$).

3.2. Changes in Iris Height in Eyes with and without Peripheral Iridectomy (PI)

The age, sex distribution, axial length, and heights of temporal and nasal sectors of the iris were not significantly different between the eyes with and without PI in the ISF group (Table 2). However, the ACD in eyes without PI was significantly deeper than that in eyes with PI.

Table 2. Baseline characteristics between the eyes after intrascleral fixation with or without peripheral iridectomy.

	PI (+)	PI (−)	p-Value
Eyes	20	9	-
Age	66.9 ± 18.9	64.6 ± 15.4	0.594 *
Sex (M/W)	15/5	7/2	0.631 **
Laterality (R/L)	11/9	3/6	0.250 **
Axial length (mm)	25.52 ± 1.82	24.87 ± 1.48	0.390 *
Nasal height of iris (mm)	−0.24 ± 0.13	−0.14 ± 0.20	0.317 *
Temporal height of iris (mm)	−0.25 ± 0.11	−0.17 ± 0.15	0.116 *
ACD (mm)	5.67 ± 0.46	6.17 ± 0.69	0.030 *

PI = peripheral iridectomy, M = man, W = female, ACD = anterior chamber depth, * = Mann–Whitney test, ** = Fisher's exact probability test.

The height of the nasal sector in eyes with PI decreased significantly to −0.88 ± 0.40 mm from the baseline (−0.24 ± 0.13 mm, $p \leq 0.001$, Wilcoxon signed-rank test, $p < 0.01$ was taken to be significant with Bonferroni correction) at 0 s and returned to −0.32 ± 0.28 mm at 0.2 s ($p = 0.131$), −0.29 ± 0.23 mm at 0.4 s ($p = 0.117$), −0.25 ± 0.17 mm at 0.6 s ($p = 0.67$), and −0.24 ± 0.16 mm at 0.8 s ($p = 0.981$). The height of the nasal sector of the iris in eyes without PI decreased significantly to −0.88 ± 0.42 mm at 0 s from the baseline (−0.14 ± 0.20 mm, $p = 0.008$, Wilcoxon signed-rank test, $p < 0.01$ was taken to be significant with Bonferroni correction). Then, the height of the nasal iris returned to −0.16 ± 0.30 mm at 0.2 s ($p = 1.0$), −0.13 ± 0.17 mm at 0.4 s ($p = 0.859$), −0.15 ± 0.17 mm at 0.6 s ($p = 0.362$), and −0.13 ± 0.17 mm at 0.8 s ($p = 1.0$, Figure 5).

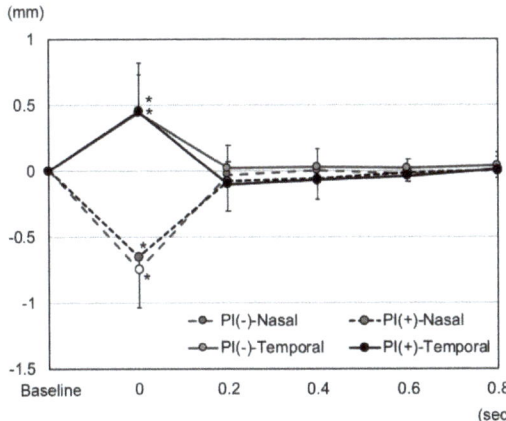

Figure 5. Changes in the height of the iris in the eyes after intrascleral fixation with and without peripheral iridectomy (PI). The nasal height of the iris in eyes with and without PI is significantly lower than the baseline position at 0 s and returned to the baseline position at 0.2 s (* $p < 0.01$). The temporal height in eyes with and without PI was significantly higher than the baseline position and also returned to the baseline position at 0.2 s. The nasal and temporal height of the iris in eyes with PI was not significantly different from that without PI at any time point.

The height of the temporal sector of the iris in the eyes with PI increased to 0.20 ± 0.26 mm at 0 s from the baseline (-0.25 ± 0.11 mm, $p < 0.001$, Wilcoxon signed-rank test, $p < 0.01$ was taken to be significant with Bonferroni correction). The height of the temporal iris then decreased significantly to -0.35 ± 0.22 mm at 0.2 s ($p = 0.025$), -0.32 ± 0.18 mm at 0.4 s ($p = 0.017$), -0.29 ± 0.15 mm at 0.6 s ($p = 0.015$), and returned to -0.24 ± 0.16 mm at 0.8 s ($p = 0.827$, Figure 5). The height of the temporal iris in eyes without PI increased significantly to 0.26 ± 0.43 mm from the baseline (-0.17 ± 0.15 mm, $p = 0.008$, Wilcoxon signed-rank test, $p < 0.01$ was taken to be significant with Bonferroni correction) at 0 s. The height of the temporal iris then returned to -0.15 ± 0.14 mm at 0.2 s ($p = 0.858$), -0.14 ± 0.11 mm at 0.4 s ($p = 0.477$), -0.16 ± 0.12 mm at 0.6 s ($p = 0.574$), and -0.13 ± 0.17 mm at 0.8 s ($p = 0.249$).

The height change of the nasal iris from the baseline in eyes with PI was not significantly different from that of eyes without PI at 0 s ($p = 0.982$), 0.2 s ($p = 0.444$), 0.4 s ($p = 0.417$), 0.6 s ($p = 0.764$), and 0.8 s ($p = 0.594$). The amount of height change of the temporal iris in eyes with PI was not significantly different from that without PI at 0 s ($p = 0.627$), 0.2 s ($p = 0.153$), 0.4 s ($p = 0.069$), 0.6 s ($p = 0.062$), and 0.8 s ($p = 0.417$).

4. Discussion

During saccadic eye movements of normal eyes, the iris, crystalline lens capsule, and anterior vitreous cortex form a barrier that prevents the aqueous humor and vitreous humor from flowing into the other chamber. These barriers then prevent iris flutter. The absence of the vitreous gel after vitrectomy is believed to enhance the flow of vitreous humor into the anterior chamber during eye movements. Silva and associates [13] reported that the computational fluid dynamics of the vitreous humor during saccadic eye movements were different for the gel phase in the vitreous cavity than that with the liquid phase because the inertial effects were more significant with the liquid vitreous. In contrast, the shear stress produced by the gel phase of vitreous humor was more than twice that of the liquid phase. In this study, all eyes were vitrectomized. However, it has been described that vitrectomy without gas tamponade is not associated with changes in anterior chamber morphology evaluated with AS-OCT [26].

After an intrascleral fixation of an IOL without a lens capsular support, the height of the temporal sector of the iris increased, and the nasal sector decreased immediately after the eye moved from a temporal gaze to the primary position. The aqueous humor is more susceptible to inertia moments than the vitreous fluid in vitrectomized eyes during eye movements because the aqueous humor is located further from the center of the eye. When the eye moves from a temporal gaze to the primary position and comes to rest at the primary position, the nasal sector of the iris is pushed posteriorly by the movement of the aqueous humor toward the posterior chamber, and the height of the nasal sector of the iris is pushed downward, i.e., decreased height. At the same time, the temporal sector of the iris is pushed upward and anteriorly toward the anterior chamber as the aqueous humor moves nasally and the vitreous liquid flows into the anterior chamber and the temporal height of the iris increases.

When the nasal sector of the iris is pushed posteriorly, the pupil margins contact the anterior surface of the IOL, and the flow of the aqueous humor stops as if a valve was closed (attachment of the pupil margin to the IOL). On the other hand, even if the temporal sector of the iris is lifted due to the inflow of vitreous humor into the anterior chamber, the pupil margin does not contact the IOLs. Thus, the flow of the vitreous humor into the anterior chamber on the temporal side is enhanced more than the outflow of aqueous humor on the nasal side as the valve is opened. These movements change the iris height, which then returns to the baseline level after 0.2 s. However, the heights of both the nasal and temporal sectors of the iris remain lower than the baseline and gradually return to the baseline level after 0.4 s. The decreased height of the iris indicates the process of recovery from the influx of vitreous humor into the anterior chamber.

A reverse pupillary block occurs when either side of the iris is pushed posteriorly during eye movements and the pupillary margin does not stay on the anterior surface of

IOL but is pushed behind the IOL by the flow of aqueous humor. A PI was thought to be able to prevent a reverse pupillary block [10,27,28]. In our cohort, we found that PI did not block the inflow of vitreous humor and the outflow of aqueous humor through the PI. The flow of fluid through the PI was expected to alter the amount of decrease in the height of the nasal sector of the iris and increase the height of the temporal sector at 0 s, but the differences were not significant. However, the ACD was shallower in the ISF group with PI at the baseline. There was one eye with an impending pupillary block that had a history of occasional pupillary blockage and spontaneous recovery in which the iris retracted posteriorly and contacted the anterior surface of IOL even at the stationary baseline position in an eye after ISF without PI (Figure 6). This case was excluded from the analyses, but the iris retracted excessively, and the ACD was deep with the angle widely opened, as described in eyes with reverse pupillary block [12]. These cases are believed to be due to an excessive inflow of vitreous humor into the anterior chamber caused by eye movements. Such cases were not seen in the ISF group with PI. To repair the excess angle recession due to the iris retraction, suturing the iris has been described to prevent pupillary capture by the IOL [9].

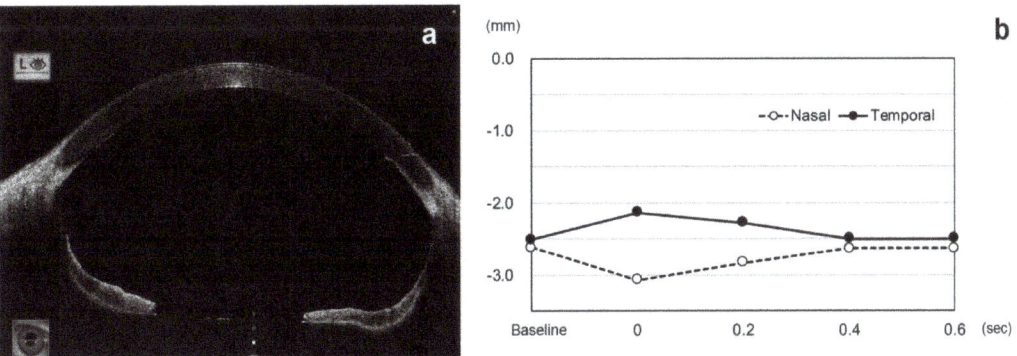

Figure 6. AS-OCT images of a 55-year-old man with an impending pupillary block after intrascleral fixation of an IOL without a peripheral iridectomy. (**a**). AS-OCT image indicates that there is an excessive iris retraction and the anterior chamber depth is 7.07 mm. (**b**). Analysis of the AS-OCT images indicates that the nasal and temporal heights of the iris changes induced by the eye movements, but the height is maintained very low.

The results indicated that the PI did not reduce iris fluttering due to eye movements; however, it is assumed the PI prevented a reverse pupillary block by blocking a homeostatic backward movement of the iris. We believe that a simulation of fluid dynamics can be reproduced using a computational model. However, in vivo and live evaluations by AS-OCT are probably more important because the conditions can vary in each case.

Our study has several limitations. First, the number of patients was too few to perform meaningful statistical analyses. In addition, the types of patients in the two groups varied because of their retrospective design. Second, the AS-OCT analyses were performed one month after the surgery and lacked data for longer postoperative follow-up times. Third, we evaluated the iris height with AS-OCT, and we did not evaluate the intracameral flow directly.

5. Conclusions

In conclusion, iris fluttering can be detected and quantified by examining consecutive swept-source AS-OCT images. Iris fluttering can act as a check valve for aqueous and vitreous humor movements. The greater amount of iris fluttering by eye movements in eyes after intrascleral fixation of the IOL may cause reverse pupillary block because of the absence of a lens capsular support behind the iris. A PI does not reduce the fluttering of the iris caused by eye movements, but it stabilizes the iris height to prevent a pupillary block.

Supplementary Materials: The following supporting information can be downloaded at: https://www.mdpi.com/xxx/s1, the video images of consecutive AS-OCT scans during the sequence of eye movements of an eye of the ISF group (Video S1: the same eye in Figure 3) and the control group (Video S2: the same eye in Figure 4).

Author Contributions: Conceptualization, M.I. and T.K.; methodology, M.I. and T.K.; validation, M.I. and T.K.; formal analysis, M.I. and T.K.; investigation. M.I., T.K. and A.H.; resources, M.I. and A.H.; data curation, M.I. and T.K.; writing-original draft preparation, M.I. and T.K.; writing-review and editing, M.I.; supervision, A.H.; project administration, M.I. and T.K. All authors have read and agreed to the published version of the manuscript.

Funding: This research received no external funding.

Institutional Review Board Statement: This study was approved by the Institutional Review Committee of the Kyorin University School of Medicine (1507).

Informed Consent Statement: All of the patients received a detailed explanation of the surgical and ophthalmic procedures, and all signed an informed consent form. All of the patients consented to our review of their medical records and their anonymized use in medical publications. The patient consent for this study was obtained in an opt-out format.

Data Availability Statement: The data presented in this study are available on request from the corresponding author (M.I.).

Acknowledgments: The authors thank Duco Hamasaki, Emeritus of the Bascom Palmer Eye Institute, University of Miami, Miami, Florida, for discussions and thorough editing of the manuscript. The corresponding author (M.I.) had full access to all the data in the study and takes responsibility for the integrity of the data and the accuracy of the data analysis.

Conflicts of Interest: M.I.: research grants from Alcon Laboratories, Inc., and personal fees (lecture fees) from Alcon Laboratories, Inc., Novartis Pharma K.K., Bayer AG, Carl Zeiss Meditec AG, Novartis Pharma K.K., Santen Pharmaceutical Co., Ltd., and Senju Pharmaceutical Co., Ltd. AMO, Logitec and Design, outside the submitted work. T.K.: research grants from Ellex, and personal fees (lecture fees) from Alcon Laboratories, Inc., Novartis Pharma K.K., Bayer AG, Carl Zeiss Meditec AG, Novartis Pharma K.K., Santen Pharmaceutical Co., Ltd., and Senju Pharmaceutical Co., Ltd. AMO., outside the submitted work. A.H.: research grants from Santen Pharmaceutical Co., Ltd., personal fees (lecture fees) from Santen Pharmaceutical Co., Ltd., Alcon Laboratories, Inc., Novartis Pharma K.K., Bayer AG, Sanwagkagaku, KOWA, Senju Pharmaceutical Co., Ltd., outside the submitted work.

References

1. Wagoner, M.D.; Cox, T.A.; Ariyasu, R.G.; Jacobs, D.S.; Karp, C.L.; American Academy of Ophthalmology. Intraocular lens implantation in the absence of capsular support: A report by the American Academy of Ophthalmology. *Ophthalmology* **2003**, *110*, 840–859. [CrossRef]
2. Monteiro, M.; Marinho, A.; Borges, S.; Ribeiro, L.; Correia, C. Scleral fixation in eyes with loss of capsule or zonule support. *J. Cataract Refract. Surg.* **2007**, *33*, 573–576. [CrossRef] [PubMed]
3. Vote, B.J.; Tranos, P.; Bunce, C.; Charteris, D.G.; Da Cruz, L. Long-term outcome of combined pars plana vitrectomy and scleral fixated sutured posterior chamber intraocular lens implantation. *Am. J. Ophthalmol.* **2006**, *141*, 308–312. [CrossRef] [PubMed]
4. Gabor, S.G.; Pavlidis, M.M. Sutureless intrascleral posterior chamber intraocular lens fixation. *J. Cataract Refract. Surg.* **2007**, *33*, 1851–1854. [CrossRef] [PubMed]
5. Scharioth, G.B.; Prasad, S.; Georgalas, I.; Tatarum, C.; Pavlidism, M. Intermediate results of sutureless intrascleral posterior chamber intraocular lens fixation. *J. Cataract Refract. Surg.* **2010**, *36*, 254–259. [CrossRef] [PubMed]
6. Ohta, T.; Toshida, H.; Murakami, A. Simplified and safe method of sutureless intrascleral posterior chamber intraocular lens fixation: Y-fixation technique. *J. Cataract Refract. Surg.* **2014**, *40*, 2–7. [CrossRef]
7. Yamane, S.; Inoue, M.; Arakawa, A.; Kadonosono, K. Sutureless 27-gauge needle-guided intrascleral intraocular lens implantation with lamellar scleral dissection. *Ophthalmology* **2014**, *121*, 61–66. [CrossRef]
8. Yamane, S.; Sato, S.; Maruyama-Inoue, M.; Kadonosono, K. Flanged Intrascleral Intraocular Lens Fixation with Double-Needle Technique. *Ophthalmology* **2017**, *124*, 1136–1142. [CrossRef]

9. Kujime, Y.; Akimoto, M. Repair of angle recession prevents pupillary capture of intrasclerally fixed intraocular lenses. *Int. Ophthalmol.* **2019**, *39*, 1163–1168. [CrossRef]
10. Bang, S.P.; Joo, C.K.; Jun, J.H. Reverse pupillary block after implantation of a scleral-sutured posterior chamber intraocular lens: A retrospective, open study. *BMC Ophthalmol.* **2017**, *17*, 35. [CrossRef] [PubMed]
11. Kim, S.I.; Kim, K. Tram-Track Suture Technique for Pupillary Capture of a Scleral Fixated Intraocular Lens. *Case Rep. Ophthalmol.* **2016**, *7*, 290–295. [CrossRef] [PubMed]
12. Higashide, T.; Shimizu, F.; Nishimura, A.; Sugiyama, K. Anterior segment optical coherence tomography findings of reverse pupillary block after scleral-fixated sutured posterior chamber intraocular lens implantation. *J. Cataract Refract. Surg.* **2009**, *35*, 1540–1547. [CrossRef] [PubMed]
13. Silva, A.F.; Pimenta, F.; Alves, M.A.; Oliveira, M.S.N. Flow dynamics of vitreous humour during saccadic eye movements. *J. Mech. Behav. Biomed. Mater.* **2020**, *110*, 103860. [CrossRef] [PubMed]
14. Abouali, O.; Modareszadeh, A.; Ghaffariyeh, A.; Tu, J. Numerical simulation of the fluid dynamics in vitreous cavity due to saccadic eye movement. *Med. Eng. Phys.* **2012**, *34*, 681–692. [CrossRef]
15. Abouali, O.; Modareszadeh, A.; Ghaffarieh, A.; Tu, J. Investigation of saccadic eye movement effects on the fluid dynamic in the anterior chamber. *J. Biomech. Eng.* **2012**, *134*, 021002. [CrossRef]
16. Modarreszadeh, S.; Abouali, O.; Ghaffariehm, A.; Ahmadim, G. Physiology of aqueous humor dynamic in the anterior chamber due to rapid eye movement. *Physiol. Behav.* **2014**, *135*, 112–118. [CrossRef]
17. Fitt, A.D.; Gonzalez, G. Fluid Mechanics of the Human Eye: Aqueous Humour Flow in The Anterior Chamber. *Bull. Math. Biol.* **2006**, *68*, 53–71. [CrossRef]
18. Radhakrishnan, S.; Yarovoy, D. Development in anterior segment imaging for glaucoma. *Curr. Opin. Ophthalmol.* **2014**, *25*, 98–103. [CrossRef]
19. Angmo, D.; Nongpiur, M.E.; Sharma, R.; Sidhu, T.; Sihota, R.; Dada, T. Clinical utility of anterior segment swept-source optical coherence tomography in glaucoma. *Oman J. Ophthalmol.* **2016**, *9*, 3–10. [CrossRef]
20. Zarei, M.; KhaliliPour, E.; Ebrahimiadib, N.; Riazi-Esfahani, H. Quantitative Analysis of the Iris Surface Smoothness by Anterior Segment Optical Coherence Tomography in Fuchs Uveitis. *Ocul. Immunol. Inflamm.* **2022**, *30*, 697–702. [CrossRef]
21. Zarei, M.; Mahmoudi, T.; Riazi-Esfahani, H.; Mousavi, B.; Ebrahimiadib, N.; Yaseri, M.; Khalili Pour, E.; Arabalibeik, H. Automated measurement of iris surface smoothness using anterior segment optical coherence tomography. *Sci. Rep.* **2021**, *11*, 8505. [CrossRef] [PubMed]
22. Yu, B.; Wang, K.; Zhang, X.; Xing, X. Biometric indicators of anterior segment parameters before and after laser peripheral iridotomy by swept-source optical coherent tomography. *BMC. Ophthalmol.* **2022**, *22*, 222. [CrossRef] [PubMed]
23. Ikegawa, W.; Suzuki, T.; Namiguchi, K.; Mizoue, S.; Shiraishi, A.; Ohashi, Y. Changes in Anterior Segment Morphology of Iris Bombe before and after Laser Peripheral Iridotomy in Patients with Uveitic Secondary Glaucoma. *J. Ophthalmol.* **2016**, *2016*, 8496201. [CrossRef] [PubMed]
24. Panda, S.K.; Tan, R.K.Y.; Tun, T.A.; Buist, M.L.; Nongpiur, M.; Baskaran, M.; Aung, T.; Girard, M.J.A. Changes in Iris Stiffness and Permeability in Primary Angle Closure Glaucoma. *Investig. Ophthalmol. Vis. Sci.* **2021**, *62*, 29. [CrossRef]
25. Ye, S.; Bao, C.; Chen, Y.; Shen, M.; Lu, F.; Zhang, S.; Zhu, D. Identification of Peripheral Anterior Synechia by Corneal Deformation Using Air-Puff Dynamic Anterior Segment Optical Coherence Tomography. *Front. Bioeng. Biotechnol.* **2022**, *10*, 856531. [CrossRef]
26. Khodabande, A.; Mohammadi, M.; Riazi-Esfahani, H.; Karami, S.; Mirghorbani, M.; Modjtahedi, B.S. Changes in anterior segment optical coherence tomography following pars plana vitrectomy without tamponade. *Int. J. Retin. Vitr.* **2021**, *7*, 15. [CrossRef]
27. Singh, H.; Modabber, M.; Safran, S.G.; Ahmed, I.I. Laser iridotomy to treat uveitis-glaucoma-hyphema syndrome secondary to reverse pupillary block in sulcus-placed intraocular lenses: Case series. *J. Cataract Refract. Surg.* **2015**, *41*, 2215–2223. [CrossRef]
28. Bharathi, M.; Balakrishnan, D.; Senthil, S. "Pseudophakic Reverse Pupillary Block" Following Yamane Technique Scleral-fixated Intraocular Lens. *J. Glaucoma* **2020**, *29*, e68–e70. [CrossRef]

Article

Correlation between Choroidal Vascularity Index and Outer Retina in Patients with Diabetic Retinopathy

Patryk Sidorczuk *, Iwona Obuchowska, Joanna Konopinska and Diana A. Dmuchowska *

Ophthalmology Department, Medical University of Bialystok, 24a M. Sklodowskiej-Curie, 15-276 Bialystok, Poland; iwonaobu@wp.pl (I.O.); joannakonopinska@o2.pl (J.K.)
* Correspondence: patryk.sidorczuk@gmail.com (P.S.); diana.dmuchowska@umb.edu.pl (D.A.D.)

Abstract: The choroid supplies blood to the outer retina. We quantified outer retinal and choroidal parameters to understand better the pathogenesis of diabetic retinopathy (DR) and diabetic macular edema (DME). The retrospective cross-sectional single-center study included 210 eyes from 139 diabetic patients and 76 eyes from 52 healthy controls. Spectral-domain optical coherence tomography (OCT) was carried out with a Spectralis HRA + OCT imaging device. The outer retinal layer (ORL), outer nuclear layer (ONL), and choroidal thicknesses were assessed along with the choroidal vascularity index (CVI). The presence of DR, whether with DME or without, was associated with choroidal thinning ($p < 0.001$). Compared with the controls, patients with DR without DME presented with lower ORL and ONL thickness ($p < 0.001$), whereas those with DR and DME had higher values of both parameters ($p < 0.001$). Significant correlations between outer retinal and choroidal parameters were found only in patients with DR without DME (ORL with choroidal thickness: $p = 0.003$, rho = 0.34; ORL with CVI: $p < 0.001$, rho = 0.49, ONL with CVI: $p < 0.027$, rho = 0.25). No correlations between choroidal and outer retinal parameters were observed in the controls and patients with DR and concomitant DME. Aside from diabetic choroidopathy, other pathogenic mechanisms seem to predominate in the latter group.

Keywords: choroid; choroidal thickness; choroidal vascularity index; diabetic macular edema; OCT; outer retina; outer retinal layer; outer nuclear layer

1. Introduction

The macula is supplied with blood from two independent sources. The inner retina, located between the internal limiting membrane (ILM) and the outer plexiform layer (OPL), is perfused by the central retinal artery, whereas the outer retina, spreading between the outer border of the OPL and the Bruch's membrane (BM), is supplied mainly by the choroid [1,2]. Since no retinal vasculature exists in the foveal region, compromised choroidal blood flow may lead to photoreceptor dysfunction [3–6]. Many previous studies demonstrated that in patients with diabetic macular edema (DME), the integrity of the ellipsoid zone and external limiting membrane (ELM) is closely associated with visual function [7–10]. Furthermore, the thickness of some outer retinal layers, e.g., total outer retina [11–13], photoreceptor outer segments [14,15], retinal pigment epithelium (RPE) [16,17], and retinal tissue between the plexiform layers [18], was shown to correlate with visual acuity.

Diabetes may lead to choroidal abnormalities similar to those observed in the retina, such as microaneurysms, dilatation and obstruction of the vessels, vascular remodeling with increased vascular tortuosity, vascular dropout, focal vascular non-perfusion, atrophy of Sattler's layer and Haller's layer, and choroidal vascularization [19–22]. Choroidopathy may trigger the development of retinopathy due to retinal tissue hypoxia and overexpression of vascular endothelial growth factor (VEGF); this contributes to further retinal damage and DME [5,20]. However, it is still unclear whether choroidopathy precedes, accompanies, or follows the retinal changes [3,22–24]. Moreover, the exact contribution of diabetic choroidopathy to the diabetes-associated damage of the neuroretina and occurrence of DME remains poorly understood [22].

DME, the major cause of severe vision loss in patients with diabetes, can occur at any stage of diabetic retinopathy (DR) and affects both the outer and inner retina [25,26]. DME is defined as an abnormal increase in intra- and extracellular fluid volume in the macula. This multifactorial condition involves many complex mechanisms, including the breakdown of the inner- and outer blood-retinal barrier (BRB) [27,28]. Other underlying pathomechanisms of DME include ischemia, neurodegeneration, and edema [29].

Optical coherence tomography (OCT) is the primary tool to visualize the retina and choroid in healthy persons and diabetic patients with DME or without. To assess the relationship between the OCT-based characteristics of the choroid and outer retina, we divided the latter into the outer retinal layer (ORL) and outer nuclear layer (ONL), with the ELM as a border separating the two. ELM is a marker of photoreceptor integrity, and its disruption is associated with visual impairment in DME [7–10]. ELM is an intercellular junction between the Müller cells and photoreceptor cells, constituting a barrier for macromolecules [30]; a disruption of ELM may result in the migration of blood components into the outer retinal layers and resultant exacerbation of photoreceptor damage. ELM can be altered due to hyperglycemia [24]. ORL includes outer and inner segments of photoreceptors and RPE. The outer segments contain discs filled with opsin, responsible for absorbing photons for later signal transduction, whereas the inner segments are a reservoir of mitochondria needed for energy supply. Consequently, both inner and outer segments have an essential function in the visual pathway [11]. RPE constitutes the outer BRB. It removes the waste that remained after the phagocytosis of photoreceptors' outer segments, provides nutrients for photoreceptors, absorbs light, pumps the fluid towards choriocapillaris, and controls retinal oxidative stress [24].

In the present study, we focused on choroidopathy, a component of DR and DME pathogenesis [3,5,20,22–24]. We aimed to explain the relationship between outer retinal and choroidal parameters. Aside from determining the choroidal thickness, we also calculated the choroidal vascularity index (CVI). CVI is a novel, OCT-based choroidal quantitative parameter providing more detailed information about the vascular component of the choroid across all its layers, i.e., choriocapillaris, Sattler's layer, and Haller's layer [31,32]. CVI has been proposed as a marker for early diagnosis, progression monitoring, and stratification of patients with various retinal and choroidal diseases and systemic conditions, including those of vascular or inflammatory origin [31]. Unlike the choroidal thickness, which depends on multiple physiological and pathological factors [31–35], CVI is considered a relatively stable parameter to evaluate changes in choroidal vasculature [36].

A number of previous studies analyzed either choroidal [6,17,34,37–43] or retinal characteristics [11–18,44] in diabetic patients with DR with concomitant DME or without. However, to the best of our knowledge, this is the first study to explore the link between the choroidal parameters (CVI and choroidal thickness) and the parameters of outer retinal thickness in such patients. A better insight into the pathogenesis of DR and DME may facilitate the stratification of patients in terms of prognosis and their qualification for novel treatments from the spectrum of personalized medicine.

2. Materials and Methods

The retrospective single-center cross-sectional study included 286 eyes from 191 patients (139 with DR and 52 controls). Medical records were analyzed for the period between 28 February 2017 and 20 February 2021. In 210 eyes from patients with diabetes, DR was confirmed by fluorescein angiography. The DR group was divided into two subgroups based on the presence of DME (DR + DME+) or lack thereof (DR + DME−). The control group (76 eyes) consisted of patients scheduled for routine ocular examination at the Department of Ophthalmology, University Teaching Hospital of Bialystok.

All patients underwent spectral-domain OCT examination. DME was diagnosed whenever the retinal thickness in the central macular subfield (1 mm in diameter) of the Early Treatment Diabetic Retinopathy Study (ETDRS) grid sector was ≥300 μm and excluded if the thickness was <300 μm [45].

The exclusion criteria of the study were: prior posterior segment surgery or intravitreal injections, macular laser photocoagulation, ametropia ≥ 3.0 diopters, macular changes resulting from other ocular diseases, glaucoma, known ocular or systemic pathology potentially able to affect the choroidal vasculature, and insufficient quality of OCT images.

The study was conducted in line with the provisions of the Declaration of Helsinki and approved by the Ethics Committee at the Medical University of Bialystok (approval number APK.002.216.2020). Written informed consent was provided by all patients involved in the study.

2.1. Optical Coherence Tomography Images Acquisition and Analysis

The protocol of the study was described elsewhere [46]. The OCT images were taken in mydriasis between 8 a.m. and 11 a.m. to avoid diurnal variation in the choroidal thickness. The images were independently assessed by two investigators (P.S. and D.A.D.) blinded to the clinical characteristics of examined eyes.

Spectral-domain OCT was carried out with a Spectralis HRA + OCT imaging device with eye tracking (Heidelberg Engineering, Heidelberg, Germany). The protocol of the OCT imaging comprised of 25 horizontal raster scans (20 × 20°) and a linear B-scan centered at the fovea. The segmentation of the retinal layers was carried out automatically with the Spectralis software (version 6.7, Heidelberg Engineering, Heidelberg, Germany), as shown in Figure 1. The internal limiting membrane (ILM), outer plexiform layer (OPL), external limiting membrane (ELM), and Bruch's membrane (BM) were detected automatically, and the choroidal–scleral junction was marked manually on each scan by shifting the BM line to the choroidal–scleral junction, as described previously [46]. Manual measurements were reviewed by the authors, and disagreements were resolved through discussion.

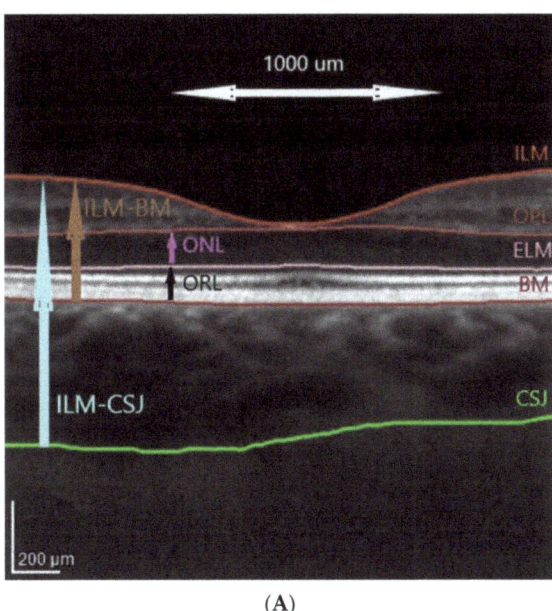

(A)

Figure 1. *Cont.*

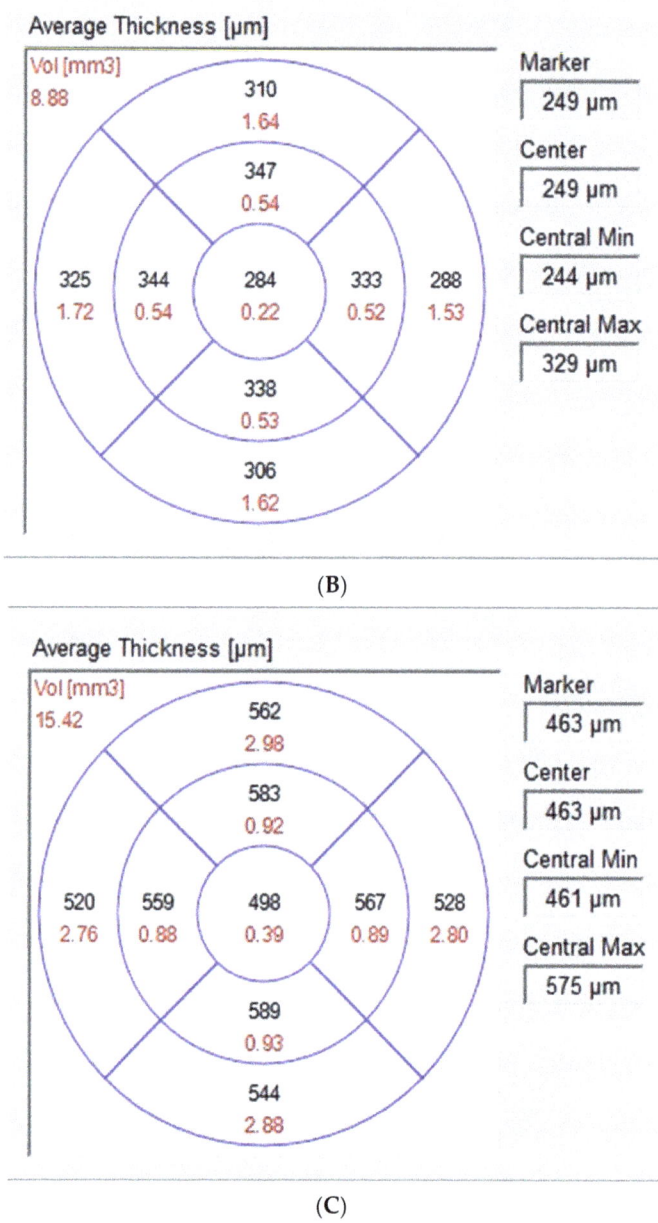

Figure 1. (**A**) Retinal layer segmentation and marking of the choroidal–scleral junction. (**B**) An ETDRS macular map showing retinal thickness (ILM-BM) and volume in 10 subfields. (**C**) An ETDRS macular map showing total thickness (ILM-CSJ) and volume in 10 subfields. Abbreviations: ILM, internal limiting membrane; OPL, outer plexiform layer; ELM, external limiting membrane; BM, Bruch's membrane; CSJ, choroidal–scleral junction; ONL, outer nuclear layer; ORL, outer retinal layer; ETDRS, Early Treatment Diabetic Retinopathy Study.

Based on ETDRS macular maps the values of choroidal parameters were obtained by subtracting retinal parameters (calculated automatically from the ILM to the BM, Figure 1A,B) from total parameters (calculated automatically from the ILM to the manually marked choroidal–scleral junction, Figure 1C). The fovea was checked and, if necessary, manually replotted. The outer retina was defined as the ONL and the ORL sum. The ONL and the ORL were defined according to the Heidelberg Spectralis HRA-OCT software, with the ONL as an area between the outer border of the OPL and the ELM and the outer retinal layer (ORL) as an area between the ELM and the BM (Figure 1A). The choroid was defined as an area between the BM and the choroidal–scleral junction.

The values for the central 1 mm ring (within a 500 μm radius from the center of the macula) were extracted from the ETDRS macular map. Average central macular thickness at the ONL and ORL was calculated by the OCT software. Choroidal central macular thickness was calculated by subtraction, as described above.

2.2. Binarization of Subfoveal Choroidal Images

Binarization and segmentation of the images were done with ImageJ software (http://imagej.nih.gov/ij, accessed on 5 May 2021, version 1.49, U. S. National Institutes of Health, Bethesda, MD, USA), using the protocol proposed by Sonoda [32,47]. Briefly, the area within a 500 μm distance nasally and temporally from the fovea was analyzed on the horizontal scan across the fovea using the polygon selection tool, with the BM as the upper margin and the choroidal–scleral junction as the lower margin. Luminal area (LA) and total choroidal area (TCA) were measured. Stromal area (SA) was calculated, and CVI was determined as the LA to TCA ratio [31,32] (Supplementary Figure S1A–D). The inter-grader reliability was measured by the absolute agreement model of the intraclass correlation coefficient (ICC). ICC values for choroidal parameters were greater than 0.8, which indicated good agreement. With Bland–Altman plot analyses, the fixed and proportional bias were excluded.

2.3. Fluorescein Angiograms Acquisition and Analysis

Fluorescein angiography was performed with a Spectralis HRA + OCT imaging device (Heidelberg Engineering, Heidelberg, Germany) according to the standard procedure. The images were used to assess the severity of DR according to the ETDRS criteria [48,49].

2.4. Statistical Analysis

Statistical analyses were carried out with R software (version 3.5.1, R Foundation for Statistical Computing, Vienna, Austria). Descriptive statistics included numbers (percentages within each group) for nominal variables and means ± standard deviations (SD) for continuous variables. The normality of the distribution was verified with the Shapiro–Wilk test, on the basis of skewness and kurtosis values, as well as based on visual inspection of histograms. Between-group comparisons were carried out with a chi-square test or Fisher exact test for nominal variables and one-way ANOVA for continuous variables, whichever appropriate. Whenever the result of the ANOVA was statistically significant, Tukey post hoc test was applied. The relationships between pairs of continuous variables were verified based on Spearman's correlation analysis. Linear univariate and multivariate regression analysis was carried out to assess relationship between choroidopathy and outer retinal thickness. Multivariate models were based on stepwise approach with AIC criterium, and independent variables with $p < 0.157$ in univariate analysis were included into multivariate models [50]. Both univariate and multivariate models were adjusted for covariates: age, sex, DR severity, and PRP. All tests were two-tailed with $\alpha = 0.05$.

3. Results

3.1. Baseline Characteristics

The study included a total of 191 patients (286 eyes). Patients with DR with concomitant DME (DR + DME+) or without (DR + DME−) and the controls did not differ significantly in terms of age, sex, and spherical equivalent. Baseline characteristics of both groups of patients with DR and the controls are presented in Table 1.

Table 1. Baseline characteristics of patients with DR with concomitant DME or without and healthy controls.

	Overall	Group			p
		DR + DME+	DR + DME−	Controls	
Number of patients	191	49	90	52	
Number of eyes	286	76	134	76	
Age, years, mean ± SD	59.24 ± 14.43	61.50 ± 11.92	60.03 ± 13.19	55.73 ± 17.87	0.103
Sex, female, n (%)	100 (52.4)	25 (51.0)	47 (52.2)	28 (53.8)	0.960
Spherical equivalent, mean ± SD	0.32 ± 1.10	0.43 ± 1.07	0.23 ± 0.99	0.39 ± 1.28	0.371
DR severity, n (%)					
NPDR	135 (47.2)	50 (65.8)	85 (63.4)	-	0.766 [1]
PDR	75 (26.2)	26 (34.2)	49 (36.6)	-	
PRP, n (%)					
No	138 (48.3)	48 (63.2)	90 (67.2)	-	0.650 [1]
Yes	72 (25.2)	28 (36.8)	44 (32.8)	-	

Notes: Groups compared with chi-square test or Fisher exact test [1] for nominal variables and with ANOVA for continuous variables. DME defined as present (DME+) when central macular subfield retinal thickness ≥ 300 μm and absent (DME−) when central macular subfield retinal thickness < 300 μm. Abbreviations: DME, diabetic macular edema; DR, diabetic retinopathy; NPDR, non-proliferative diabetic retinopathy; PDR, proliferative diabetic retinopathy; PRP, panretinal photocoagulation.

3.2. Between-Group Comparison of Outer Retinal and Choroidal Parameters

Healthy controls presented with significantly higher choroidal thickness and CVI values than patients with DR (Table 2). However, the three groups did not differ significantly in terms of other choroidal parameters, i.e., luminal area (LA), stromal area (SA), and total choroidal area (TCA).

Table 2. Choroidal and outer retinal parameters in patients with DR with concomitant DME or without and healthy controls.

	DR + DME+	DR + DME−	Controls	p	Post Hoc		
					DR + DME+ vs. DR + DME−	DR + DME− vs. Controls	DR + DME+ vs. Controls
Choroidal parameters							
CVI	0.62 ± 0.05	0.63 ± 0.05	0.65 ± 0.05	0.001	0.576	0.089	**<0.001**
LA (mm^2)	0.24 ± 0.05	0.25 ± 0.08	0.25 ± 0.06	0.266			
SCA (mm^2)	0.15 ± 0.03	0.14 ± 0.04	0.14 ± 0.03	0.204			
TCA (mm^2)	0.39 ± 0.08	0.40 ± 0.01	0.39 ± 0.08	0.773			
Choroid (μm)	250.75 ± 45.61	265.34 ± 60.91	303.64 ± 72.77	**<0.001**	0.218	**<0.001**	**<0.001**
Central macular thickness (1 mm diameter)							
ORL (μm)	92.58 ± 24.10	84.20 ± 4.97	87.64 ± 3.52	**<0.001**	**<0.001**	0.157	0.052
ONL (μm)	141.70 ± 85.70	82.38 ± 18.03	92.13 ± 10.81	**<0.001**	**<0.001**	0.306	**<0.001**

Notes: Data presented as mean ± SD. Groups compared with ANOVA. In cases of statistically significant differences, Tukey post hoc test was applied. Significant p values in bold. Abbreviations: DME, diabetic macular edema; DR, diabetic retinopathy; CVI, choroidal vascularity index; LA, luminal area; SA, stromal area; TCA, total choroidal area; ORL, outer retinal layer; ONL, outer nuclear layer.

Compared with healthy controls, patients from the DR + DME− group presented with a lower thickness of both components of the outer retina, ORL and ONL. Meanwhile, the values of both these parameters in patients from the DR + DME+ group were significantly higher than in the control group.

3.3. Intra-Group Correlations and Regressions between Outer Retinal and Choroidal Parameters

We analyzed correlations between the outer retinal (ONL and ORL) and choroidal parameters (choroidal thickness, CVI, LA, SA, and TCA) within each of the three groups

(Table 3). No significant correlations between the choroidal and outer retinal parameters were found in the controls and DR + DME+ group. In DR + DME− group, however, ORL correlated positively with choroidal central macular thickness, CVI, and LA, and a positive correlation was found between ONL and CVI.

Table 3. Correlations between outer retinal and choroidal parameters in patients with DR with concomitant DME or without and healthy controls.

Correlation:	DR + DME+		DR + DME−		Controls	
	Rho	p	Rho	p	Rho	p
ORL central macular thickness (1 mm diameter)						
Choroidal central macular thickness (μm)	0.23	0.160	**0.34**	**0.003**	0.27	0.069
CVI	−0.01	0.953	**0.49**	**<0.001**	0.12	0.426
LA (mm^2)	0.23	0.171	**0.41**	**<0.001**	0.19	0.191
SA (mm^2)	0.17	0.314	0.12	0.293	0.05	0.719
TCA (mm^2)	0.18	0.285	0.32	0.005	0.17	0.242
ONL central macular thickness (1 mm diameter)						
Choroidal central macular thickness (μm)	−0.07	0.683	0.01	0.932	−0.27	0.058
CVI	0.35	0.031	**0.25**	**0.027**	0.14	0.336
LA (mm^2)	0.08	0.641	0.09	0.430	−0.02	0.871
SA (mm^2)	−0.22	0.191	−0.20	0.077	−0.16	0.289
TCA (mm^2)	−0.03	0.856	−0.01	0.981	−0.09	0.558

Notes: rho, Spearman's correlation coefficient. Only the results for a single eye from each patient were considered during the analysis, n = 191. Since the dataset included the results for a single eye from each patient, there was no violation of the independence assumption between observations for correlation analysis. Significant p values with rho values in bold. Abbreviations: DME, diabetic macular edema; DR, diabetic retinopathy; CVI, choroidal vascularity index; LA, luminal area; SA, stromal area; TCA, total choroidal area; ORL, outer retinal layer; ONL, outer nuclear layer.

Based on univariate regression analysis (Table 4), ORL central macular thickness (1-mm diameter) was associated with choroidal central macular thickness (β = 0.03, p = 0.019), CVI (β = 43.70, p < 0.001), LA (β = 18.73, p = 0.004), and TCA (β = 10.20, p = 0.021). Multivariate model for ORL indicated that CVI alone (β = 43.70, p < 0.001) was the best determinant of ORL with R^2 = 0.26 (R^2 adj. = 0.21). Inclusion of other parameters did not increase the quality of model. Low value of R^2 indicated presence of other factors additional to this analysis impacting the thickness of ORL.

Table 4. Univariate linear regression for ORL and ONL in patients with DR without concomitant DME.

	ORL Central Macular Thickness (1 mm Diameter)				ONL Central Macular Thickness (1 mm Diameter)			
	β	SE	p	R^2/R^2 adj.	β	SE	p	R^2/R^2 adj.
Choroidal central macular thickness (μm)	0.03	0.01	**0.019**	0.14/0.08	0.03	0.04	0.395	0.23/0.18
CVI	43.70	9.93	**<0.001**	0.26/0.21	67.03	36.32	0.069	0.26/0.21
LA (mm^2)	18.73	6.22	**0.004**	0.17/0.11	7.94	21.92	0.718	0.23/0.17
SA (mm^2)	12.29	12.54	0.330		−34.52	41.74	0.411	0.23/0.18
TCA (mm^2)	10.20	4.32	**0.021**	0.13/0.07	−0.70	14.91	0.963	0.23/0.17

Notes: β, beta estimate; SE, standard error; R^2 adj., adjusted R-squared. Only the results for a single eye from each patient were considered during the analysis, n = 90. All models were adjusted for covariates: age, sex, DR severity, and PRP. Significant p vales in bold. Abbreviations: DME, diabetic macular edema; DR, diabetic retinopathy; CVI, choroidal vascularity index; LA, luminal area; SA, stromal area; TCA, total choroidal area; ORL, outer retinal layer; ONL, outer nuclear layer.

For ONL univariate regression analysis did not identify significant associations.

4. Discussion

As the demand of the outer retina for oxygen and nutrients is primarily covered by diffusion from the choroidal circulation [5], we decided to quantify outer retinal and choroidal parameters in patients with DR. Our study showed that patients with DR had the lower choroidal thickness and CVI than healthy controls. While the thickness of two components of the outer retina, ORL and ONL, in patients from the DR + DME− group was lower than in the controls, patients from the DR + DME+ group presented with higher values of these parameters than persons from the control group. Additionally, in patients from the DR + DME− group, ORL correlated positively with choroidal central macular thickness and LA; furthermore, both ORL and ONL correlated positively with CVI in this group of patients.

Choroidal thickness varies depending on multiple physiological and pathological factors, such as age, sex, refraction, axial length, time of the day, DME, DR severity and PRP, duration, and control of DM [31–35,40]. Our study groups did not differ significantly in terms of age, sex, spherical equivalent, DR severity, and PRP rate, and hence, a confounding effect of these variables was unlikely. CVI is a more independent measure [31,36] and therefore was considered a primary variable analyzed in this study.

In our study, healthy controls presented with significantly higher choroidal thickness than patients with DR, whether with concomitant DME or without. Although published data in this matter are inconclusive, our findings are in line with most previous studies [6,17,34,37–39]. Wang et al. observed increased choroidal thickness at the early stages of DR, followed by a decrease in this parameter with DR progression; meanwhile, DME was not significantly associated with choroidal thickness. Those findings suggest that alterations in choroidal parameters may play a role in the pathogenesis of DR [51]. In our study, the presence of DR was associated with a substantial decrease in CVI, with a statistically significant difference in this parameter observed between the DR + DME+ group and the controls; this observation is consistent with the results of previous studies [40–43]. However, we found no significant between-group differences in other choroidal parameters, LA, SA, and TCA. In our previous study, which centered around the choroid but not the outer retina, patients with various types of DME (cystoid, diffuse, with subretinal fluid) presented with lower CVI and choroidal thickness than the controls [46].

Both components of the outer retina, ORL and ONL, were thinner in the DR + DME− group and thicker in the DR + DME+ group when compared with healthy controls. Our findings are consistent with the results published by Sim et al., who reported outer retinal thinning in eyes with diabetic macular ischemia without macular edema and found outer retinal thickening in eyes with macular edema [12]. According to those authors, the ischemic thinning might be masked by coexisting edema. Our findings seem to support this hypothesis. We found significant differences in ORL and ONL thickness in patients with DR with concomitant DME and without. Thinning of the outer retina reflects neurodegeneration, which might be a reason behind the reduced outer retinal thickness in the DR + DME− group. Reduced choroidal thickness associated with DR may lead to the hypoxia of retinal tissues, resultant impairment of outer BRB, development of DME, and further progression thereof [6]. At a molecular level, hyperglycemia is associated with the activation of various pathways, including polyol pathway, protein kinase C pathway, generation of advanced glycation end-products, inflammation, and oxidative stress [24,52]. Activation of those pathways affects retinal and choroidal vessels and neurons, RPE cells, and glial cells [26,53].

Our findings are partly in agreement with the results published by Wang et al., according to whom DR patients presented with significantly lower choroidal, ORL, and RPE thickness than the controls, without significant differences observed between patients with concomitant DME and without [17]. Damian et al. found thinner ONL and ORL in patients in whom diabetes coexisted with mild DR or lack thereof, without concomitant DME [54]. Other authors reported outer retinal atrophic changes in DME [13] with PROS (photoreceptor outer segment) shortening [13,44].

In the present study, ORL thickness in the DR + DME− group correlated significantly with choroidal central macular thickness, CVI, and LA; a significant correlation between ONL and CVI was found in this group as well. Multivariate model for ORL indicated that CVI alone was the best determinant of ORL. To the best of our knowledge, none of the previous studies documented such correlations in patients with DR and concomitant DME. Damian et al. analyzed correlations between choroidal and outer retinal parameters in diabetic patients with mild DR or lack thereof, without concomitant DME. They found significant correlations between CVI and RPE thickness as well as between choroidal thickness and photoreceptor layer thickness [54]. While the results of that study could be partially consistent with our findings in the DR + DME− group, the analyzed cohort differed considerably, as it included patients with mild or absent DR.

Consistently with previous reports [54,55], we found no significant correlations between choroidal parameters (CVI and choroidal thickness) and outer retinal parameters in healthy controls.

Similarly, no significant correlations between retinal and choroidal parameters were observed in the DR + DME+ group. Gerendas et al. analyzed total retinal thickness and choroidal thickness in patients with DME and also did not find a significant correlation between these parameters [56]. However, in our present study, we considered outer retinal thickness rather than total retinal thickness, and hence, our findings should not necessarily be directly compared with those reported by Gerendas et al. [56] The lack of correlation between outer retinal parameters and choroidal parameters in patients with DME might reflect complex pathogenesis of this condition. All cells maintain internal homeostasis due to the existence of membrane transport systems that control the inflow and outflow of ions from the cell. Many pathological conditions (e.g., ischemia) are not only associated with the disruption of the BRB but may also lead to the damage of membrane ionic channels and resultant cellular swelling. Thus, neuronal and/or glial swelling may often be a component of retinal edema; probably, this refers in particular to the areas of ischemic capillary loss where severe metabolic insult occurs, and no viable capillaries survive to generate extracellular fluid [57]. Consequently, different stages of macular edema, i.e., cytotoxic (intracellular) versus vasogenic (extracellular), need to be considered and analyzed separately [58]. Moreover, patients may differ in terms of the disease pathways involved. Finally, ischemia, neurodegeneration, and edema can occur independently from one another [29,59,60].

In summary, we cautiously hypothesize that the blood supply is more than sufficient in healthy controls even with a variable flow through the choroid. However, this is not the case in patients with DR, as shown by decreased choroidal thickness and lower CVI values. The choroidal atrophy may lead to ischemia as a predominant pathogenetic mechanism of DR at this stage. Hypoxia may, in turn, cause RPE and photoreceptor degeneration, with resultant thinning of the outer retina. Further stages of the disease, when the disruption of the BRB occurs, and DME develops, involve multiple and complex pathogenetic mechanisms, and as a result, the relationship between choroidal circulation and outer retinal thickness is not that evident.

This study has some strengths, among them the inclusion of DME treatment-naïve patients and the analysis of age-, sex-, and refractive error-matched groups. All measurements were taken between 8 a.m. and 11 a.m. to avoid diurnal variations. The study included a homogenous group consisting solely of patients with spherical equivalent refractive error < 3.0 diopters. Compared with previous studies, we analyzed a larger number of patients with proliferative DR, often underrepresented in clinical research. Notably, we considered multiple choroidal parameters rather than only thickness. Further, this is the first published study to analyze a correlation between CVI and outer retinal thickness in such a group of patients.

We are well-aware of the potential limitations of this study. Due to the retrospective design of the study, the information about the type of diabetes, laboratory values, and the time of the onset of DME was unavailable. It also needs to be stressed that CVI was determined based on a 1 mm single foveal scan; this is a relatively common practice given that CVI is similar across all the ETDRS subfields [35]. Future advances in automated three-dimensional CVI evaluation may address this limitation. Furthermore, we focused solely on anatomical parameters; meanwhile, the analysis of correlations between functional parameters seems to be an interesting direction for future research. Additionally, we analyzed only a single mechanism involved in DR/DME development, i.e., choroidopathy, whereas the pathogenesis of these conditions is complex. We did not consider a recently discovered role of previously underappreciated, deep capillary plexus in satisfying the metabolic requirements of the outer retina [2]. Future studies may address this limitation by introducing OCT angiography in the study design. Unfortunately, the analysis of OCT angiographic images in patients with DME still constitutes a problem nowadays.

5. Conclusions

In conclusion, the presence of DR with concomitant DME or without is associated with changes in choroidal and outer retinal parameters. However, a significant correlation between outer retinal parameters and choroidal parameters was found only in the DR + DME− group, and no link between these parameters was observed in healthy controls and patients from the DR + DME+ group.

Supplementary Materials: The following supporting information can be downloaded at: https://www.mdpi.com/article/10.3390/jcm11133882/s1, Figure S1. Image binarization of the choroid and calculation of choroidal vascularity index (CVI).

Author Contributions: P.S. and D.A.D. worked on the conception, study design, data analysis, and main text; P.S. worked on execution, acquisition of data, and figures and tables; I.O. and J.K. reviewed the whole article. All authors are accountable for the accuracy of the contents, and will ensure that questions related to the accuracy or integrity of any part of the work are appropriately investigated, resolved, and the resolution documented in the literature. All authors have read and agreed to the published version of the manuscript.

Funding: This work was supported by the Medical University of Bialystok, Poland (grant no. SUB/1/DN/21/002/1157).

Institutional Review Board Statement: The study was conducted in line with the provisions of the Declaration of Helsinki and approved by the Ethics Committee at the Medical University of Bialystok (approval number APK.002.216.2020). Written informed consent was provided by all patients involved in the study.

Informed Consent Statement: Informed consent was obtained from all subjects involved in the study.

Data Availability Statement: All the materials and information will be available upon an e-mail request to the corresponding author. Names and exact data of the participants of the study may not be available owing to patient confidentiality and privacy policy.

Conflicts of Interest: The authors declare no conflict of interest.

References

1. Linsenmeier, R.A.; Padnick-Silver, L. Metabolic dependence of photoreceptors on the choroid in the normal and detached retina. *Investig. Ophthalmol. Vis. Sci.* **2000**, *41*, 3117–3123.
2. Scarinci, F.; Nesper, P.L.; Fawzi, A.A. Deep Retinal Capillary Nonperfusion Is Associated with Photoreceptor Disruption in Diabetic Macular Ischemia. *Am. J. Ophthalmol.* **2016**, *168*, 129–138. [CrossRef] [PubMed]
3. Cao, J.; McLeod, S.; Merges, C.A.; Lutty, G.A. Choriocapillaris degeneration and related pathologic changes in human diabetic eyes. *Arch. Ophthalmol.* **1998**, *116*, 589–597. [CrossRef] [PubMed]
4. Parravano, M.; Ziccardi, L.; Borrelli, E.; Costanzo, E.; Frontoni, S.; Picconi, F.; Parisi, V.; Sacconi, R.; Di Renzo, A.; Varano, M.; et al. Outer retina dysfunction and choriocapillaris impairment in type 1 diabetes. *Sci. Rep.* **2021**, *11*, 15183. [CrossRef]
5. Borrelli, E.; Palmieri, M.; Viggiano, P.; Ferro, G.; Mastropasqua, R. Photoreceptor damage in diabetic choroidopathy. *Retina* **2020**, *40*, 1062–1069. [CrossRef]
6. Querques, G.; Lattanzio, R.; Querques, L.; Del Turco, C.; Forte, R.; Pierro, L.; Souied, E.H.; Bandello, F. Enhanced depth imaging optical coherence tomography in type 2 diabetes. *Investig. Ophthalmol. Vis. Sci.* **2012**, *53*, 6017–6024. [CrossRef]

7. Maheshwary, A.S.; Oster, S.F.; Yuson, R.M.; Cheng, L.; Mojana, F.; Freeman, W.R. The association between percent disruption of the photoreceptor inner segment-outer segment junction and visual acuity in diabetic macular edema. *Am. J. Ophthalmol.* **2010**, *150*, 63–67.e1. [CrossRef]
8. Alasil, T.; Keane, P.A.; Updike, J.F.; Dustin, L.; Ouyang, Y.; Walsh, A.C.; Sadda, S.R. Relationship between optical coherence tomography retinal parameters and visual acuity in diabetic macular edema. *Ophthalmology* **2010**, *117*, 2379–2386. [CrossRef]
9. Otani, T.; Yamaguchi, Y.; Kishi, S. Correlation between visual acuity and foveal microstructural changes in diabetic macular edema. *Retina* **2010**, *30*, 774–780. [CrossRef]
10. Murakami, T.; Nishijima, K.; Sakamoto, A.; Ota, M.; Horii, T.; Yoshimura, N. Association of pathomorphology, photoreceptor status, and retinal thickness with visual acuity in diabetic retinopathy. *Am. J. Ophthalmol.* **2011**, *151*, 310–317. [CrossRef]
11. Wong, R.L.; Lee, J.W.; Yau, G.S.; Wong, I.Y. Relationship between Outer Retinal Layers Thickness and Visual Acuity in Diabetic Macular Edema. *Biomed. Res. Int.* **2015**, *2015*, 981471. [CrossRef] [PubMed]
12. Sim, D.A.; Keane, P.A.; Fung, S.; Karampelas, M.; Sadda, S.R.; Fruttiger, M.; Patel, P.J.; Tufail, A.; Egan, C.A. Quantitative analysis of diabetic macular ischemia using optical coherence tomography. *Investig. Ophthalmol. Vis. Sci.* **2014**, *55*, 417–423. [CrossRef] [PubMed]
13. Lee, D.H.; Kim, J.T.; Jung, D.W.; Joe, S.G.; Yoon, Y.H. The relationship between foveal ischemia and spectral-domain optical coherence tomography findings in ischemic diabetic macular edema. *Investig. Ophthalmol. Vis. Sci.* **2013**, *54*, 1080–1085. [CrossRef]
14. Yuodelis, C.; Hendrickson, A. A qualitative and quantitative analysis of the human fovea during development. *Vision Res.* **1986**, *26*, 847–855. [CrossRef]
15. Forooghian, F.; Stetson, P.F.; Meyer, S.A.; Chew, E.Y.; Wong, W.T.; Cukras, C.; Meyerle, C.B.; Ferris, F.L. Relationship between photoreceptor outer segment length and visual acuity in diabetic macular edema. *Retina* **2010**, *30*, 63–70. [CrossRef]
16. Damian, I.; Nicoara, S.D. Optical Coherence Tomography Biomarkers of the Outer Blood-Retina Barrier in Patients with Diabetic Macular Oedema. *J. Diabetes Res.* **2020**, *2020*, 8880586. [CrossRef]
17. Wang, X.N.; Li, S.T.; Li, W.; Hua, Y.J.; Wu, Q. The thickness and volume of the choroid, outer retinal layers and retinal pigment epithelium layer changes in patients with diabetic retinopathy. *Int. J. Ophthalmol.* **2018**, *11*, 1957–1962.
18. Pelosini, L.; Hull, C.C.; Boyce, J.F.; McHugh, D.; Stanford, M.R.; Marshall, J. Optical coherence tomography may be used to predict visual acuity in patients with macular edema. *Investig. Ophthalmol. Vis. Sci.* **2011**, *52*, 2741–2748. [CrossRef]
19. Lutty, G.A. Diabetic choroidopathy. *Vision Res.* **2017**, *139*, 161–167. [CrossRef]
20. Melancia, D.; Vicente, A.; Cunha, J.P.; Abegão Pinto, L.; Ferreira, J. Diabetic choroidopathy: A review of the current literature. *Graefes. Arch. Clin. Exp. Ophthalmol.* **2016**, *254*, 1453–1461. [CrossRef]
21. Sun, Z.; Yang, D.; Tang, Z.; Ng, D.S.; Cheung, C.Y. Optical coherence tomography angiography in diabetic retinopathy: An updated review. *Eye* **2021**, *35*, 149–161. [CrossRef]
22. Brinks, J.; van Dijk, E.H.C.; Klaassen, I.; Schlingemann, R.O.; Kielbasa, S.M.; Emri, E.; Quax, P.H.A.; Bergen, A.A.; Meijer, O.C.; Boon, C.J.F. Exploring the choroidal vascular labyrinth and its molecular and structural roles in health and disease. *Prog. Retin. Eye Res.* **2022**, *87*, 100994. [CrossRef] [PubMed]
23. Sidorczuk, P.; Pieklarz, B.; Konopinska, J.; Saeed, E.; Mariak, Z.; Dmuchowska, D. Foveal avascular zone does not correspond to choroidal characteristics in patients with diabetic retinopathy: A single-center cross-sectional analysis. *Diabetes Metab. Syndr. Obes. Targets Ther.* **2021**, *14*, 2893–2903. [CrossRef] [PubMed]
24. Țălu, Ș.; Nicoara, S.D. Malfunction of outer retinal barrier and choroid in the occurrence and progression of diabetic macular edema. *World J. Diabetes* **2021**, *12*, 437–452. [CrossRef] [PubMed]
25. Klein, R.; Klein, B.E.; Moss, S.E.; Cruickshanks, K.J. The Wisconsin Epidemiologic Study of Diabetic Retinopathy: XVII. The 14-year incidence and progression of diabetic retinopathy and associated risk factors in type 1 diabetes. *Ophthalmology* **1998**, *105*, 1801–1815. [CrossRef]
26. Daruich, A.; Matet, A.; Moulin, A.; Kowalczuk, L.; Nicolas, M.; Sellam, A.; Rotschild, P.-R.; Omri, S.; Gelize, E.; Jonet, L.; et al. Mechanisms of macular edema: Beyond the surface. *Prog. Retin. Eye Res.* **2018**, *63*, 20–68. [CrossRef]
27. Xu, H.Z.; Le, Y.Z. Significance of outer blood-retina barrier breakdown in diabetes and ischemia. *Investig. Ophthalmol. Vis. Sci.* **2011**, *52*, 2160–2164. [CrossRef]
28. Rangasamy, S.; McGuire, P.G.; Franco Nitta, C.; Monickaraj, F.; Oruganti, S.R.; Das, A. Chemokine mediated monocyte trafficking into the retina: Role of inflammation in alteration of the blood-retinal barrier in diabetic retinopathy. *PLoS ONE* **2014**, *9*, e108508. [CrossRef]
29. Marques, I.P.; Alves, D.; Santos, T.; Mendes, L.; Santos, A.R.; Lobo, C.; Durbin, M.; Cunha-Vaz, J. Multimodal Imaging of the Initial Stages of Diabetic Retinopathy: Different Disease Pathways in Different Patients. *Diabetes* **2019**, *68*, 648–653. [CrossRef]
30. Murakami, T.; Yoshimura, N. Structural changes in individual retinal layers in diabetic macular edema. *J. Diabetes Res* **2013**, *2013*, 920713. [CrossRef]
31. Agrawal, R.; Ding, J.; Sen, P.; Rousselot, A.; Chan, A.; Nivison-Smith, L.; Wei, X.; Mahajan, S.; Kim, R.; Mishra, C.; et al. Exploring choroidal angioarchitecture in health and disease using choroidal vascularity index. *Prog. Retin. Eye Res.* **2020**, *77*, 100829. [CrossRef] [PubMed]
32. Sonoda, S.; Sakamoto, T.; Yamashita, T.; Uchino, E.; Kawano, H.; Yoshihara, N.; Terasaki, H.; Shirasawa, M.; Tomita, M.; Ishibashi, T. Luminal and stromal areas of choroid determined by binarization method of optical coherence tomographic images. *Am. J. Ophthalmol.* **2015**, *159*, 1123–1131.e1. [CrossRef] [PubMed]

33. Agrawal, R.; Salman, M.; Tan, K.A.; Karampelas, M.; Sim, D.A.; Keane, P.A.; Pavesio, C. Choroidal Vascularity Index (CVI)–A Novel Optical Coherence Tomography Parameter for Monitoring Patients with Panuveitis? *PLoS ONE* **2016**, *11*, e0146344. [CrossRef] [PubMed]
34. Campos, A.; Campos, E.J.; Martins, J.; Ambrósio, A.F.; Silva, R. Viewing the choroid: Where we stand, challenges and contradictions in diabetic retinopathy and diabetic macular oedema. *Acta Ophthalmol.* **2017**, *95*, 446–459. [CrossRef] [PubMed]
35. Singh, S.R.; Vupparaboina, K.K.; Goud, A.; Dansingani, K.K.; Chhablani, J. Choroidal imaging biomarkers. *Surv. Ophthalmol.* **2019**, *64*, 312–333. [CrossRef]
36. Iovino, C.; Pellegrini, M.; Bernabei, F.; Borrelli, E.; Sacconi, R.; Govetto, A.; Vaggo, A.; Di Zazzo, A.; Forlini, M.; Finocchio, L.; et al. Choroidal Vascularity Index: An In-Depth Analysis of This Novel Optical Coherence Tomography Parameter. *J. Clin. Med.* **2020**, *9*, 595. [CrossRef]
37. Esmaeelpour, M.; Považay, B.; Hermann, B.; Hofer, B.; Kajic, V.; Hale, S.L.; North, R.V.; Drexler, W.; Sheen, N.J.L. Mapping choroidal and retinal thickness variation in type 2 diabetes using three-dimensional 1060-nm optical coherence tomography. *Investig. Ophthalmol. Vis. Sci.* **2011**, *52*, 5311–5316. [CrossRef]
38. Esmaeelpour, M.; Brunner, S.; Ansari-Shahrezaei, S.; Shahrezaei, S.A.; Nemetz, S.; Povazay, B.; Kajic, V.; Drexler, W.; Binder, S. Choroidal thinning in diabetes type 1 detected by 3-dimensional 1060 nm optical coherence tomography. *Investig. Ophthalmol. Vis. Sci.* **2012**, *53*, 6803–6809. [CrossRef]
39. Endo, H.; Kase, S.; Takahashi, M.; Yokoi, M.; Isozaki, C.; Katsuta, S.; Kase, M. Alteration of layer thickness in the choroid of diabetic patients. *Clin. Exp. Ophthalmol.* **2018**, *46*, 926–933. [CrossRef]
40. Tan, K.A.; Laude, A.; Yip, V.; Loo, E.; Wong, E.P.; Agrawal, R. Choroidal vascularity index—A novel optical coherence tomography parameter for disease monitoring in diabetes mellitus? *Acta Ophthalmol.* **2016**, *94*, e612–e616. [CrossRef]
41. Kim, M.; Ha, M.J.; Choi, S.Y.; Park, Y.H. Choroidal vascularity index in type-2 diabetes analyzed by swept-source optical coherence tomography. *Sci. Rep.* **2018**, *8*, 70. [CrossRef] [PubMed]
42. Gupta, C.; Tan, R.; Mishra, C.; Khandelwal, N.; Raman, R.; Kim, R.; Agrawal, R.; Sen, P. Choroidal structural analysis in eyes with diabetic retinopathy and diabetic macular edema-A novel OCT based imaging biomarker. *PLoS ONE* **2018**, *13*, e0207435. [CrossRef] [PubMed]
43. Markan, A.; Agarwal, A.; Arora, A.; Bazgain, K.; Rana, V.; Gupta, V. Novel imaging biomarkers in diabetic retinopathy and diabetic macular edema. *Ther. Adv. Ophthalmol.* **2020**, *12*, 2515841420950513. [CrossRef] [PubMed]
44. Ozkaya, A.; Alkin, Z.; Karakucuk, Y.; Karatas, G.; Fazil, K.; Gurkan Erdogan, M.; Parente, I.; Taskapili, M. Thickness of the retinal photoreceptor outer segment layer in healthy volunteers and in patients with diabetes mellitus without retinopathy, diabetic retinopathy, or diabetic macular edema. *Saudi J. Ophthalmol.* **2017**, *31*, 69–75. [CrossRef]
45. Virgili, G.; Menchini, F.; Casazza, G.; Hogg, R.; Das, R.R.; Wang, X.; Michelessi, M. Optical coherence tomography (OCT) for detection of macular oedema in patients with diabetic retinopathy. *Cochrane Database Syst. Rev.* **2015**, *1*, CD008081. [CrossRef]
46. Dmuchowska, D.A.; Sidorczuk, P.; Pieklarz, B.; Konopińska, J.; Mariak, Z.; Obuchowska, I. Quantitative Assessment of Choroidal Parameters in Patients with Various Types of Diabetic Macular Oedema: A Single-Centre Cross-Sectional Analysis. *Biology* **2021**, *10*, 725. [CrossRef]
47. Sonoda, S.; Sakamoto, T.; Yamashita, T.; Shirasawa, M.; Uchino, E.; Terasaki, H.; Tomita, M. Choroidal structure in normal eyes and after photodynamic therapy determined by binarization of optical coherence tomographic images. *Investig. Ophthalmol. Vis. Sci.* **2014**, *55*, 3893–3899. [CrossRef]
48. Early Treatment Diabetic Retinopathy Study Research Group. Grading diabetic retinopathy from stereoscopic color fundus photographs—An extension of the modified Airlie House classification. ETDRS report number 10. *Ophthalmology* **1991**, *98* (Suppl. 5), 786–806. [CrossRef]
49. Early Treatment Diabetic Retinopathy Study Research Group. Classification of diabetic retinopathy from fluorescein angiograms. ETDRS report number 11. *Ophthalmology* **1991**, *98* (Suppl. 5), 807–822. [CrossRef]
50. Heinze, G.; Dunkler, D. Five myths about variable selection. *Transpl. Int.* **2017**, *30*, 6–10. [CrossRef]
51. Wang, W.; Liu, S.; Qiu, Z.; He, M.; Wang, L.; Li, Y.; Huang, W. Choroidal Thickness in Diabetes and Diabetic Retinopathy: A Swept Source OCT Study. *Investig. Ophthalmol. Vis. Sci.* **2020**, *61*, 29. [CrossRef] [PubMed]
52. Pietrowska, K.; Dmuchowska, D.A.; Krasnicki, P.; Bujalska, A.; Samczuk, P.; Parfieniuk, E.; Kowalczyk, T.; Wojnar, M.; Mariak, Z.; Kretowski, A.; et al. An exploratory LC-MS-based metabolomics study reveals differences in aqueous humor composition between diabetic and non-diabetic patients with cataract. *Electrophoresis* **2018**, *39*, 1233–1240. [CrossRef] [PubMed]
53. Krasnicki, P.; Dmuchowska, D.A.; Proniewska-Skretek, E.; Dobrzycki, S.; Mariak, Z. Ocular haemodynamics in patients with type 2 diabetes and coronary artery disease. *Br. J. Ophthalmol.* **2014**, *98*, 675–678. [CrossRef] [PubMed]
54. Damian, I.; Roman, G.; Nicoară, S.D. Analysis of the Choroid and Its Relationship with the Outer Retina in Patients with Diabetes Mellitus Using Binarization Techniques Based on Spectral-Domain Optical Coherence Tomography. *J. Clin. Med.* **2021**, *10*, 210. [CrossRef]
55. Karahan, E.; Zengin, M.O.; Tuncer, I. Correlation of choroidal thickness with outer and inner retinal layers. *Ophthalmic Surg. Lasers Imaging Retin.* **2013**, *44*, 544–548. [CrossRef]
56. Gerendas, B.S.; Waldstein, S.M.; Simader, C.; Deak, G.; Hajnajeeb, B.; Zhang, L.; Bogunovic, H.; Abramoff, M.D.; Kundi, M.; Sonka, M.; et al. Three-dimensional automated choroidal volume assessment on standard spectral-domain optical coherence tomography and correlation with the level of diabetic macular edema. *Am. J. Ophthalmol.* **2014**, *158*, 1039–1048. [CrossRef]
57. Marmor, M.F. Mechanisms of fluid accumulation in retinal edema. *Doc. Ophthalmol.* **1999**, *97*, 239–249. [CrossRef]

58. Santos, A.R.; Santos, T.; Alves, D.; Marques, I.P.; Lobo, C.; Cunha-Vaz, J. Characterization of Initial Stages of Diabetic Macular Edema. *Ophthalmic Res.* **2019**, *62*, 203–210. [CrossRef]
59. Cunha-Vaz, J.; Ribeiro, L.; Lobo, C. Phenotypes and biomarkers of diabetic retinopathy. *Prog. Retin. Eye Res.* **2014**, *41*, 90–111. [CrossRef]
60. Dmuchowska, D.A.; Krasnicki, P.; Mariak, Z. Can optical coherence tomography replace fluorescein angiography in detection of ischemic diabetic maculopathy? *Graefes Arch. Clin. Exp. Ophthalmol.* **2014**, *252*, 731–738. [CrossRef]

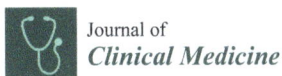

Article

Evaluation of Radial Peripapillary Capillary Density in G6PD Deficiency: An OCT Angiography Pilot Study

Rita Serra [1,2,3,*], Giuseppe D'Amico Ricci [4], Stefano Dore [4], Florence Coscas [3] and Antonio Pinna [4]

1. Department of Biomedical Sciences, University of Sassari, Viale San Pietro 43, 07100 Sassari, Italy
2. Istituto di Ricerca Genetica e Biomedica (IRGB), CNR, Cittadella Universitaria di Cagliari, 09042 Monserrato, Italy
3. Centre Ophtalmologique de l'Odeon, 113 bd Saint Germain, 75006 Paris, France; coscas.f@gmail.com
4. Ophthalmology Unit, Department of Medical, Surgical, and Experimental Sciences, University of Sassari, 07100 Sassari, Italy; giuseppedamicoricci@icloud.com (G.D.R.); stefanodore@hotmail.com (S.D.); apinna@uniss.it (A.P.)
* Correspondence: rita.serra@ymail.com

Abstract: Glucose-6-phosphate-dehydrogenase (G6PD) deficiency is an inherited enzymatic disorder causing hemolytic anemia. The purpose of this pilot study was to compare vascular density (VD) values of the radial peripapillary capillary (RPC) plexus in G6PD-deficient and G6PD-normal men, using optical coherence tomography angiography (OCTA). Methods: 46 G6PD-deficient men and 23 age-matched male controls were included. A complete ophthalmological evaluation, consisting of slit-lamp biomicroscopy, best-corrected visual acuity, intra-ocular pressure measurement, structural optical coherence tomography, and OCTA scanning of the optic nerve head, was performed. The en-face angioflow images were carefully analyzed and the VD values of the RPC plexus were measured using the AngioAnalytics™ software embedded in the OCTA device. Medical conditions, including systemic hypertension, hypercholesterolemia, and diabetes mellitus, were also investigated. Results: G6PD-deficient eyes showed higher values of VD in all peripapillary sectors, but a statistical significance ($p = 0.03$) was reached only in the infero-temporal sector. There were no significant differences in terms of hypercholesterolemia, systemic arterial hypertension, and diabetes mellitus between the two study groups. Conclusion: Results show that VD values of the RPC plexus are higher in G6PD-deficient men than in G6PD-normal subjects, but a statistically significant difference was found only in the inferior temporal sector. Overall, our preliminary findings support the hypothesis that the RPC layer of G6PD-deficient men consists of a denser vascular network, which may contribute to offering protection against ocular atherosclerotic vasculopathies.

Keywords: glucose-6-phosphate-dehydrogenase deficiency; optic nerve head; optical coherence tomography angiography; radial peripapillary capillary; vascular density

1. Introduction

With a worldwide prevalence of approximately 500 million people affected, glucose-6-phosphate-dehydrogenase (G6PD) deficiency is an inherited enzymatic disorder causing hemolytic anemia [1].

G6PD is a ubiquitous cytoplasmatic enzyme implicated in the regulation of carbon flow through the pentose phosphate pathway, essential for cell protection against oxidative stress. G6PD plays a crucial role in the conversion of glucose-6-phosphate into 6-phosphogluconate, a biochemical reaction associated with the simultaneous synthesis of reduced nicotinamide adenine dinucleotide phosphate (NADPH), essential for the proper functioning of glutathione reductase, an enzyme that transforms glutathione disulfide (GSSG) into reduced glutathione (GSH) [2,3]. Hemizygous males have uniformly deficient erythrocytes, whereas heterozygous females have mosaic populations of G6PD-deficient and normal red blood cells because of random inactivation of the X chromosome.

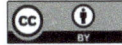

In red blood cells, NADPH production and, therefore, protection against oxidative stress are strongly related to G6PD activity [2]. Consequently, in G6PD-deficient patients, the ingestion of agents with oxidant properties, such as broad bean (*Vicia faba*) or some drugs (e.g., quinine derivatives, sulphonamides, and several anti-inflammatory agents), may trigger a decreased availability of GSH that may cause oxidation of hemoglobin and peroxidation of membrane lipids, thus leading to erythrocyte lysis and jaundice, which are typical clinical manifestations of hemolytic anemia [4].

In Sardinia (Italy), a major Mediterranean island, G6PD deficiency represents a real public health issue, since over 10% of the population shows the G6PD-deficient genotype [4].

It has been supposed that the high prevalence of this inherited enzymopathy may derive from the natural selection induced by Plasmodium falciparum malaria, endemic in Sardinia until the 1950s. In fact, G6PD deficiency, associated with increased oxidative stress in red blood cells, impairs plasmodium growth, offering protection against the development of severe malaria [5].

Previous studies have highlighted that G6PD deficiency seems also to be associated with a decreased risk of developing several systemic and ophthalmological conditions, including cardiovascular and cerebrovascular diseases, colorectal cancer, retinal vein occlusion (RVO), and nonarteritic anterior ischemic optic neuropathy (NA-AION) [2,4,6,7]. G6PD deficiency also shows a trend for protection against severe proliferative diabetic retinopathy (PDR) [8]. Although some hypotheses have been proposed, how exactly G6PD deficiency may be involved in protecting against the occurrence of RVO, NA-AION, and perhaps severe PDR is still not known [4].

The retina is a highly metabolic tissue requiring tight regulation of blood perfusion and redox homeostasis for normal functioning. Cumulative oxidative stress causes damage to the retinal microvasculature and ganglion cells. Evidence from animal models indicates that endothelial Nox2, an NADPH-dependent enzyme, contributes to age-related capillary rarefaction in nervous tissue by increasing the production of reactive oxygen species [9]. Theoretically, G6PD deficiency, characterized by decreased NADPH production and, consequently, Nox2 activity, might be associated with a better capillary network.

In the past, our knowledge and understanding of the pathophysiological mechanisms underlying retinal vascular diseases were limited to traditional angiography, an invasive imaging technique allowing only a two-dimensional en-face analysis of the retinal vasculature [10]. The recent introduction of optical coherence tomography angiography (OCTA) in clinical practice has revolutionized our approach to retinal and optic nerve head (ONH) assessment [11]. Indeed, this novel imaging technique generates high-resolution images of retinal and ONH plexuses [11,12]. Specifically, OCTA has made possible the detailed in vivo visualization of the radial peripapillary capillary (RPC) plexus, which is not feasible with traditional imaging techniques [11,13].

Recent research has focused on the RPC plexus, which plays a crucial role in the nourishment of retinal ganglion cells and, as a result, is involved in the pathogenesis of several retinal disorders [14–16]. The embedded OCTA software, by automatically providing quantitative parameters (e.g., vascular density [VD]), allows for the objective evaluation of the blood flow and circulation in the RPC plexus, opening new areas of interesting research [16].

The number of studies assessing the RPC plexus of the ONH is limited [13]. Furthermore, we are unaware of any previous published report investigating the RPC plexus in G6PD-deficient patients. Therefore, the aim of the present study was to determine the VD values of the RPC plexus in G6PD-deficient and G6PD-normal patients and ascertain whether, or not, there were significant differences in terms of peripapillary microvascular changes between the two study groups.

2. Materials and Methods

This was a case–control study, enrolling 46 consecutive G6PD-deficient men and 23 apparently healthy G6PD-normal male controls, who were examined at the Ophthalmology Unit, Department of Medical, Surgical, and Experimental Sciences, University of Sassari, Sassari, Italy, from January to June 2017. Women were excluded due to the small number of homozygote subjects with a total lack of erythrocyte G6PD activity.

This observational study was performed according to the tenets of the Declaration of Helsinki for research involving human subjects. Institutional ethics review board approval was obtained. Each participant was given detailed information and provided written consent before inclusion.

The inclusion criteria for cases were male gender, G6PD deficiency, clear ocular media, and intra-ocular pressure (IOP) <20 mm Hg. Exclusion criteria included a history of ocular trauma, retinal and optic disc disease, uveitis, high myopia ($\geq$6 diopters), intraocular surgery (apart from phacoemulsification performed at least 6 months before the study entry), diabetes mellitus, thalassemia trait, and kidney failure.

Apart from the presence of normal G6PD activity, the inclusion and exclusion criteria for the controls were the same as those for the cases.

Blood samples were collected from each participant. Erythrocyte G6PD activity was analyzed using a quantitative assay (G6PD/6PGD, Biomedic snc, Sassari, Italy), as described previously [4].

All participants underwent a full ophthalmological examination and optic disc imaging. This included measurement of best-corrected visual acuity (BCVA), slit-lamp biomicroscopy with dilated indirect ophthalmoscopy, Goldmann applanation tonometry, B-scan OCT (Topcon OCT-2000), and OCTA (AngioVue XRTVue Avanti, Optovue, Fremont, CA, USA).

The OCTA scanning area was centered on the ONH. The AngioVue disc mode automatically segmented the ONH into four layers: ONH, vitreous, RPC plexus, and choroid. We assessed 4.5×4.5 mm OCTA scans of the RPC plexus, which extended from the inner limiting membrane (ILM) to 100 µm under the ILM, which we set as the lower boundary.

Each scan was reviewed to confirm the correct segmentation and sufficient image quality, as confirmed by the signal strength index (>55), and was repeated when necessary.

Furthermore, VD values of the RPC plexus, provided using the AngioAnalytics software embedded in the OCTA device, were recorded and compared with those of healthy eyes.

Color-coded perfusion maps were automatically generated using the flow density map software AngioAnalytics, which provided the VD values of the nine different peripapillary sectors (grid-based flow density) of the entire ONH scan. In brief, bright red stood for perfused vessel density of >50%, dark blue meant no perfusion, and intermediate perfusion densities were color-coded accordingly.

Medical conditions such as diabetes mellitus, systemic hypertension, and hypercholesterolemia were assessed. Specifically, participants were classified as hypertensive if they were receiving antihypertension drugs or if their blood pressure was >140 mm Hg systolically or >90 mm Hg diastolically (according to the WHO/International Society of Hypertension). Participants were considered to be diabetic if they were under treatment for insulin- or non-insulin-dependent diabetes mellitus, or if their fasting plasma glucose level was >126 mg/dL and/or their plasma glucose level was >200 mg/dL 2 h after a 75 g oral glucose load in a glucose tolerance test (as defined by the WHO). Hypercholesterolemia was defined by the intake of lipid-lowering drugs or a fasting plasma cholesterol level of >220 mg/dL [4].

The statistical software package Minitab 19 for macOS (Statistical Software. [Computer software]. State College, PA, USA: Minitab, Inc. www.minitab.com; accessed on 5 June 2022) and/or Stata 14 for Mac OS X (StataCorp. 2015. Stata Statistical Software: Release 14. College Station, Texas, U.S.: StataCorp LP) were used to perform data processing, summaries, and analyses. Missing data were not replaced. Summary statistics, including the number of subjects (N), number of observations (Obs), mean, median, standard deviation (SD), minimum (Min), and maximum (Max), were calculated for continuous variables. Frequencies and percentages were calculated for categorical data. A Wilcoxon rank-sum test was performed between groups for each variable. A multivariate analysis of covariance (MANCOVA) test was used to examine statistical differences between groups with regards to the flow density maps of the RPC plexus. Statistical tests were two-sided at the 0.05 significance level with 95% confidence intervals.

3. Results

Our study included 46 eyes of 46 G6PD-deficient men (mean age 43.93 ± 15.79 years) and 23 eyes of 23 apparently healthy G6PD-normal men (mean age 45.30 ± 18.02 years). The mean BCVA was 0.07 ± 0.12 LogMAR in the G6PD-defient group and −0.1 ± 0.1 LogMAR in the controls, which is not a statistically significant difference. In the G6PD-deficient group, three eyes were pseudophakic, whereas there were five pseudophakic eyes in the control group. The refractive error (spherical equivalent) was −0.69 ± 2.01 diopters in G6PD-deficient patients and −0.55 ± 1.05 diopters in the controls, which again is not a significant difference. No significant differences were found as well in terms of hypercholesterolemia, systemic hypertension, and diabetes between the two groups. All demographic and clinical data of both study groups are shown in Table 1.

Table 1. Demographic and clinical data of glucose-6-phosphate-dehydrogenase (G6PD)-deficient patients and G6PD-normal controls.

	G6PD-Deficient Subjects	G6PD-Normal Controls
Total eyes, n	46	23
Total patients, n	46	23
Age, mean ± SD (years)	43.93 ± 15.79	45.30 ± 18.02
BCVA, mean ± SD (LogMAR)	0.07 ± 0.12	−0.10 ± 0.10
Refractive error, mean ± SD (spherical equivalent)	−0.69 ± 2.01	−0.55 ± 1.05

Categorical variables are shown as numbers. Continuous variables are shown as mean ± standard deviation (SD). BCVA = best-corrected visual acuity.

The VD values of the RPC plexus in G6PD-deficient and G6PD-normal individuals are summarized in Table 2. G6PD-deficient eyes showed higher values of VD in all peripapillary sectors, but a statistical significance ($p = 0.03$) was reached only in the infero-temporal sector.

Table 2. Radial peripapillary capillary (RPC) vascular density (VD) values in glucose-6-phosphate-dehydrogenase (G6PD)-deficient patients and G6PD-normal controls.

Peripapillary SECTORS	G6PD-Deficient Subjects	G6PD-Normal Controls	p Value
Supero-temporal	57.71 ± 4.27	56.49 ± 4.29	>0.05
Supero-middle	58.43 ± 4.08	58.08 ± 3.35	>0.05
Supero-nasal	50.02 ± 4.68	49.33 ± 5.37	>0.05
Intermediate-temporal	55.56 ± 3.99	55.30 ± 3.68	>0.05
Intermediate-nasal	50.13 ± 4.50	50.10 ± 4.00	>0.05
Inferior-temporal	58.75 ± 4.79	57.06 ± 4.27	**0.03**
Inferior-middle	59.79 ± 4.38	59.03 ± 4.14	>0.05
Inferior-nasal	46.75 ± 4.53	45.79 ± 4.17	>0.05

Continuous variables are shown as mean ± standard deviation (SD).

Representative images of the RPC plexus in G6PD-deficient and G6PD-normal individuals are shown in Figure 1.

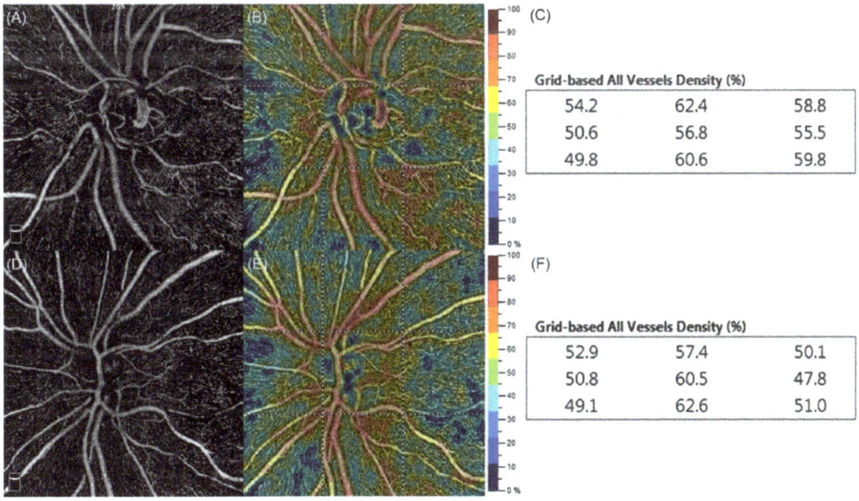

Figure 1. Optical coherence tomography angiography (OCTA) of the radial peripapillary capillary (RPC) plexus in Glucose-6-Phosphate-Dehydrogenase (G6PD)-deficient and G6PD-normal individuals of the same age (55 years). RPC en-face angiograms (**A,D**), corresponding color-coded perfusion maps (**B,E**), and grid-based vessels density (VD; **C,F**) from a G6PD-deficient man (**A–C**) and a G6PD-normal control (**D–F**). In (**C**), VD values are higher than in (**F**) in six out of nine quadrants.

4. Discussion

In this case–control study, we compared ONH findings in G6PD-deficient and G6PD-normal individuals. Specifically, we focused on the VD of the RPC plexus as automatically detected by OCTA. Interestingly, in G6PD-deficient subjects, the VD values of the RPC plexus were higher, reaching a statistically significant difference in the inferior temporal sector ($p = 0.03$).

RPCs are the innermost layer of capillaries surrounding the ONH and extending straight along the course of the retinal nerve fiber layer (RNFL) to the posterior pole [13,16–19]. Light microscope observations have highlighted that RPCs do not derive from ONH arterioles or retinal arteries [18]; rather, they seem to arise from deeper arterial vessels located in the ganglion cell layer or in the outer RNFL and then extend to the superficial RNFL, where they form parallel rows, with rare anastomoses and bifurcations [13,14].

Recent OCTA reports on the appearance of RPCs have confirmed that these capillaries have a peculiar distribution and arrangement that runs along the paths of the major temporal vessels up to 4–5 mm from the ONH, and that they form the most superficial vascular layer located within the RNFL [16–19]. RPCs, which are easy to identify via OCTA by their typical features, seem to be specialized in the nourishment of the RNFL, especially the most superficial nerve fibers, which subserve the peri-central visual field [15].

Bjerrum scotoma is a peri-central visual field defect strongly related to selective damage to RPCs, which are more vulnerable to increased IOP than other retinal capillaries, probably because of their peculiar distribution and vascular pattern [14,16]. Therefore, it has been supposed that RPCs may represent the first damage site in glaucomatous eyes [13,16].

OCTA has revolutionized the vascular imaging approach towards the ONH, allowing for visualization and qualitative/quantitative assessment of the RPC plexus. Noteworthy recent research has focused on the study of the RPC plexus because injuries at this level seem to play a key role, not only in glaucoma, but also in retinal vascular disorders (e.g., RVO, PDR) [15,18].

Histopathological evidence indicates that occlusion of linear blood vessels parallel to RNFL axons, corresponding to the RPC plexus, translates into the occurrence of flame-shaped hemorrhages and cotton wool spots due to stagnant axonal flow in the RNFL [20]. The exact pathogenetic mechanism behind RVO remains elusive; however, intraluminal thrombus formation has been associated with venous stasis, endothelial damage, and hypercoagulability. A strong correlation between RVO and typical atherosclerosis risk factors, including systemic hypertension, hypercholesterolemia, and diabetes mellitus, has widely been documented [4,21,22].

In two former studies on Sardinian patients with RVO and NA-AION, the frequency of G6PD deficiency was found to be significantly lower than expected, suggesting that G6PD-deficient subjects may have a decreased risk of developing RVO and NA-AION [4,7]. Why and how G6PD deficiency may offer protection against RVO and NA-AION is still a matter of debate. Batetta et al. [23] have demonstrated that G6PD-deficient patients show decreased cholesterol synthesis and esterification due to peculiar alterations in lipid metabolism, which is likely to be responsible for reduced cholesterol accumulation in the arteries of these subjects. Therefore, the slower progression of the atherosclerotic process in G6PD-deficient patients may translate into a reduced risk of atherosclerotic vascular disorders, including RVO and NA-AION. Furthermore, this theory may explain why G6PD-deficient patients show low mortality rates from cardiovascular and cerebrovascular diseases [2].

In our study, G6PD-deficient men had significantly higher VD values of the RPC plexus than age-matched G6PD-normal controls, suggesting the presence of a denser vascular network in the former. Theoretically, this OCTA finding may represent an advantage in protection against retinal vascular disorders.

The NADPH oxidase (Nox) family catalyzes the reduction of O_2 to reactive oxygen species, coupled with NADPH oxidation. Seven isoforms of Nox (Nox1-5 and Duox1-2) have been identified so far. Among them, Nox2 is highly expressed in cells throughout the central nervous system and retina, including endothelial cells [8,24]. There is evidence from mouse studies that endothelial Nox2 activity increases with age in the brain and contributes to age-related capillary rarefaction [8]. Since Nox2 is an NADPH-dependent enzyme, G6PD-deficient individuals might experience reduced endothelial Nox2 activity and reduced age-related capillary rarefaction.

The balance between the activity of nitric oxide synthase (NOS), an NAPDH-dependent enzyme, and concentrations of glutathione (GSH), a physiological NO scavenger, may play a crucial role in preventing the development of vascular disorders [25,26]. It is not known whether NOS and GSH are out of balance in G6PD-deficient subjects; however, experimental evidence indicates that G6PD deficiency may lead to decreased NO production [27]. In G6PD deficiency, it is possible that the combined action of NO and GSH may be responsible for inhibiting low-density lipoprotein esterification, smooth muscle cell proliferation, and platelet aggregation, which may lead to vessel dilation and a slow-down of the atherosclerotic process.

The present study has some important limitations, principally related to the small number of eyes examined. In total, 69 male patients were enrolled, and the G6PD-deficient group was chosen to be twice as large as the control group. Furthermore, no women were included in this study due to a lack of homozygote female subjects available. Nevertheless, we are unaware of any previously published report assessing the VD of the RPC plexus in G6PD-deficient and G6PD-normal individuals.

In conclusion, our results show that G6PD-deficient men have higher VD values in the RPC plexus, although a statistically significant difference was found only in the inferior temporal sector ($p = 0.03$). A denser vascular network at this level, together with decreased cholesterol synthesis and esterification, may contribute to explaining why G6PD-deficient men seem to have a reduced risk of ocular vascular diseases, such as RVO and NA-AION.

Further larger studies are necessary to confirm these preliminary findings and establish the potential protective role of G6PD deficiency against ocular diseases.

Author Contributions: Conceptualization, R.S. and A.P.; formal analysis, R.S., G.D.R., S.D. and A.P.; methodology, R.S. and A.P.; supervision, A.P. and F.C.; writing—original draft, R.S.; and writing—review and editing, R.S., A.P. and F.C. All authors have read and agreed to the published version of the manuscript.

Funding: This research received no external funding.

Institutional Review Board Statement: This study was approved by the Ethical Committee, ASL-Sassari, Sassari, Italy; Protocol n. 1162L 28 June 2013.

Informed Consent Statement: Informed consent was obtained from all subjects involved in the study.

Data Availability Statement: Not applicable.

Conflicts of Interest: The authors declare no conflict of interest.

References

1. Luzzatto, L.; Poggi, V. Glucose-6-phosphate dehydrogenase deficiency. In *Nathan and Oski's Hematology of Infancy and Childhood*, 7th ed.; Orkin, S.H., Nathan, D.G., Ginsburg, D., Look, A.T., Fisher, D.E., Lux, S.E., Eds.; Saunders Elsevier: Philadelphia, PA, USA, 2009; Volume 1, pp. 883–907.
2. Cocco, P.; Todde, P.; Fornera, S.; Manca, M.B.; Manca, P.; Sias, A.R. Mortality in a cohort of men expressing the glucose-6-phosphate dehydrogenase deficiency. *Blood* **1998**, *91*, 706–709. [CrossRef]
3. Beutler, E. G6PD deficiency. *Blood* **1994**, *84*, 3613. [CrossRef]
4. Pinna, A.; Carru, C.; Solinas, G.; Zinellu, A.; Carta, F. Glucose-6-Phosphate Dehydrogenase Deficiency in Retinal Vein Occlusion. *Investig. Opthalmol. Vis. Sci.* **2007**, *48*, 2747–2752. [CrossRef]
5. Siniscalco, M.; Bernini, L.; Latte, B.; Motulsky, A.G. Favism and Thalassæmia and their Relationship to Malaria. *Nature* **1961**, *190*, 1179–1180. [CrossRef]
6. Dore, M.P.; Davoli, A.; Longo, N.; Marras, G.; Pes, G.M. Glucose-6-phosphate dehydrogenase deficiency and risk of colorectal cancer in Northern Sardinia: A retrospective observational study. *Medicine* **2016**, *95*, e5254. [CrossRef]
7. Pinna, A.; Solinas, G.; Masia, C.; Zinellu, A.; Carru, C.; Carta, A. Glucose-6-Phosphate Dehydrogenase (G6PD) Deficiency in Nonarteritic Anterior Ischemic Optic Neuropathy in a Sardinian Population, Italy. *Investig. Opthalmol. Vis. Sci.* **2008**, *49*, 1328–1332. [CrossRef]
8. Pinna, A.; Contini, E.L.; Carru, C.; Solinas, G. Glucose-6-Phosphate Dehydrogenase Deficiency and Diabetes Mellitus with Severe Retinal Complications in a Sardinian Population, Italy. *Int. J. Med. Sci.* **2013**, *10*, 1907–1913. [CrossRef]
9. Fan, L.M.; Geng, L.; Cahill-Smith, S.; Liu, F.; Douglas, G.; Mckenzie, C.A.; Smith, C.; Brooks, G.; Channon, K.M.; Li, J.M. Nox2 contributes to age-related oxidative damage to neurons and the cerebral vasculature. *J Clin. Investig.* **2022**, *51*, 3374–3386. [CrossRef]
10. Serra, R.; Coscas, F.; Boulet, J.F.; Cabral, D.R.; Lupidi, M.; Coscas, G.J.; Souied, E.H. Predictive Activation Biomarkers of Treatment-Naive Asymptomatic Choroidal Neovascularization in Age-Related Macular Degeneration. *Retina* **2020**, *40*, 1224–1233. [CrossRef]
11. Spaide, R.F.; Klancnik, J.M.; Cooney, M.J. Retinal Vascular Layers Imaged by Fluorescein Angiography and Optical Coherence Tomography Angiography. *JAMA Ophthalmol.* **2015**, *133*, 45–50. [CrossRef]
12. Serra, R.; Sellam, A.; Coscas, F.; Bruyère, E.; Sieiro, A.; Coscas, G.J.; Souied, E.H. Evaluation of pseudophakic cystoid macular edema using optical coherence tomography angiography. *Eur. J. Ophthalmol.* **2018**, *28*, 234–240. [CrossRef]
13. Scoles, D.; Gray, D.C.; Hunter, J.J.; Wolfe, R.; Gee, B.P.; Geng, Y.; Masella, B.D.; Libby, R.T.; Russell, S.; Williams, D.R.; et al. In-Vivo imaging of retinal nerve fiber layer vasculature: Imaging histology comparison. *BMC Ophthalmol.* **2009**, *23*, 9. [CrossRef]
14. Alterman, M.; Henkind, P. Radial peripapillary capillaries of the retina. II. Possible role in Bjerrum scotoma. *Br. J. Ophthalmol.* **1968**, *52*, 26–31. [CrossRef]
15. Kornzweig, A.L.; Eliasoph, I.; Feldstein, M. Selective Atrophy of the Radial Peripapillary Capillaries in Chronic Glaucoma. *Arch. Ophthalmol.* **1968**, *80*, 696–702. [CrossRef]
16. Mansoori, T.; Sivaswamy, J.; Gamalapati, J.S.; Balakrishna, N. Radial Peripapillary Capillary Density Measurement Using Optical Coherence Tomography Angiography in Early Glaucoma. *J. Glaucoma* **2017**, *26*, 438–443. [CrossRef]
17. Michaelson, I. *Retinal Circulation in Man and Animals*; Charles C Thomas: Springfield, IL, USA, 1954.
18. Henkind, P. Radial peripapillary capillaries of the retina. I. Anatomy: Human and comparative. *Br. J. Ophthalmol.* **1967**, *51*, 115–123. [CrossRef]
19. Yu, P.K.; Balaratnasingam, C.; Xu, J.; Morgan, W.H.; Mammo, Z.; Han, S.; MacKenzie, P.; Merkur, A.; Kirker, A.; Albiani, D.; et al. Label-Free Density Measurements of Radial Peripapillary Capillaries in the Human Retina. *PLoS ONE* **2015**, *10*, e0135151. [CrossRef]

20. Ip, M.; Hendrick, A. Retinal Vein Occlusion Review. *Asia Pac. J. Ophthalmol. (Phila)* **2018**, *7*, 40–45. [CrossRef]
21. Clarkson, J.G. Central retinal vein occlusion. In *Medical Retina*, 3rd ed.; Ryan, S.J., Ed.; Mosby Inc.: St. Louis, MO, USA, 2001; Volume 2, pp. 1368–1375.
22. Fekrat, S.; Finkelstein, D. Branch retinal vein occlusion. In *Medical Retina*, 3rd ed.; Ryan, S.J., Ed.; Mosby Inc.: St. Louis, MO, USA, 2001; Volume 2, pp. 1376–1381.
23. Batetta, B.; Bonatesta, R.R.; Sanna, F.; Putzolu, M.; Mulas, M.F.; Collu, M.; Dessì, S. Cell growth and cholesterol metabolism in human glucose- 6-phosphate dehydrogenase deficient lymphomononuclear cells. *Cell Prolif.* **2002**, *35*, 143–154. [CrossRef]
24. Kowluru, R.A.; Radhakrishnan, R.; Mohammad, G. Regulation of Rac1 transcription by histone and DNA methylation in diabetic retinopathy. *Sci. Rep.* **2021**, *11*, 14097. [CrossRef]
25. Wallace, M. NADPH diaphorase activity in activated astrocytes representing inducible nitric oxide synthase. *Methods Enzym.* **1996**, *268*, 497–503. [CrossRef]
26. Li, H.; Poulos, T.L. Structure–function studies on nitric oxide synthases. *J. Inorg. Biochem.* **2005**, *99*, 293–305. [CrossRef]
27. Stanton, R.C. Glucose-6-phosphate dehydrogenase, NADPH, and cell survival. *IUBMB Life* **2012**, *64*, 362–369. [CrossRef]

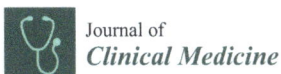

Journal of Clinical Medicine

Article

Correlating Ocular Physiology and Visual Function with Mild Cognitive Loss in Senior Citizens in Taiwan

Kuo-Chen Su [1,2], Hong-Ming Cheng [3,†], Yu Chu [2], Fang-Chun Lu [2], Lung-Hui Tsai [2,*,†] and Ching-Ying Cheng [1,2,*]

1. Department of Ophthalmology, Chung Shan Medical University Hospital, Taichung 402, Taiwan; jimmysu8@csmu.edu.tw
2. Department of Optometry, Chung Shan Medical University, Taichung 402, Taiwan; tom830107@gmail.com (Y.C.); lu700112@gmail.com (F.-C.L.)
3. Department of Optometry, Asia University, Taichung 413, Taiwan; hm_cheng@yahoo.com
* Correspondence: x8c032@yahoo.com.tw (L.-H.T.); ldiioul.tw@gmail.com (C.-Y.C.); Tel.: +886-4-2473-0022 (C.-Y.C.)
† These authors contributed equally to this work.

Abstract: Purpose: The transition of Taiwan from an aging to a super-aging society has come with a cost as more elderly now suffer from cognitive impairment. The main purpose of our study was to investigate if early detection can be developed so that timely intervention can be instituted. We analyzed the correlation of cognitive function with ocular physiology and visual functions between senior citizens aged 60 years or older in Taiwan. **Methods:** Thirty-six healthy subjects were recruited for the study. Addenbrooke's cognitive examination III (ACE-III), binocular functions (including objective and subjective refraction, distance and near dissociated phoria, stereopsis, contrast sensitivity, adult developmental eye movement (ADEM), and ocular physiology (by using optical coherence tomography, OCT, and macular pigment measurement, MPS) were performed, and the data were analyzed via independent *t*-test, chi-square test, Pearson correlation, linear regression, and ROC (receiver operating characteristic) curve. **Results:** Data analysis showed that (1) patients with poor eye movement had a strong correlation with the total score and all dimensions of cognitive functions, (2) the thickness of the macula had a strong correlation with attention and memory, and (3) patients with poor eye movement and poor stereopsis in combination with thinner inferior macula appeared to have lower cognitive abilities. **Discussion and Conclusions:** Cognitive dysfunction is not readily identified during the early stage of cognitive decline. The use of simple and inexpensive ADEM or stereopsis test and comparing the OCT results that are popular in optometry clinics for reference can be diagnostic in identifying patients with mild cognitive impairments. With the combined use of macular pigment density or retinal thickness measurements, it was possible to effectively predict the early degradation of cognition.

Keywords: cognitive function; binocular vision; mild cognitive impairment; ocular physiology; dementia

Citation: Su, K.-C.; Cheng, H.-M.; Chu, Y.; Lu, F.-C.; Tsai, L.-H.; Cheng, C.-Y. Correlating Ocular Physiology and Visual Function with Mild Cognitive Loss in Senior Citizens in Taiwan. *J. Clin. Med.* **2022**, *11*, 2624. https://doi.org/10.3390/jcm11092624

Academic Editors: Jay Chhablani and Sumit Randhir Singh

Received: 7 March 2022
Accepted: 5 May 2022
Published: 6 May 2022

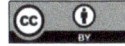

Copyright: © 2022 by the authors. Licensee MDPI, Basel, Switzerland. This article is an open access article distributed under the terms and conditions of the Creative Commons Attribution (CC BY) license (https://creativecommons.org/licenses/by/4.0/).

1. Introduction

Alzheimer's disease is the most common type of dementia [1–3]. Studies have shown that many patients with Alzheimer's disease (AD) have reading difficulties resulting from line skipping, mainly because of degeneration in fixation, saccadic pursuit, or vergence capabilities [4,5]. Although such changes are usually subtle in the early stages of dementia, or mild cognitive impairment (MCI), they can still be detected through a functional vision assessment [5]. In terms of saccades, Pirozzolo and Hansch compared 12 Alzheimer's patients with a control group, and found that the saccadic efficiency of Alzheimer's patients increased significantly [4], which suggests a change in higher cortical regulatory roles in sensory-motor integration. Although Alzheimer's patients have normal amplitudes in visual evoked potential (VEP) examination, the change in latency shows that the patients have difficulty interpreting visual information to some extent [6]. Additional studies have also demonstrated that contrast sensitivity, pupil response, color vision, fixation, saccadic eye movement, etc. are implicated in functional deficits in the early stages of dementia [7–10]. Furthermore, while binocular vision problems are already common in the elderly population [11], relevant studies have pointed out that the visual function of the elderly with MCI is even worse [12].

In terms of visual physiology, retinal examination can provide a non-invasive method which is similar to the examination of brain pathology [13]; previous literature has pointed out that the reduction in macular thickness [14,15], thinning of retinal nerve fiber layers, changes in the optic nerve or optic disc [16,17], and macular pigment density [18] are closely related to dementia progression. Kim and Kang's 2019 study [19] showed that the macular ganglion intracellular plexiform layer (GC-IPL) and total macular and peripheral retinal nerve fiber layer (RNFL) in the Alzheimer's group were significantly thinner than those in the control group [19]; Claire and Michèle [20] also indicated that, when comparing with the control group, the thickness of RNFL in patients with MCI, mild AD, or moderate to severe AD was significantly decreased.

To summarize, the degradation of cognition may have a causal relationship with the overall binocular visual functions and ocular physiology that is yet to be explicitly explored. The purpose of our study was to demonstrate, for the first time, that the decline in visual function and ocular physiology may be correlated and even interact significantly with MCI.

2. Materials and Methods

The study was a cross-sectional study that was conducted from 20 November 2020 to 30 March 2021 at Chung Shan Medical University Hospital (CSMUH)-affiliated Dementia Intergraded Care Center. All the procedures were conducted in accordance with the Declaration of Helsinki. Approval was obtained from the Institutional Review Board of CSMUH (Taichung, Taiwan) (approval number: CS19110). The age and physical, spirit, and compliance situations may have determined the duration for each subject to complete the entire examination. The manuscript is reported according to the STROBE guideline [21,22].

2.1. Research Subjects

All participants had binocular and monocular distance and near visual acuity of 0.8 or better, spherical power ranged from −5.00 D to +2.00 D, and astigmatism was <1.00 D. Twenty-three subjects were already excluded at the recruiting stage owing to eye and/or mental problems. Those with an optic disc ratio not within the normal range could be a high-risk group with high myopia or glaucoma, and were also excluded and referred. A total of 40 people eventually participated and four were later dismissed, one with poor communication because of auditory nerve damage, and three others simply dropped out. Finally, the effective sample was 36 with 6 men and 30 women, and the average age was for men: 68.83 ± 9.07, for women: 73.67 ± 9.44 years, and for all subjects was 72.86 ± 9.43 years. An independent t-test indicated no significant difference in age and ACE-III cognitive score as far as sex; therefore, the results were analyzed with all 36 subjects combined.

2.2. Research Materials

Addenbrooke's cognitive examination III (ACE-III, Chinese version) was performed for differentiating patients with or without cognitive impairment. The sensitive of ACE-III is reported to be trustworthy for detecting early stages of dementia, and is available in different languages [23]. ACE-III contains 5 sub-tests with a total of 100 questions, including attention (18 questions), memory (26 questions), language fluency (14 questions), language comprehension (26 questions), and visuospatial ability (16 questions). The criteria of ACE-III is 83 [23], i.e., subjects who finish with 83 points or less are regarded as being ACE-abnormal.

Binocular visual function examination included subjective refraction (Shin-Nippon Wide-View Refraction NVision-K 5001, Tokyo, Japan), distance and near visual acuity

(View-M digital visual acuity chart and TMVC near point test card), phoria (Howell card for distance and near), adult developmental eye movement test (ADEM), Stereo-Fly for stereo acuity test, and the low contrast flip chart for near and distance contrast sensitivity. In order to avoid potential bias, each test was performed by the same optometrist. ADEM was developed by Gené-Sampedro et al. [24] which was modified from the DEM test [25], and although DEM has been suggested to be potentially useful for adults [26], the norm of DEM was only constructed up to the age of 14, and modification was therefore necessary [27,28]. Subjects were asked to read a series of numbers as fast as possible which were arranged either horizontally or vertically. Four possible behavioral types can be found with the ADEM test: normal, ocular movement dysfunction, naming disorder, and combined.

Ocular physiology examination included optical coherence tomography (OCT, Topcon, MAESTRO2, Tokyo, Japan) and macular pigment measurement (Macular Pigment Screener II, MPS-II), both of which were performed on patients without mydriasis, in a dim light room. In the examination of macular thickness with OCT within the center area (recorded as a circle with a diameter of 1 mm), the inner area (a circle with a diameter of 1 mm to 3 mm), and the outer area (a circle with a diameter of 3 mm to 6 mm). With OCT, the retinal thickness of the inner and outer area was divided into four quadrants: superior, inferior, nasal, and temporal. Macular pigment is believed to play a beneficial role in visual performance [29,30]; therefore, subjects were asked to perform three times and were first instructed to push a button as soon as a flicker was perceived.

2.3. Data Analysis and Statistical Analysis

G* Power analysis was used to determine the sample size in this study, in which the condition was set at the effect size d = 0.8, α = 0.05, power $(1 - \beta)$ = 0.95. Data were analyzed by using SPSS 26.0 statistical software (IBM, Armonk, NY, USA). For the statistics including (1) independent t-test for comparing binocular visual functions and ocular physiology between ACE groups; (2) chi-square analysis between the ACE group and ADEM types, distance, and near phoria; (3) linear regression analysis about cognitive function, visual function, and ocular physiology; (4) ROC curve between significant variables; and (5) Pearson correlation analysis between OCT, ADEM, MPS, and stereopsis, a value of $p < 0.05$ was considered statistically significant.

3. Results

The ACE-III test contains attention, memory, language fluency, language comprehension, and visuospatial categories, and the reliability of the ACE-III cognitive examination was excellent with Cronbach's alpha coefficient = 0.82. In addition, 15 ACE-normal and 21 ACE-abnormal subjects were found by the ACE score. G* Power analysis showed that there was still enough power after recalculation and adjustment.

The results of the independent t-test showed that cognitive function showed significant differences not only in the total score of ACE ($t = -8.93$, $p = 0.00$) but also in all subtests: attention ($t = -4.54$, $p = 0.00$), memory ($t = -9.89$, $p = 0.00$), language fluency ($t = -5.06$, $p = 0.00$), language comprehension ($t = -5.26$, $p = 0.00$), and visuospatial ($t = -6.58$, $p = 0.00$), indicating that the degradation of cognitive function had a wide range of effects (Table 1).

3.1. Ocular Physiology between ACE-Abnormal and ACE-Normal Groups

All data were collected after confirming that subjects had no existing eye diseases and risks; at the same time, all participants had eligible refractive errors and visual acuity. In analyzing visual physiology, because the data from the left and right eyes were not significantly different, the data shown here are from the right eye. The density of macular pigment was significantly different ($t = -2.50$, $p = 0.02$) where that in the ACE-abnormal group was lower than that in the ACE-normal group (Table 2).

Table 1. Independent *t*-test of ACE-III total score and subtests between ACE groups.

	ACE-Abnormal N = 21/M (SD)	ACE-Normal N = 15/M (SD)	Levene F Value	*t*	*p*
ACE Total score	63.00 (12.64)	88.93 (3.51)	19.24	−8.93	0.000 **
ACE Attention	13.57 (3.71)	17.40 (0.91)	19.21	−4.54	0.000 **
ACE Memory	14.05 (2.78)	22.60 (2.20)	0.07	−9.89	0.000 **
ACE Language fluency	5.14 (2.73)	9.33 (1.99)	2.66	−5.06	0.000 **
ACE Language comprehension	19.95 (4.40)	25.13 (0.83)	20.53	−5.27	0.000 **
ACE Visuospatial	10.29 (2.24)	14.47 (1.19)	4.03	−6.58	0.000 **

** $p < 0.01$.

Table 2. Independent *t*-test of ocular physiology between ACE-normal and -abnormal subjects.

	ACE-Abnormal N = 21/M (SD)	ACE-Normal N = 15/M (SD)	Levene F Value	*t*	*p*
MPS	0.27 (0.22)	0.49 (0.30)	1.17	−2.50	0.02 *
OCT-Center-Fovea	250.05 (35.55)	257.07 (26.01)	0.11	−0.65	0.52
OCT-Inner-Temporal	296.52 (27.12)	311.40 (18.63)	1.74	−1.83	0.08
OCT-Inner-Superior	305.52 (27.79)	330.00 (20.04)	1.23	−2.91	0.01 *
OCT-Inner-Nasal	310.29 (26.84)	324.93 (24.54)	0.10	−1.67	0.10
OCT-Inner-Inferior	301.14 (24.63)	320.53 (18.30)	0.74	−2.58	0.01 **
OCT-Outer-Temporal	251.00 (32.74)	270.40 (13.55)	4.84	−2.44	0.02 *
OCT-Outer-Superior	260.15 (34.32)	293.13 (24.52)	1.85	−3.16	0.003 **
OCT-Outer-Nasal	278.38 (26.63)	307.13 (16.32)	2.96	−3.70	0.001 **
OCT-Outer-Inferior	252.95 (23.70)	273.07 (16.78)	2.73	−2.82	0.008 **

* $p < 0.05$, ** $p < 0.01$.

In the OCT examination of the macula, except for the central area (OCT-Center-Fovea: $t = -0.65$, $p = 0.52$), the inner area of temporal (OCT-Inner-Temporal: $t = -1.83$, $p = 0.08$) and nasal (OCT-Inner-Nasal: $t = -1.67$, $p = 0.10$) quadrants were not significantly different, but the rest of the macular thickness was significantly different between the two groups: there were obvious differences in the peripheral part of the macula, especially thickness of the outer, the inferior, and the superior areas (Table 2, Figure 1).

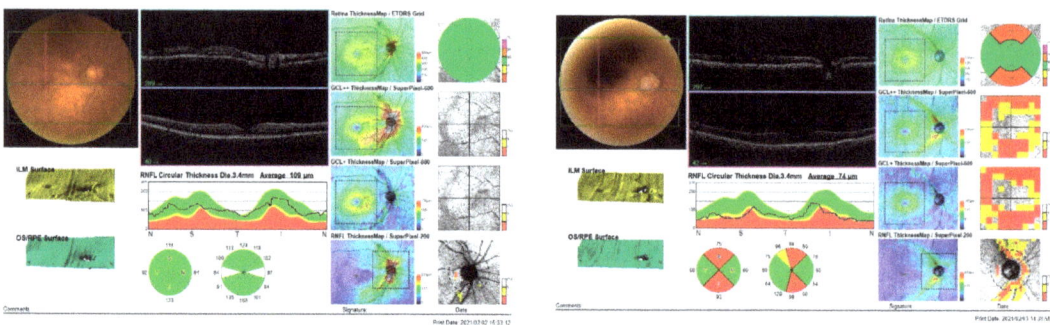

Figure 1. OCT measurement: examples of one ACE-normal case (**left**) and an ACE-abnormal case (**right**).

3.2. Visual Functions between ACE-Abnormal and ACE-Normal Groups

In term of visual functions, eye movement (ADEM), stereopsis, contrast sensitivity, distance phoria, and near phoria were performed. The difference and the analysis results with the independent sample *t*-test are listed in Table 3. The performance of the two groups in ADEM_V was significantly different ($t = -5.70$, $p = 0.000$), and the ADEM_V of the ACE-abnormal group was significantly less than the ACE-normal group; the same results also appeared in ADEM_H ($t = 6.24$, $p = 0.000$), ADEM_Ratio ($t = 5.63$, $p = 0.000$), and stereopsis

(t = 5.95, p = 0.006). Only contrast sensitivity (t = 1.45, p = 0.16) did not reach a significant difference between the two groups.

Table 3. Independent t-test of visual function between ACE-normal and -abnormal subjects.

	ACE-Abnormal N = 21/M (SD)	ACE-Normal N = 15/M (SD)	Levene F Value	t	p
ADEM_V	60.86 (23.42)	30.20 (6.50)	27.51	5.70	0.000 **
ADEM_H	84.38 (37.41)	31.87 (8.03)	33.45	6.24	0.000 **
ADEM_Ratio	1.35 (0.20)	1.06 (0.12)	5.07	5.63	0.000 **
Stereo	2.40 (0.55)	1.93 (0.41)	4.23	2.95	0.006 **
Contrast sensitivity	1.37 (0.38)	1.25 (0.00)	7.45	1.45	0.16

ADEM: adult developmental eye movement; VT vertical time; and HT: horizontal time. ** $p < 0.01$.

3.2.1. ACE Cognitive Function and ADEM Eye Movement

Adult saccade eye movement, including vertical time, horizontal time, and ADEM ratio: in the ACE-abnormal group, 3 patients had the normal type, 2 had difficulty in naming, 16 had combined disorder, and none had only eye movement disorder. In the ACE-normal group, 17 had the normal type of ADEM, and 1 had difficulty in naming (as shown in Figure 2). Chi-square analysis was used to analyze the differences between ADEM types and the cognitive function, and the results showed that eye movement abilities had significant difference (Chi-square = 21.96, p = 0.000) in cognitive function, i.e., there was a strong correlation between eye movement and cognitive functions. It is worthwhile to mention that the proportion of ADEM combined disorders in the ACE-abnormal group was much higher than the ACE-normal group, which showed that in the ADEM of patients with cognitive dysfunction, the probability of combined naming and eye movement difficulties was significantly higher in the ACE-abnormal group.

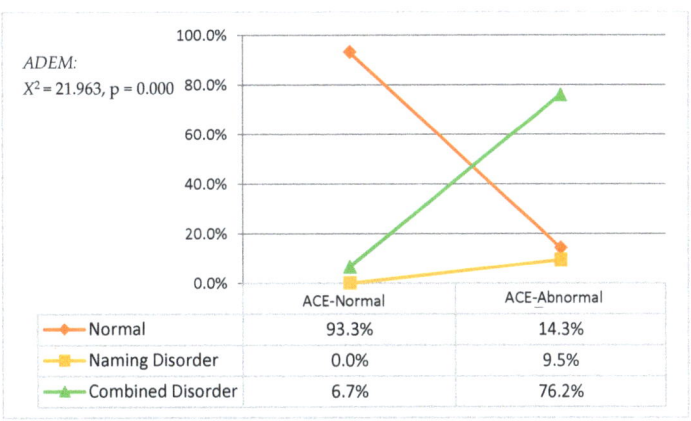

Figure 2. ADEM types between ACE-normal and -abnormal subjects.

3.2.2. ACE Cognitive Function and Phoria

Distant phoria test showed: in the ACE-abnormal group, there were seven patients with orthophoria, five with esophoria, seven with exophoria, and two with monovision; in the ACE-normal group, six patients were with orthophoria, six with esophoria, and three with exophoria. (as shown in Figure 3). Chi-square analysis showed that ACE cognition was not correlated with phoria (Chi-square = 2.847, p = 0.416). The near phoria test showed: in the ACE-abnormal group, there were 4 patients with orthophoria, 3 with esotropia, 12 with exophoria, and 2 with monovision; in the ACE-normal group, 3 patients have esophoria and 12 patients with exophoria (as shown in Figure 3). Same as distance phoria, near phoria also showed no significant difference (Chi-square = 4.261, p = 0.235) in cognitive function. The results indicated that there was no correlation between eye position and cognitive function [31].

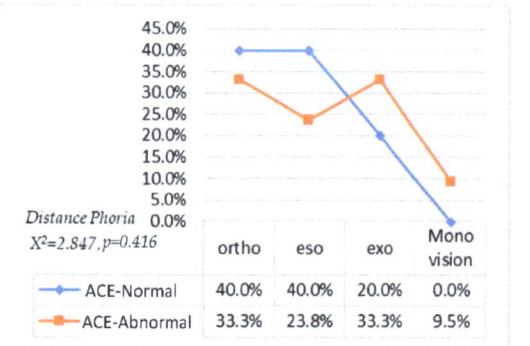
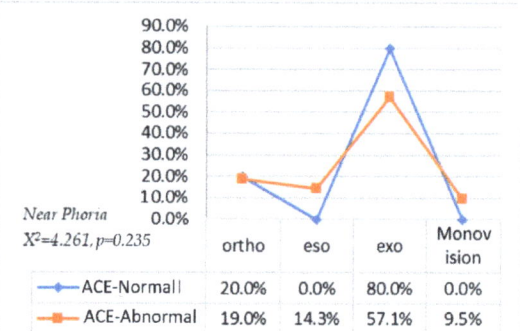

Figure 3. Distance phoria and near phoria between ACE-normal and -abnormal subjects.

3.3. Indicator for Cognitive Function

3.3.1. Linear Regression Analysis on Significant Variables

According to the analysis above, there were significant differences between normal and abnormal cognitive groups in macular pigment, retinal thickness, eye movement ability, and stereopsis. If the ACE total score was taken as the dependent variable, and macular pigment, retinal thickness, eye movement ability, and stereopsis were all taken as independent variables for linear regression analysis, the results showed that ADEM horizonal, stereopsis, and retinal thickness (outer layer, inferior quadrant) had a high ability to predict and explain cognition decline. The three independent variables could be used to explain up to 82.1% (adjusted to 80.4%) of the explained variation generated by the cognitive ability dependent variables (Table 4).

Furthermore, ADEM-V and retinal thickness (outer layer, inferior quadrant, OCT_O_I) also had a high ability to predict and explain ACE attention (71.6%), ADEM-Ratio and OCT_O_I could predict ACE memory for up to 81.0%, ADEM-H and stereopsis could explain 55.5% of ACE language fluency, ADEM-V and stereopsis could explain 68.1% of ACE language comprehension, and ADEM-H could explain 43.8% of ACE visuospatial.

The data showed that horizontal eye movement was related to language fluency and visuospatial abilities; vertical eye movement to attention and language comprehension; the overall eye movement ability to memory; the thickness of the retina (OCT_O_I) was related to attention, memory, and overall cognitive ability; and stereopsis to language fluency, language comprehension, and overall cognitive ability.

3.3.2. ROC Curve Analysis about Significant Variables

Since eye movement, stereopsis, and retinal thickness showed good explanatory capabilities for cognitive ability, the critical criteria (cut-off point) value of various tests in clinical examination was worthy of further discussion. The results of the ROC curve analysis showed that eye movement examination had the most discriminative ability of clinical screening, the AUC (area under the curve) of horizontal eye movement (ADEM_H) was 0.924 ($p = 0.000$), sensitivity = 0.857, and specificity = 0.867, and clinical identification could set the cut-off point at 38.5 s. Similarly, other eye movement examinations (vertical eye movement: AUC = 0.914, $p = 0.000$, cut-off point = 35.5; eye movement ratio: AUC = 0.902, $p = 0.000$, cut-off point = 1.12) could also be used as clinically important reference values.

Table 4. Linear regression analysis on significant variables.

Dependent Variables		R	R^2	Adjusted R^2	SE	Change Value			F	Sig.
						R^2 Change	F Change	p for F Change		
ACE total score	1. ADEM-H	0.841	0.707	0.698	9.03	0.707	79.638	0.000	79.638	0.000 **
	2. 1 + Stereopsis	0.890	0.792	0.779	7.72	0.085	13.158	0.001	61.069	0.000 **
	3. 2 + OCT-O-I	0.906	0.821	0.804	7.29	0.029	4.946	0.034	47.382	0.000 **
ACE attention	1. ADEM-V	0.824	0.679	0.670	2.00	0.679	69.930	0.000	69.930	0.000 **
	2. 1 + OCT-O-I	0.846	0.716	0.699	1.91	0.037	4.178	0.049	40.422	0.000 **
ACE memory	1. ADEM-Ratio	0.825	0.681	0.672	2.85	0.681	70.564	0.000	70.564	0.000 **
	2. 1 + OCT-O-I	0.900	0.810	0.698	2.23	0.129	21.633	0.000	68.159	0.000 **
ACE language fluency	1. ADEM-H	0.674	0.455	0.438	2.35	0.455	27.538	0.000	27.538	0.000 **
	2. 1 + Stereopsis	0.745	0.555	0.528	2.15	0.101	7.238	0.011	19.990	0.000 **
ACE language	1. ADEM-V	0.777	0.603	0.591	2.75	0.603	50.216	0.000	50.216	0.000 **
	2. 1 + Stereopsis	0.825	0.681	0.661	2.51	0.077	7.729	0.009	34.092	0.000 **
ACE visuospatial	1. ADEM-H	0.662	0.438	0.421	2.16	0.438	25.721	0.000	25.721	0.000 **

** $p < 0.01$.

In addition, the thickness of the retina (OCT_O_I) and stereopsis also showed good to excellent discriminative abilities, with which OCT-O-I performed at AUC = 0.795, $p = 0.009$, cut-off point = 243 mm, and stereopsis performed at AUC = 0.794, $p = 0.012$, the cut-off point = 100. All variables could be cross-validated before referral and identification(Table 5 and Figure 4).

Table 5. ROC curve analysis about DEM, stereopsis, and OCT.

Variable	AUC	SE	p	95%CI		Sensitivity	Specificity	Cut-Off Point
				Lower	Upper			
ADEM_V	0.914	0.047	0.000 **	0.823	1.00	0.857	0.867	35.5
ADEM_H	0.924	0.047	0.000 **	0.831	1.00	0.905	0.933	38.5
ADEM_Ratio	0.902	0.049	0.000 **	0.806	0.997	0.762	0.933	1.21
OCT_O_I	0.795	0.079	0.009 **	0.604	0.913	1	0.429	243
Stereopsis	0.794	0.084	0.012 *	0.585	0.913	0.857	0.733	100

* $p < 0.05$, ** $p < 0.01$.

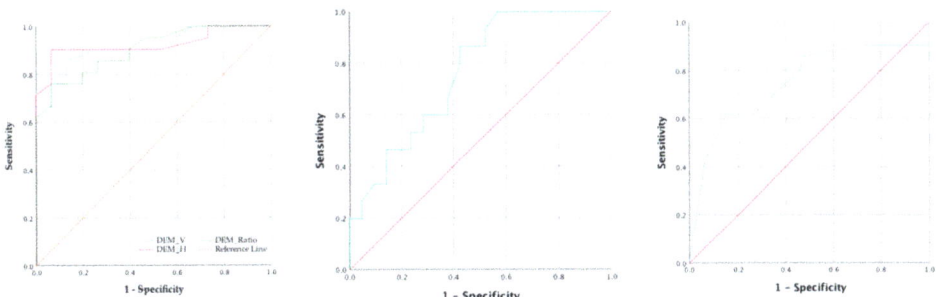

Figure 4. ROC curve analysis about ADEM, OCT_O_I, and stereopsis.

4. Discussion

In this study, an ACE score of 83 was used as the cut-off point, and all subjects were divided into either the ACE-normal (>83) or ACE-abnormal (≤83) group. There were significant differences in the performance of the total score and six cognitive dimensions. On the whole, this cognitive screening questionnaire showed great reliability and validity, and it could effectively identify patients with mild cognitive impairments. However, ACE examination was time-consuming, and subjects were required to have sufficient cooperation.

Despite these shortcomings, the biggest difference between the ACE-normal cognitive function group and the abnormal group was the proportion of eye movement disorders. With the ADEM test, for patients with abnormal cognitive function, the probability of combined naming and eye movement difficulty was significantly higher than that in the normal group. ADEM has excellent discriminative power in predicting cognitive states under the linear regression and ROC curve, so ADEM can effectively identify the presence of cognitive impairment [25]; in addition, ADEM is inexpensive, rapid, and simple, and it is an ideal tool for the screening of cognitive impairment.

Our present study further pointed to two possibly simpler and more effective screening methods that can be conducted in a clinical setting:

1. In terms of visual physiology, the macular pigment density of the ACE-abnormal group was significantly lower than that of the ACE-normal group, and there was a significant difference in the peripheral thickness of the macular (the superior, inferior, and temporal of the outer macular layer) between the normal and the abnormal groups. Previous studies have indicated that the superior and inferior layers are the most obvious [32] in patients with cognitive impairment. Our results further indicated the outer and inferior macular layers as having excellent discrimination ability in predicting cognitive states under the linear regression and ROC curve. Fundus examination of patients can therefore be used to effectively detect the developing decline of the cognitive state [33,34]. According to the previous studies and the results of this study, we can assume that the thinning of the ganglion cell layer leads to the disappearance of neurons, thereby affecting the dorsal and the ventral pathways; in addition, these neural changes contribute to age-related losses of low-level visual functions and even higher-order visual perceptions, including face perception [35], motion processing [36–38], and reading speed [39].
2. Moreover, linear regression indicated that ADEM, stereopsis, and macular thinness interact to some extent. For example, ADEM-V, ADEM-H, and stereopsis appeared in the cognitive function of language comprehension and language fluency, presumably because the ADEM measurement can be classified as a group of naming disorders or a combined disorder [25]. When it comes to stereopsis, the reason it is correlated with language comprehension and language fluency might be traced back to the pyramid of binocular vision development [40,41].

We should point out that procedures (1) and (2) described above, for monitoring cognitive impairment through readily available testing of eye movement and stereopsis, and OCT measurement of retinal thickness, must be performed as a whole. In a well-equipped eye clinic, this is not a problem. Otherwise, the correlation between single tests and cognitive function may not be as high as desired (see Figure 5, the correlation coefficient was between 0.40 and 0.47), and referrals for additional tests may become necessary.

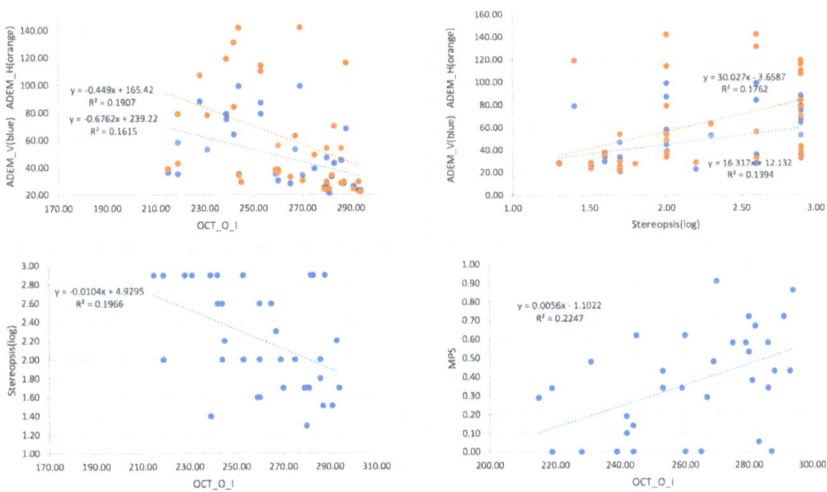

Figure 5. Correlations between OCT_O_I, MPS, Stereopsis, and ADEM values.

5. Conclusions

Mild cognitive impairment (MCI) is a sign and also a necessary process before entering dementia; in the initial stage, it is often considered to be a due phenomenon of aging and ignored. There appears concurrent drastic changes in ocular physiology and visual function. In fact, eye movement, stereo vision, macular thinness are all indicators in the beginning stage of dementia. A reliable testing for MCI should also be a non-investment, more convenient, low-cost, and less time-consuming. Our results showed that testing of visual function and ocular physiology was suitable for the rapid screening of patients with MCI before the onset of overt mobile and cognitive disabilities.

Author Contributions: Conceptualization, C.-Y.C. and L.-H.T.; investigation, data curation, and formal analysis, C.-Y.C., Y.C. and F.-C.L.; writing—original draft preparation, C.-Y.C., K.-C.S. and Y.C.; writing—review and editing, C.-Y.C., K.-C.S. and H.-M.C. All authors have read and agreed to the published version of the manuscript.

Funding: This research was funded by Chung Shan Medical University research project (CSMU-INI-108-07) in Taiwan.

Institutional Review Board Statement: The study was conducted according to the guidelines of the Declaration of Helsinki and approved by the Ethics Committee of Chung Shan Medical University Hospital (Taichung, Taiwan) (approval number: CS19110).

Informed Consent Statement: Informed consent was obtained from all subjects involved in the study.

Data Availability Statement: The datasets used during the current study are available from the corresponding author.

Conflicts of Interest: The authors declare that there are no conflict of interest regarding the publication of this paper.

References

1. Kukull, W.-A.; Bowen, J.-D. Dementia epidemiology. *Med. Clin. N. Am.* **2002**, *86*, 573–590. [CrossRef]
2. Guerreiro, R.; Bras, J. The age factor in Alzheimer's disease. *Genome Med.* **2015**, *7*, 106. [CrossRef] [PubMed]
3. Crous-Bou, M.; Minguillón, C.; Gramunt, N.; Molinuevo, J.L. Alzheimer's Disease Prevention: From Risk Factors to Early Intervention. *Alzheimer's Res. Ther.* **2017**, *9*, 71. [CrossRef]
4. Pirozzolo, F.J.; Hansch, E.C. Oculomotor Reaction Time in Dementia Reflects Degree of Cerebral Dysfunction. *Science* **1981**, *214*, 349–351. [CrossRef] [PubMed]

5. Pelak, V.S. Ocular Motility of Aging and Dementia. *Curr. Neurol. Neurosci. Rep.* 2010, *10*, 440–447. [CrossRef]
6. Leinonen, H.; Lipponen, A.; Gurevicius, K.; Tanila, H. Normal Amplitude of Electroretinography and Visual Evoked Potential Responses in AβPP/PS1 Mice. *J. Alzheimer's Dis.* 2016, *51*, 21–26. [CrossRef]
7. Armstrong, R.A. Alzheimer's disease and the eye. *J. Optom.* 2009, *2*, 103–111. [CrossRef]
8. Armstrong, R.; Kergoat, H. Oculo-visual changes and clinical considerations affecting older patients with dementia. *Ophthalmic Physiol. Opt.* 2015, *35*, 352–376. [CrossRef]
9. Willard, A.; Lueck, C. Ocular motor disorders. *Curr. Opin. Neurol.* 2014, *27*, 75–82. [CrossRef]
10. Katz, B.; Rimmer, S. Ophthalmologic manifestations of Alzheimer's disease. *Surv. Ophthalmol.* 1989, *34*, 31–43. [CrossRef]
11. Leat, S.J.; Chan, L.L.; Maharaj, P.-D.; Hrynchak, P.K.; Mittelstaedt, A.; Machan, C.M.; Irving, E.L. Binocular Vision and Eye Movement Disorders in Older Adults. *Investig. Ophthalmol. Vis. Sci.* 2013, *54*, 3798–3805. [CrossRef] [PubMed]
12. Kaido, M.; Fukui, M.; Kawashima, M.; Negishi, K.; Tsubota, K. Relationship between visual function and cognitive function in the elderly: A cross-sectional observational study. *PLoS ONE* 2020, *15*, e0233381. [CrossRef] [PubMed]
13. Ikram, M.K.; Cheung, C.Y.; Wong, T.Y.; Chen, C.P. Retinal pathology as biomarker for cognitive impairment and Alzheimer's disease. *J. Neurol. Neurosurg. Psychiatry* 2012, *83*, 917–922. [CrossRef]
14. Iseri, P.K.; Altintas, O.; Tokay, T.; Yüksel, N. Relationship between Cognitive Impairment and Retinal Morphological and Visual Functional Abnormalities in Alzheimer Disease. *J. Neuro-Ophthalmol.* 2006, *26*, 18–24. [CrossRef]
15. Ito, Y.; Sasaki, M.; Takahashi, H.; Nozaki, S.; Matsuguma, S.; Motomura, K.; Ui, R.; Shikimoto, R.; Kawasaki, R.; Yuki, K.; et al. Quantitative Assessment of the Retina Using OCT and Associations with Cognitive Function. *Ophthalmology* 2020, *127*, 107–118. [CrossRef] [PubMed]
16. Valenti, D.A. Alzheimer's disease and glaucoma: Imaging the biomarkers of neurodegenerative disease. *Int. J. Alzheimer's Dis.* 2011, *2010*, 793931. [CrossRef] [PubMed]
17. Bambo, M.P.; Garcia-Martin, E.; Pinilla, J.; Herrero, R.; Satue, M.; Otin, S.; Fuertes, I.; Marques, M.L.; Pablo, L.E. Detection of retinal nerve fiber layer degeneration in patients with Alzheimer's disease using optical coherence tomography: Searching new biomarkers. *Acta Ophthalmol.* 2014, *92*, e581–e582. [CrossRef]
18. Johnson, E.J. A possible role for lutein and zeaxanthin in cognitive function in the elderly. *Am. J. Clin. Nutr.* 2012, *96*, 1161S–1165S. [CrossRef]
19. Kim, J.-I.; Kang, B.-H. Decreased retinal thickness in patients with Alzheimer's disease is correlated with disease severity. *PLoS ONE* 2019, *14*, e0224180. [CrossRef]
20. Paquet, C.; Boissonnot, M.; Roger, F.; Dighiero, P.; Gil, R.; Hugon, J. Abnormal retinal thickness in patients with mild cognitive impairment and Alzheimer's disease. *Neurosci. Lett.* 2007, *420*, 97–99. [CrossRef]
21. Sunjic-Alic, A.; Zebenholzer, K.; Gall, W. Reporting of Studies Conducted on Austrian Claims Data. In *Navigating Healthcare Through Challenging Times*; IOS Press: Amsterdam, The Netherlands, 2021; pp. 62–69.
22. Cuschieri, S. The STROBE guidelines. *Saudi J. Anaesth.* 2019, *13* (Suppl. S1), S31–S34. [CrossRef] [PubMed]
23. Bruno, D.; Schurmann Vignaga, S. Addenbrooke's cognitive examination III in the diagnosis of dementia: A critical review. *Neuropsychiatr. Dis. Treat.* 2019, *15*, 441–447. [CrossRef]
24. Sampredo, A.; Richman, J.; Pardo, M.J. The adult developmental eye movement test (A-DEM): A tool for saccadic evaluation in adults. *J. Behav. Optom.* 2003, *4*, 1–5.
25. Garzia, R.P.; Richman, J.E.; Nicholson, S.B.; Gaines, C.S. A new visual-verbal saccade test: The Developmental Eye Movement test (DEM). *J. Am. Optom. Assoc.* 1990, *61*, 124–135. [PubMed]
26. Suchoff, I.B.; Kapoor, N.; Waxman, R.; Ference, W. The occurrence of ocular and visual dysfunctions in an acquired brain-injured patient sample. *J. Am. Optom. Assoc.* 1999, *70*, 301–308. [PubMed]
27. Sampedro, A.G.; Richman, J.E.; Pardo, M.S. The Adult Developmental Eye Movement Test (A–DEM). *J. Behav. Optom.* 2003, *14*, 101–105.
28. Gené-Sampedro, A.; Monteiro, P.M.L.; Bueno-Gimeno, I.; Gene-Morales, J.; Piñero, D.P. Validation of a modified version of the adult developmental eye movement test. *Sci. Rep.* 2021, *11*, 19759. [CrossRef]
29. Stringham, J.M.; Garcia, P.V.; Smith, P.A.; McLin, L.N.; Foutch, B.K. Macular Pigment and Visual Performance in Glare: Benefits for Photostress Recovery, Disability Glare, and Visual Discomfort. *Investig. Ophthalmol. Vis. Sci.* 2011, *52*, 7406–7415. [CrossRef]
30. Hammond, B.R.; Fletcher, L.M.; Elliott, J.G. Glare Disability, Photostress Recovery, and Chromatic Contrast: Relation to Macular Pigment and Serum Lutein and Zeaxanthin. *Investig. Ophthalmol. Vis. Sci.* 2013, *54*, 476–481. [CrossRef]
31. Chang, C.W.; Su, K.C.; Lu, F.C.; Cheng, H.M.; Cheng, C.Y. Visual Function and Visual Perception among Senior Citizens with Mild Cognitive Impairment in Taiwan. *Healthcare* 2022, *10*, 20. [CrossRef]
32. Murueta-Goyena, A.; Del Pino, R.; Galdós, M.; Arana, B.; Acera, M.; Carmona-Abellán, M.; Fernández-Valle, T.; Tijero, B.; Lucas-Jiménez, O.; Ojeda, N.; et al. Retinal Thickness Predicts the Risk of Cognitive Decline in Parkinson Disease. *Ann. Neurol.* 2021, *89*, 165–176. [CrossRef] [PubMed]
33. Cunha, L.P.; Lopes, L.C.; Costa-Cunha, L.V.; Costa, C.F.; Pires, L.A.; Almeida, A.L.; Monteiro, M.L. Macular Thickness Measurements with Frequency Domain-OCT for Quantification of Retinal Neural Loss and its Correlation with Cognitive Impairment in Alzheimer's Disease. *PLoS ONE* 2016, *11*, e0153830.
34. Mammadova, N.; Neppl, T.K.; Denburg, N.L.; West Greenlee, M.H. Reduced Retinal Thickness Predicts Age-Related Changes in Cognitive Function. *Front. Aging Neurosci.* 2020, *12*, 81. [CrossRef]

35. Konar, Y.; Bennett, P.J.; Sekuler, A.B. Effects of aging on face identification and holistic face processing. *Vis. Res.* **2013**, *88*, 38–46. [CrossRef]
36. Bennett, P.J.; Sekuler, R.; Sekuler, A.B. The effects of aging on motion detection and direction identification. *Vis. Res.* **2007**, *47*, 799–809. [CrossRef] [PubMed]
37. Betts, L.R.; Taylor, C.P.; Sekuler, A.B.; Bennett, P.J. Aging reduces center-surround antagonism in visual motion pro-cessing. *Neuron* **2005**, *45*, 361–366. [CrossRef] [PubMed]
38. Fernandez, R.; Monacelli, A.; Duffy, C.J. Visual Motion Event Related Potentials Distinguish Aging and Alzheimer's Disease. *J. Alzheimer's Dis.* **2013**, *36*, 177–183. [CrossRef]
39. Owsley, C. Aging and vision. *Vis. Res.* **2011**, *51*, 1610–1622. [CrossRef]
40. Scheiman, M.; Wick, B. *Clinical Management of Binocular Vision: Heterophoric, Accommodative, and Eye Movement Disorders*; Lippincott Williams & Wilkins: Philadelphia, PA, USA, 2008.
41. Xi, J.; Jia, W.-L.; Feng, L.-X.; Lu, Z.-L.; Huang, C.-B. Perceptual Learning Improves Stereoacuity in Amblyopia. *Investig. Opthalmol. Vis. Sci.* **2014**, *55*, 2384–2391. [CrossRef]

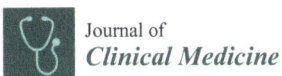

Article

OCT Angiography Fractal Analysis of Choroidal Neovessels Secondary to Central Serous Chorioretinopathy, in a Caucasian Cohort

Rita Serra [1,2,3,*,†], Antonio Pinna [4], Francine Behar-Cohen [5] and Florence Coscas [3,*,†]

1. Department of Biomedical Sciences, University of Sassari, 07100 Sassari, Italy
2. Istituto di Ricerca Genetica e Biomedica (IRGB), CNR, Cittadella Universitaria di Cagliari, 09042 Monserrato, Italy
3. Centre Ophtalmologique de l'Odeon, 113 Bd Saint Germain, 75006 Paris, France
4. Department of Medical, Surgical and Experimental Sciences, Ophthalmology Unit, University of Sassari, 07100 Sassari, Italy; apinna@uniss.it
5. Assistance Publique-Hôpitaux de Paris, Department of Ophthalmology, Ophtalmopole, Hôpital Cochin, 75014 Paris, France; francine.behar@gmail.com
* Correspondence: rita.serra@ymail.com (R.S.); coscas.f@gmail.com (F.C.); Tel.: +1-43295659 (R.S. & F.C.); Fax: +1-43291456 (R.S. & F.C.)
† These authors equally contributed to this work.

Abstract: Central serous chorioretinopathy (CSCR) can be complicated by different types of choroidal neovascularization (CNV). The purpose of this study was to investigate the incidence and quantitative optical coherence tomography angiography (OCT-A) features of CSCR-related CNVs. Methods: This was a retrospective multicenter study including 102 eyes of 102 Caucasian patients with acute or complex CSCR. All patients underwent a comprehensive ophthalmological examination. Quantitative OCT-A parameters, including vascular perfusion density (VPD), fractal dimension (FD), and lacunarity (LAC), were measured in CNV eyes. Results: Forty eyes (39.2%) had acute CSCR, whereas the remaining sixty-two (60.8%) had complex CSCR. CNV was observed in 37 (36.27%) eyes, all of which had the complex form. CNVs were classified as type 1 CNV in 11/37 (29.73%) cases and as polypoidal choroidal vasculopathy (PCV) in the remaining 26/37 (70.27%). Overall, the mean VPD, FD, and LAC of CSCR-related CNVs were 0.52 ± 0.20%, 1.44 ± 0.12, and 2.40 ± 1.1, respectively. No significant difference between type 1 CNV and PCV was found. Conclusion: Complex CSCR is often complicated by type 1 CNV and PCV with similar neovascular architecture and branching complexity, a finding supporting the idea that they might be different stages of the same neovascular process. Future OCT-A fractal analysis-based studies that also include other relevant parameters, such as demographics, presentation, morphology on multimodal imaging, and response to treatment, are necessary before drawing any definitive conclusions.

Keywords: central serous chorioretinopathy; fractal analysis; indocyanine green angiography; optical coherence tomography angiography; polypoidal choroidal vasculopathy; type 1 choroidal neovascularization

Citation: Serra, R.; Pinna, A.; Behar-Cohen, F.; Coscas, F. OCT Angiography Fractal Analysis of Choroidal Neovessels Secondary to Central Serous Chorioretinopathy, in a Caucasian Cohort. *J. Clin. Med.* **2022**, *11*, 1443. https://doi.org/10.3390/jcm11051443

Academic Editors: Giacinto Triolo and Jay Chhablani

Received: 31 January 2022
Accepted: 2 March 2022
Published: 6 March 2022

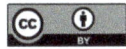

Copyright: © 2022 by the authors. Licensee MDPI, Basel, Switzerland. This article is an open access article distributed under the terms and conditions of the Creative Commons Attribution (CC BY) license (https://creativecommons.org/licenses/by/4.0/).

1. Introduction

The pachychoroid spectrum includes a group of macular disorders (pachychoroid pigment epitheliopathy, pachychoroid neovasculopathy, polypoidal choroidal vasculopathy (PCV), central serous chorioretinopathy (CSCR), and choroidal excavations), presenting a thick choroid and dilated veins facing areas of choriocapillaris attenuation ("pachyvessels") [1,2]. Choroidal neovascularization (CNV) is frequently observed in pachychoroid-associated diseases, but whether pathogenic events are similar in CSCR-related type 1 CNV and PCV is unknown.

CSCR is characterized by choroidal vascular abnormalities with subsequent episodes of serous retinal detachment at the posterior pole, typically affecting young and middle-aged adults [3]. Although the underlying pathophysiological mechanism is still not entirely clear, some risk factors, such as psychosocial stress, uncontrolled systemic hypertension, extraocular glucocorticoids, and pregnancy, have been reported [4]. Generally, the natural history of CSCR has a self-limiting course with a good visual outcome; however, a subset of patients show subretinal fluid (SRF) lasting over six months and/or multifocal sites of epitheliopathy, which predisposes to recurrence, CNV formation, and poor long-term visual outcome [3,5,6]. Recently, the later forms of the disease have been identified as "complex" CSCR [6].

CSCR may be complicated by different types of CNV [2,7]. Type 1 CNV extends below the retinal pigment epithelium (RPE), along the roof of flat irregular pigment epithelium detachments (PEDs) on spectral-domain optical coherence tomography (SD-OCT), and inconsistently shows indistinct late leakage on fluorescein angiography (FA) [2,8,9]. Indocyanine green angiography (ICG-A), thanks to its ability to image the choroidal circulation, has shown that many CSCR-related CNVs initially labeled as type 1 CNVs are instead PCVs [10,11]. Therefore, despite being more time-consuming than FA, ICG-A is currently the gold standard for studying the choroidal vasculature and distinguishing type 1 CNV from PCV [12]. Originally, type 1 CNVs and PCVs were considered two specific idiopathic entities in terms of epidemiology, natural history, prognosis, and traditional multimodal imaging [13,14]. Recently, the Consensus on Neovascular Age-Related Macular Degeneration (AMD) Nomenclature Study Group included PCV in the type 1 CNV group [15]. However, PCV and type 1 CNV may show different prognoses and responses to treatment, and whether or not they are unique clinical entities is still a matter of debate.

In the last years, OCT angiography (OCT-A), a novel non-invasive imaging technique, has become more and more popular in clinical practice. OCT-A allows for the detailed evaluation of CNVs secondary to several retinal diseases [16,17] and is particularly sensitive in the detection of angiographically silent CNVs in CSCR [2,18,19]. Furthermore, OCT-A fractal analysis may be helpful in distinguishing neovascular lesions with different natural histories and prognoses, as reported by Serra et al. [16] in a recent study comparing type 1 CNV in the remission phase versus treatment-naïve quiescent CNV in AMD patients. Similarly, Al Sheik et al. [20] demonstrated that OCT-A fractal analysis is useful for differentiating active type 1 CNV from CNV in the remission phase.

To the best of our knowledge, no study has performed OCT-A fractal analysis of type 1 CNVs and PCVs secondary to CSCR. In this context, the purpose of our investigation was to evaluate the incidence and quantitative OCT-A features of CSCR-related CNVs. Potential biomarkers associated with type 1 CNV and PCV, such as vascular perfusion density (VPD), fractal dimension (FD), and lacunarity (LAC), were analyzed.

2. Materials and Methods

This was a retrospective review of CSCR cases from two high-volume referral centers (Odeon Ophthalmology Center, Paris, France, and Ophthalmology Unit, Department of Medical, Surgical, and Experimental Sciences, University of Sassari, Sassari, Italy) between March 2018 and July 2019.

The current study was conducted in compliance with the tenets of the Declaration of Helsinki for research involving human subjects. All participants provided informed consent to participate in the present survey.

The inclusion criteria were a diagnosis of CSCR in Caucasian patients and high-quality retinal images. Acute CSCR was defined based on the detection of acute serous retinal detachments that involved the posterior pole, were unrelated to other retinal disorders i.e., dome-shaped macula or staphyloma, uveal effusion syndrome, inherited retinal diseases, acquired vitelliform lesions, tumors, inflammation (Vogt–Koyanagi–Harada disease or posterior scleritis), drug toxicity, tractional maculopathy, retinal vascular diseases, optic pit maculopathy, choroidal nevus, CNV due to other causes, or acute hypertensive retinopathy, and were associated with choroidal hyperpermeability and pachyvessels (focal or diffuse dilation of choroidal vessels in Haller's layer) [2,6,21]. Complex CSCR was defined as a condition of documented clinical CSCR features (i.e., SRF, RPE changes in the macular area on FA/ICG-A, and SD-OCT) for a duration of at least six months and/or multifocal epitheliopathy diagnosed on mid-phase ICG-A [6].

Exclusion criteria were the presence of any other concomitant ocular disease potentially affecting imaging interpretation (e.g., myopia > 6 diopters), ocular inflammation, angioid streaks, and relevant opacities of the optic media. Furthermore, eyes with poor-quality images on OCT-A (i.e., presence of artifacts secondary to eye movement or poor fixation) were also excluded.

All eligible patients underwent a complete ophthalmic examination. For each patient, all of the following were performed on the same day: best-corrected visual acuity (BCVA) measurement with Early Treatment Diabetic Retinopathy Study (ETDRS) charts, slit-lamp biomicroscopy with dilated indirect fundoscopy, multimodal retinal imaging, including fundus autofluorescence (FA) and ICG-A (Heidelberg Spectralis HRA + OCT, Heidelberg Engineering, Heidelberg, Germany), SD-OCT analysis (Spectralis Domain OCT, Heidelberg Engineering, Heidelberg, Germany) by the acquisition of a macular volume scan (49 B-scans within a $30° \times 20°$ area) centered on the fovea, and OCT-A (AngioVue XRTVue Avanti, Optovue, Fremont, CA, USA), Triton swept-source OCTA (Topcon, Tokyo, Japan), or Spectralis OCT-A (Spectralis; Heidelberg Engineering, Heidelberg, Germany).

After meticulous review of patients' records and multimodal retinal images, two masked retinal specialists (R.S. and F.C.) classified CSCR as acute or complex. We also assessed the presence of CNVs and determined their subtype according to previously described criteria for multimodal imaging evaluation. On early and intermediate ICG-A frames, type 1 CNV appeared as a hypercyanescent neovascular network, which became a plaque on late frames. PCV was characterized by a typical branching vascular network with aneurysmal dilations on early and intermediate ICG-A frames [17,22,23].

Rare disagreements over the presence or classification of CNVs in images were resolved by open adjudication between readers.

In eyes showing CSCR-related CNVs, the OCT-A angiocube was centered on the CNV, and its appearance and location were compared with ICG-A images. The automated segmentation provided by the OCT-A software was carefully adjusted for correct visualization of the capillary plexus, outer retinal layers, and choriocapillaris to better identify blood flow abnormalities suggestive of CNV and remove segmentation artifacts. Specifically, to avoid differences related to different slab positions, slabs extending from the outer boundary of the outer plexiform layer up to 8 mm beneath the Bruch's membrane were used to visualize all CNV lesions. To improve CNV visualization, the thickness between two automated segmentation lines was altered, moved through the en face layer of the OCT-A, and then correlated with the cross-sectional OCT findings on the OCT-A platform.

Two investigators (R.S. and A.P.) independently reviewed all OCT-A scans to ensure correct segmentation and image quality for post hoc analysis.

To estimate VPD, FD, and LAC, OCT-A slabs showing CNVs were exported in Tagged Image File Format (TIFF) to a previously validated custom graphical user interface built in MATLAB (v.r 2018) for fractal analysis. Images were binarized using the Otsu method [24], and the filtering of speckle noise was achieved by using a median filter with a radius of 2 pixels (small, nonconnected pixels < 10 pixels were removed). Then, the density map was computed, the highest density zone was identified, and the CNV area was calculated by setting a pixel-mm scale. Quantitative OCT-A analysis of VPD, FD, and LAC was performed using a graphical interface. The box-counting method at multiple origins was applied to the image of the binary skeleton to estimate the FD and LAC of the vascular network, which are global indices of morphological complexity and structural non-uniformity, respectively. VPD was defined as the total area of perfused vasculature (on the binarized image) per unit area in a region of measurement (Figures 1 and 2) [17].

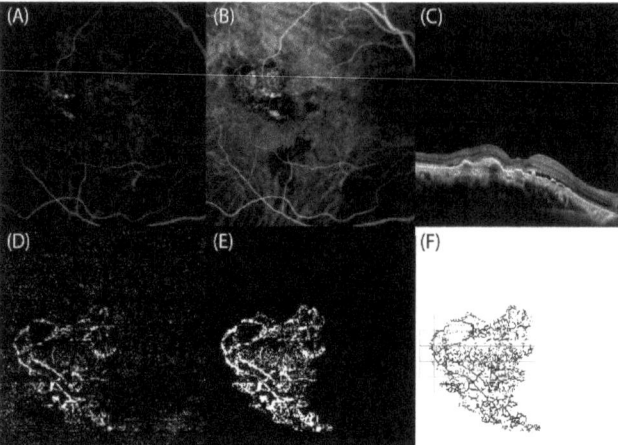

Figure 1. Right eye with polypoidal choroidal vasculopathy (PCV) secondary to complex central serous chorioretinopathy: multimodal retinal imaging and optical coherence tomography angiography (OCT-A) fractal analysis. (**A**,**B**) Indocyanine green angiography frames reveal the presence of a hypercyanescent network corresponding to the branching vascular network (BVN) associated with roundish hypercyanescent structures (polyps) at the terminal ends. (**C**) SD-OCT scan highlights the thick choroid and the subretinal fluid associated with flat irregular pigment epithelium detachments corresponding to the PCV. (**D**) OCT-A slab confirms the presence of a hyperreflective BVN ending with polyps. (**E**) Binarized and (**F**) skeletonized OCT-A image of PCV, obtained using a graphical interface to estimate quantitative fractal parameters.

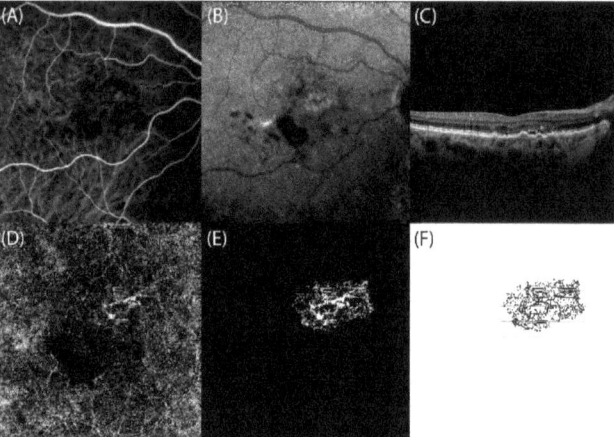

Figure 2. Right eye of type 1 choroidal neovascularization (CNV) secondary to complex central serous chorioretinopathy: multimodal retinal imaging and optical coherence tomography angiography (OCT-A) fractal analysis. (**A**,**B**) Indocyanine green angiography frames reveal the presence of a hypercyanescent network corresponding to type 1 CNV. (**C**) SD-OCT scan highlights the thick choroid and the subretinal fluid associated with flat irregular pigment epithelium detachments corresponding to type 1 CNV. (**D**) OCT-A slab confirms the presence of type 1 CNV appearing as hyperreflective network in the macula region. (**E**) Binarized and (**F**) skeletonized OCT-A image of type 1 CNV, obtained using a graphical interface to estimate quantitative fractal parameters.

The results of descriptive analysis are expressed as numbers and percentages for categorical variables and as means ± standard deviation (SD) for quantitative variables. After testing the data distribution for normality, t-test was used, as appropriate. The correlation between FD values and the area of the lesions was evaluated using Pearson's correlation test. A p value < 0.05 was considered statistically significant. The study data were analyzed using the Statistical Package for Social Sciences version 20.0 for Mac (IBM, Chicago, IL, USA).

3. Results

A total of 102 eyes of 102 Caucasian patients (72 men, 30 women; mean age: 60.23 ± 13.19 years) with CSCR were included in the study. Among patients, 40 (39.2%) patients (32 men, 8 women) had acute CSCR, whereas the remaining 62 (40 men, 22 women) had complex CSCR. Acute CSCR patients were significantly younger than those with the complex form (mean age: 52.20 ± 9.52 years vs. 68.27 ± 10 years; $p < 0.0001$). Mean BCVA was significantly higher in acute CSCR than in the complex form (87.06 ± 18.58 vs. 79.61 ± 23.32 ETDRS letters; $p = 0.03$)

All demographic and clinical data are summarized in Table 1.

Table 1. Demographic and clinical features of central serous chorioretinopathy patients ($n = 102$).

	Acute CSCR	Complex CSCR	p Value
Total eyes, n (%)	40 (39.21%)	62 (60.79%)	-
Sex			
- Male, n (%)	32 (80%)	40 (64.51%)	-
- Female, n (%)	8 (20%)	22 (35.49%)	-
Age, mean ± SD (years)	52.20 ± 9.52	68.27 ± 10	<0.0001
BCVA, mean ± SD (ETDRS letters)	87.06 ± 18.58	79.61 ± 23.32	0.03

Categorical variables are presented as n (%). Continuous variables are presented as mean ± standard deviation (SD). CSCR = central serous chorioretinopathy. BCVA = best-corrected visual acuity.

CNVs were identified in 37/102 (36.27%) eyes, all with complex CSCR. They were classified as type 1 CNV in 11/37 (29.73%) cases and as PCV in the remaining 26 (70.27%). The mean age was 65.18 ± 17.35 years in the type 1 CNV group (7 men, 4 women) and 71.50 ± 7.79 years in the PCV group (17 men, 9 women) ($p > 0.05$). The mean BCVA was 68 ± 39.46 ETDRS letters in the type 1 CNV group and 80.5 ± 15.17 ETDRS letters in the PCV group ($p > 0.05$). Both PCN and type 1 CNV eyes had previously been treated with intravitreal injections of anti-vascular endothelial growth factor (VEGF) agents (4.14 ± 2.6 vs. 6.42 ± 4.07 injections, respectively; $p > 0.05$). On SD-OCT, SRF was observed in 2/11 (18.18%) type 1 CNV eyes and in 4/26 (15.38%) PCV eyes.

Comparison of mid/late ICG-A frames and OCT-A slabs revealed a perfect correspondence in shape and location between the hypercyanescent neovascular networks of type 1 CNV and PCV and the hyperreflective network on OCT-A, appearing as a hyperreflective PED on simultaneous structural OCT. Furthermore, in 20/26 (76.9%) PCV eyes, polypoidal lesions appearing as aneurysmatic hypercyanescent dilations on ICG-A corresponded to roundish hyporeflective structures on OCT-A.

All OCT-A findings were matched with the results of multimodal imaging to ensure that the CNV location was correctly identified during segmentation analysis.

Overall, in CSCR eyes with neovascular complications, the mean CNV area, VPD, FD, and LAC were 2.33 ± 2.06 mm^2, 0.52 ± 0.20%, 1.44 ± 0.12, and 2.40 ± 1.1, respectively. No statistically significant difference was found in terms of area, VPD, FD, and LAC between type 1 CNV and PCV eyes (2.28 ± 1.93 vs. 2.35 ± 2.16 mm^2, 0.53 ± 0.23% vs. 0.52 ± 0.19%, 1.46 ± 0.15 vs. 1.43 ± 0.10, and 2.10 ± 0.49 vs. 2.53 ± 1.26, respectively). Furthermore, no statistically significant association was found between FD values and neovascular lesion size ($r = -0.056$, $p = 0.79$). All quantitative OCT-A data are summarized in Table 2.

Table 2. Quantitative optical coherence tomography angiography (OCT-A) parameters of type 1 choroidal neovascularization (CNV) and polypoidal choroidal vasculopathy (PCV) in complex central serous chorioretinopathy eyes.

	Type 1 CNV	PCV	p Value
VPD, mean ± SD (%)	0.53 ± 0.23	0.52 ± 0.19	0.98
FD, mean ± SD	1.46 ± 0.15	1.43 ± 0.10	0.61
LAC, mean ± SD	2.10 ± 0.49	2.53 ± 1.26	0.33

Continuous variables are presented as mean ± standard deviation (SD). PCV = polypoidal choroidal vasculopathy. CNV = choroidal neovascularization. VPD = vascular perfusion density. FD = fractal dimension. LAC = lacunarity.

4. Discussion

In the last decade, the use of a multimodal imaging approach has resulted in an increasing incidence of CSCR-related CNV lesions, with reported rates ranging from 20% to 58% [2,25].

Similarly, we found a CNV in 37 (36.27%) out of 102 CSCR eyes, all of which had the complex form. Overall, a CNV was identified in 59.6% of eyes with complex CSCR. This high rate can be explained by the use of multimodal imaging in the diagnosis of CNV. The significant correlation between CNV lesions and complex CSCR is likely to depend on the associated epitheliopathy, as suggested by numerous reports identifying epitheliopathy and long-lasting SRF as important predisposing factors for CNV development [2,7,26]. Epitheliopathy, underlying choroidal abnormalities, and choroidal blood flow deregulation seem to play critical roles [25,27,28]. Vascular remodeling in the context of venous overload may also predispose to CNV occurrence [28]. Other authors have postulated that pachyvessels develop when there is increased choroidal perfusion, which promotes oxidative stress, Bruch's membrane injury, and diffuse RPE changes, usually seen above mid-phase hyperpermeability plaques [29]. In eyes with long-lasting CSCR, the CNV is frequently silent for several years and is only diagnosed when OCT-A is performed [18,19].

In CSCR, the prevalent pattern is type 1 CNV [26], although type 2 CNV extending through Bruch's membrane towards the subretinal space has also been described [7]. In this regard, Lee et al. [7] recently described a surprisingly high incidence (76.7%) of type 2 CNV. This discrepancy may be due to the different retinal imaging approaches used to classify CSCR-related CNVs. Alternatively, as previously demonstrated by Chhablani et al. [30], the proportion of type 1 and 2 CNVs may vary, depending on whether or not PCVs are included.

In our study, no type 2 CNV was found. Of the 37/102 (36.27%) eyes with CNVs, 11 (29.73%) had type 1 CNV, and 26 (70.27%) had PCV. Although PCV is relatively uncommon in eyes with wet AMD, with incidence rates ranging from 4% to 9.8% [31,32], in our survey, almost two-thirds of CNVs were PCVs, suggesting a strong correlation between complex CSCR and PCV development. This correlates well with the high incidence of PCV in the Asiatic population, which seems to be unaffected by choroidal thinning with aging [33]. This finding suggests that PCV, which is an aneurysmal dilation of the neovascular process, may also result from choroidal vascular congestion. Another possible explanation for the high rate of PCV in complex CSCR is the long evolution period of silent CNVs, because type 1 CNVs may acquire aneurysmal dilations over time [13,28]. In our Caucasian cohort, PCV patients were approximately 10 years older than those with type 1 CNVs; therefore, we cannot exclude that the former had had CNVs for many years before multimodal retinal imaging could visualize them.

Recently, several reports have highlighted the efficacy of OCT-A in detecting different CNV types associated with AMD. Indeed, OCT-A may provide detailed images of the different retinal layers, thus allowing the identification of morphological characteristics typical of each CNV type [16,17,21]. Furthermore, Coscas et al. demonstrated that morphological CNV features on OCT-A, such as the presence of a branching vascular network, tiny vessels, and peripheral arcade, are related to the activity status of the CNV [34].

Although quantitative OCT-A parameters are useful biomarkers to objectively distinguish AMD-related CNVs with different natural histories and prognoses [16], we failed to find any statistical difference in terms of VPD, FD, and LAC between type 1 CNV and PCV in CSCR eyes. This result might imply that type 1 CNV and PCV in CSCR eyes share similar neovascular architecture and complexity, thus supporting the idea that they are two stages of the same neovascular process, as suggested by Siedlecki et al. [35] and Hua et al. [36].

Our study has several limitations, mainly due to its retrospective nature and the relatively small number of eyes analyzed.

It is also important to acknowledge that the presence of serous PEDs, SRF, and RPE changes, all typical CSCR features, might have somewhat influenced fractal analysis results. Furthermore, we cannot exclude that fractal analysis results may have been affected by the intrinsic limitations of OCT-A instruments. Indeed, the ability of OCT-A to visualize blood flow is limited to a certain range of flow velocities (minimum, 0.5–2 mm/s; saturation, 9 mm/s estimated for current devices) [37]. Therefore, it is theoretically possible that certain neovascular networks, or parts of them, are not detected by OCT-A, because their flow speed is below the instrument detection limit [17]. Evidence indicates that PCVs can show different flow speeds within the same lesion, which may result in a turbulent flow with minimal or no signal on OCT-A. In fact, PCV consists of a branching vascular network, generally appearing on OCT-A as a hyperreflective network terminating with hyporeflective aneurysmal dilations [38].

Finally, we also acknowledge that OCT-A angiocubes provided with the different devices used in this study are characterized by a different number of B-scans, which may lead to a different representation of CNV lesions. However, Munk et al. revealed that no significant differences exist in terms of CNV detection and VD value computation among different OCT-A modules if the correct OCT-A segmentation is used [39]. A similar result was reported by Mastropasqua et al. [40], who failed to find any statistical difference among CNV measurements obtained by different OCT-A devices [40]. By contrast, other authors have reported statistically significant differences between OCT-A devices in terms of CNV area computations, but they argued that such differences may depend on projection artifacts [41].

In summary, our results show that complex CSCR is often complicated by the occurrence of type 1 CNV and PCV with similar neovascular architecture and branching complexity, a finding supporting the idea that they might be different stages of the same neovascular process. However, future studies based on OCT-A fractal analysis but also including other relevant parameters, such as demographics, presentation, morphology on multimodal imaging, and response to treatment, are necessary before drawing any definitive conclusions on whether PCV in CSCR eyes is a specific clinical entity or a variant of type 1 CNV.

Author Contributions: Conceptualization, R.S. and F.C.; formal analysis, R.S., A.P. and F.B.-C.; methodology, R.S., A.P. and F.C.; supervision, F.B.-C. and F.C.; writing—original draft, R.S.; writing—review and editing, R.S., A.P., F.B.-C. and F.C. All authors have read and agreed to the published version of the manuscript.

Funding: This research received no external funding.

Institutional Review Board Statement: Not applicable.

Informed Consent Statement: Informed consent was obtained from all subjects involved in the study.

Data Availability Statement: Not applicable.

Acknowledgments: The authors are sincerely grateful to Sergio Pilia for his assistance in image processing.

Conflicts of Interest: The authors declare no conflict of interest.

References

1. Dansingani, K.K.; Balaratnasingam, C.; Naysan, J.; Freund, K.B. En face imaging of pachychoroid spectrum disorders with swept-source optical coherence tomography. *Retina* **2016**, *36*, 499–516. [CrossRef]
2. Savastano, M.C.; Rispoli, M.; Lumbroso, B. The incidence of neovascularization in central serous chorioretinopathy by optical coherence tomography angiography. *Retina* **2021**, *41*, 302–308. [CrossRef]
3. Spaide, R.F.; Campeas, L.; Haas, A.; Yannuzzi, L.A.; Fisher, Y.L.; Guyer, D.R.; Slakter, J.S.; Sorenson, J.A.; Orlock, D.A. Central Serous Chorioretinopathy in Younger and Older Adults. *Ophthalmology* **1996**, *103*, 2070–2080. [CrossRef]
4. Haimovici, R.; Koh, S.; Gagnon, D.; Lehrfeld, T.; Wellik, S. Risk factors for central serous chorioretinopathy: A case–control study. *Ophthalmology* **2004**, *111*, 244–249. [CrossRef] [PubMed]
5. Piccolino, F.C.; De La Longrais, R.R.; Manea, M.; Cicinelli, S. Posterior Cystoid Retinal Degeneration in Central Serous Chorioretinopathy. *Retina* **2008**, *28*, 1008–1012. [CrossRef] [PubMed]
6. Chhablani, J.; Behar-Cohen, F.; Central Serous Chorioretinopathy International Group. Validation of central serous chorioretinopathy multimodal imaging-based classification system. *Graefes Arch. Clin. Exp. Ophthalmol.* 2021, *online ahead of print*. [CrossRef]
7. Lee, G.-I.; Kim, A.Y.; Kang, S.W.; Cho, S.C.; Park, K.H.; Kim, S.J.; Kim, K.T. Risk Factors and Outcomes of Choroidal Neovascularization Secondary to Central Serous Chorioretinopathy. *Sci. Rep.* **2019**, *9*, 3927. [CrossRef]
8. Fung, A.T.; Yannuzzi, L.A.; Freund, K. Type 1 (sub-retinal pigment epithelial) neovascularization in central serous chorioretinopathy masquerading as neovascular age-related macular degeneration. *Retina* **2012**, *32*, 1829–1837. [CrossRef]
9. Biçer, Ö; Batıoğlu, F.; Demirel, S.; Özmert, E. Multimodal Imaging in Pachychoroid Neovasculopathy: A Case Report. *Turk. J. Ophthalmol.* **2018**, *48*, 262–266. [CrossRef] [PubMed]
10. Ahuja, R.M.; Downes, S.M.; Stanga, P.E.; Koh, A.H.; Vingerling, J.R.; Bird, A.C. Polypoidal choroidal vasculopathy and central serous chorioretinopathy. *Ophthalmology* **2001**, *108*, 1009–1010. [CrossRef]
11. Guyer, D.R.; Yannuzzi, L.A.; Slakter, J.S.; Sorenson, J.A.; Ho, A.; Orlock, D. Digital Indocyanine Green Videoangiography of Central Serous Chorioretinopathy. *Arch. Ophthalmol.* **1994**, *112*, 1057–1062. [CrossRef]
12. Anantharaman, G.; Sheth, J.; Bhende, M.; Narayanan, R.; Natarajan, S.; Rajendran, A.; Manayath, G.; Sen, P.; Biswas, R.; Banker, A.; et al. Polypoidal choroidal vasculopathy: Pearls in diagnosis and management. *Indian J. Ophthalmol.* **2018**, *66*, 896–908. [CrossRef] [PubMed]
13. Yannuzzi, L.A.; Sorenson, J.; Spaide, R.F.; Lipson, B. Idiopathic polypoidal choroidal vasculopathy (IPCV). *Retina* **1990**, *10*, 1–8. [CrossRef] [PubMed]
14. Wong, C.W.; Wong, T.Y.; Cheung, C.M.G. Polypoidal Choroidal Vasculopathy in Asians. *J. Clin. Med.* **2015**, *4*, 782–821. [CrossRef]
15. Spaide, R.F.; Jaffe, G.J.; Sarraf, D.; Freund, K.B.; Sadda, S.R.; Staurenghi, G.; Waheed, N.K.; Chakravarthy, U.; Rosenfeld, P.J.; Holz, F.G.; et al. Consensus Nomenclature for reporting neovascular age-related macular degeneration data: Consensus on neovascular age related macular degeneration nomenclature study group. *Ophthalmology* **2020**, *127*, 616–636. [CrossRef]
16. Serra, R.; Coscas, F.; Pinna, A.; Cabral, D.; Coscas, G.; Souied, E.H. Quantitative optical coherence tomography angiography features of inactive macular neovascularization in age-related macular degeneration. *Retina* **2021**, *41*, 93–102. [CrossRef] [PubMed]
17. Serra, R.; Coscas, F.; Pinna, A.; Cabral, D.; Coscas, G.; Souied, E.H. Fractal analysis of polypoidal choroidal neovascularisation in age-related macular degeneration. *Br. J. Ophthalmol.* **2021**, *105*, 1421–1426. [CrossRef]
18. Romdhane, K.; Zola, M.; Matet, A.; Daruich, A.; Elalouf, M.; Behar-Cohen, F.; Mantel, I. Predictors of treatment response to intravitreal anti-vascular endothelial growth factor (anti-VEGF) therapy for choroidal neovascularisation secondary to chronic central serous chorioretinopathy. *Br. J. Ophthalmol.* **2020**, *104*, 910–916. [CrossRef] [PubMed]
19. Romdhane, K.; Mantel, I. Choroidal Neovascularisation Complicating Chronic Central Serous Chorioretinopathy: The Discovery Rate on Multimodal Imaging. *Klin. Mon. Für Augenheilkd.* **2019**, *236*, 536–541. [CrossRef] [PubMed]
20. Al-Sheikh, M.; Iafe, N.A.; Phasukkjiwatana, N.; Sadda, S.R.; Sarraf, D. Biomarkers of neovascular activity in age-related macular degeneration using optical coherence tomography angiography. *Retina* **2018**, *38*, 220–230. [CrossRef] [PubMed]
21. Forte, R.; Coscas, F.; Serra, R.; Cabral, D.; Colantuono, D.; Souied, E.H. Long-term follow-up of quiescent choroidal neovascularisation associated with age-related macular degeneration or pachychoroid disease. *Br. J. Ophthalmol.* **2020**, *104*, 1057–1063. [CrossRef] [PubMed]
22. Garrity, S.T.; Sarraf, D.; Freund, K.B.; Sadda, S.R. Multimodal Imaging of Nonneovascular Age-Related Macular Degeneration. *Investig. Opthalmol. Vis. Sci.* **2018**, *59*, AMD48–AMD64. [CrossRef] [PubMed]
23. Pece, A.; Bolognesi, G.; Introini, U.; Pacelli, G.; Calori, G.; Brancato, R. Indocyanine green angiography of well-defined plaque choroidal neovascularization in age-related macular degeneration. *Arch. Ophthalmol.* **2000**, *118*, 630–634. [CrossRef] [PubMed]
24. Otsu, N. A Threshold Selection Method from Gray-Level Histograms. *IEEE Trans. Syst. Man. Cybern.* **1979**, *9*, 62–66. [CrossRef]
25. Maftouhi, M.Q.-E.; El Maftouhi, A.; Eandi, C.M. Chronic Central Serous Chorioretinopathy Imaged by Optical Coherence Tomographic Angiography. *Am. J. Ophthalmol.* **2015**, *160*, 581.e1–587.e1. [CrossRef]
26. Manayath, G.J.; Ranjan, R.; Shah, V.S.; Karandikar, S.S.; Saravanan, V.R.; Narendran, V. Central serous chorioretinopathy: Current update on pathophysiology and multimodal imaging. *Oman J. Ophthalmol.* **2018**, *11*, 103–112. [CrossRef]
27. Sartini, F.; Figus, M.; Casini, G.; Nardi, M.; Posarelli, C. Pachychoroid neovasculopathy: A type-1 choroidal neovascularization belonging to the pachychoroid spectrum—Pathogenesis, imaging and available treatment options. *Int. Ophthalmol.* **2020**, *40*, 3577–3589. [CrossRef]

28. Spaide, R.F.; Cheung, C.M.G.; Matsumoto, H.; Kishi, S.; Boon, C.J.; van Dijk, E.H.; Mauget-Faysse, M.; Behar-Cohen, F.; Hartnett, M.E.; Sivaprasad, S.; et al. Venous overload choroidopathy: A hypothetical framework for central serous chorioretinopathy and allied disorders. *Prog. Retin. Eye Res.* **2022**, *86*, 100973. [CrossRef] [PubMed]
29. Bousquet, E.; Provost, J.; Zola, M.; Spaide, R.F.; Mehanna, C.; Behar-Cohen, F. Mid-Phase Hyperfluorescent Plaques Seen on Indocyanine Green Angiography in Patients with Central Serous Chorioretinopathy. *J. Clin. Med.* **2021**, *10*, 4525. [CrossRef] [PubMed]
30. Chhablani, J.; Kozak, I.; Pichi, F.; Chenworth, M.; Berrocal, M.H.; Bedi, R.; Singh, R.P.; Wu, L.; Meyerle, C.; Casella, A.M.; et al. Outcomes of treatment of choroidal neovascularization associated with central serous chorioretinopathy with intravitreal antiangiogenic agents. *Retina* **2015**, *35*, 2489–2497. [CrossRef]
31. Lafaut, B.A.; Leys, A.M.; Snyers, B.; Rasquin, F.; De Laey, J.J. Polypoidal choroidal vasculopathy in Caucasians. *Graefe's Arch. Clin. Exp. Ophthalmol.* **2000**, *238*, 752–759. [CrossRef]
32. Scassellati-Sforzolini, B.; Mariotti, C.; Bryan, R.; Yannuzzi, L.A.; Giuliani, M.; Giovannini, A. Polypoidal choroidal vasculopathy in Italy. *Retina* **2001**, *21*, 121–125. [CrossRef]
33. Lee, W.K.; Baek, J.; Dansingani, K.K.; Lee, J.H.; Freund, K.B. Choroidal morphology in eyes with polypoidal choroidal vasculopathy and normal or subnormal subfoveal choroidal thickness. *Retina* **2016**, *36* (Suppl. 1), S73–S82. [CrossRef] [PubMed]
34. Coscas, F.; Lupidi, M.; Boulet, J.F.; Sellam, A.; Cabral, D.R.; Serra, R.; Français, C.; Souied, E.H.; Coscas, G. Optical coherence tomography angiography in exudative age-related macular degeneration: A predictive model for treatment decisions. *Br. J. Ophthalmol.* **2019**, *103*, 1342–1346. [CrossRef] [PubMed]
35. Siedlecki, J.; Schworm, B.; Priglinger, S.G. The Pachychoroid Disease Spectrum—And the Need for a Uniform Classification System. *Ophthalmol. Retin.* **2019**, *3*, 1013–1015. [CrossRef] [PubMed]
36. Hua, R.; Duan, J.; Zhang, M. Pachychoroid Spectrum Disease: Underlying Pathology, Classification, and Phenotypes. *Curr. Eye Res.* **2021**, *46*, 1437–1448. [CrossRef] [PubMed]
37. Serra, R.; Coscas, F.; Boulet, J.F.; Cabral, D.R.; Lupidi, M.; Coscas, G.J.; Souied, E.H. Predictive activation biomarkers of treatment-naive asymptomatic choroidal neovascularization in age-related macular degeneration. *Retina* **2020**, *40*, 1224–1233. [CrossRef] [PubMed]
38. Rebhun, C.B.; Moult, E.M.; Novais, E.A.; Moreira-Neto, C.; Ploner, S.B.; Louzada, R.N.; Lee, B.; Baumal, C.R.; Fujimoto, J.G.; Duker, J.S.; et al. Polypoidal Choroidal Vasculopathy on Swept-Source Optical Coherence Tomography Angiography with Variable Interscan Time Analysis. *Transl. Vis. Sci. Technol.* **2017**, *6*, 4. [CrossRef]
39. Munk, M.R.; Giannakaki-Zimmermann, H.; Berger, L.; Huf, W.; Ebneter, A.; Wolf, S.; Zinkernagel, M.S. OCT-angiography: A qualitative and quantitative comparison of 4 OCT-A devices. *PLoS ONE* **2017**, *12*, e0177059. [CrossRef]
40. Mastropasqua, R.; Evangelista, F.; Amodei, F.; D'Aloisio, R.; Pinto, F.; Doronzo, E.; Viggiano, P.; Porreca, A.; Di Nicola, M.; Parravano, M.; et al. Optical Coherence Tomography Angiography in Macular Neovascularization: A Comparison Between Different OCTA Devices. *Transl. Vis. Sci. Technol.* **2020**, *9*, 6. [CrossRef]
41. Corvi, F.; Cozzi, M.; Barbolini, E.; Nizza, D.; Belotti, M.; Staurenghi, G.; Giani, A. Comparison between several optical coherence tomography angiography devices and indocyanine green angiography of choroidal neovascularization. *Retina* **2020**, *40*, 873–880. [CrossRef]

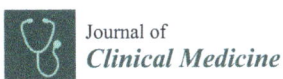

Article

Topographic Relationships among Deep Optic Nerve Head Parameters in Patients with Primary Open-Angle Glaucoma

Do-Young Park [1], Hoon Noh [2], Changwon Kee [2] and Jong-Chul Han [2,3,*]

[1] Department of Ophthalmology, Yeungnam University Hospital, Yeungnam University College of Medicine, Daegu 42415, Korea; dypark@ynu.ac.kr
[2] Department of Ophthalmology, Samsung Medical Center, Sungkyunkwan University School of Medicine, Seoul 06351, Korea; appletea06@gmail.com (H.N.); ckee@skku.edu (C.K.)
[3] Department of Medical Device, Management and Research, SAIHST, Sungkyunkwan University, Seoul 06355, Korea
* Correspondence: heartmedic79@gmail.com

Abstract: Purpose: To investigate the topographic relationships among the deep optic nerve head (ONH) parameters representing myopic axial elongation or changes in the lamina cribrosa (LC) in patients with primary open-angle glaucoma (POAG). Methods: Among patients with POAG who visited the clinic between January 2015 and March 2017, the following deep ONH parameters were measured using spectral-domain optical coherence tomography (SD-OCT): externally oblique border tissue (EOBT) length, ONH tilt angle, optic canal (OC) obliqueness, and anterior LC insertion depth (ALID). In addition, the angular locations of the maximal value of each parameter were measured. We analyzed the correlations between the parameters, correlations with axial length (AL), and the spatial correspondence with glaucomatous ONH damage. Results: A total of 100 eyes with POAG were included in the analysis. The EOBT length, ONH tilt angle, and OC obliqueness were correlated with each other and with AL, whereas ALID showed less correlation with the other parameters and AL. The angular location where the three AL-related parameters had maximum values was also correlated with the predominant region of the glaucomatous ONH damage, while the angular location of the deepest ALID showed less correlation. Conclusions: Among the deep ONH parameters, the AL-related parameters EOBT length, ONH tilt angle, and OC obliqueness showed strong spatial correspondence with glaucomatous ONH damage, whereas the LC-related parameter ALID was less correlated with both AL and the region with glaucomatous ONH damage. Further studies are needed to determine how these differences affect glaucomatous ONH change.

Keywords: open-angle glaucoma; myopia; optic nerve head parameter; lamina cribrosa; optical coherence tomography

Citation: Park, D.-Y.; Noh, H.; Kee, C.; Han, J.-C. Topographic Relationships among Deep Optic Nerve Head Parameters in Patients with Primary Open-Angle Glaucoma. *J. Clin. Med.* **2022**, *11*, 1320. https://doi.org/10.3390/jcm11051320

Academic Editors: Jay Chhablani and Sumit Randhir Singh

Received: 30 December 2021
Accepted: 25 February 2022
Published: 27 February 2022

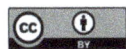

Copyright: © 2022 by the authors. Licensee MDPI, Basel, Switzerland. This article is an open access article distributed under the terms and conditions of the Creative Commons Attribution (CC BY) license (https://creativecommons.org/licenses/by/4.0/).

1. Introduction

Deep optic nerve head (ONH) structures such as the parapapillary sclera, scleral canal wall, and lamina cribrosa are known to be closely related to the development of glaucomatous optic disc damage [1–3]. Although intraocular pressure (IOP) plays the most important role in glaucomatous ONH injury, the location of optic disc damage cannot be predicted by IOP. On the other hand, the deep ONH structures and their locational properties are deeply associated with the site of the glaucomatous ONH damage [4–7]. Visualization of deep ONH structures such as Bruch's membrane (BM) openings or border tissue of Elschnig using optical coherence tomography (OCT) has made it possible to evaluate the association between deep ONH structures and glaucomatous damage by objectively measuring the ONH parameters [8–11].

In our prior studies, we measured deep ONH parameters including externally oblique border tissue (EOBT) length, ONH tilt angle, and optic canal (OC) obliqueness and found that these characteristics were associated with the presence of glaucoma and the location of glaucomatous damage in eyes with myopic normal tension glaucoma [6,7]. In addition to these parameters, anterior lamina cribrosa insertion depth (ALID) has recently been demonstrated to represent the posterior migration of the laminar insertion and is displaced more posteriorly in eyes with POAG than in healthy eyes [12–16]. However, how the LC-related parameter ALID is associated with other deep ONH parameters such as EOBT length, ONH tilt angle, and OC obliqueness, or myopic axial elongation, remains unclear.

Thus, we measured four deep ONH parameters in this study: EOBT length, ONH tilt angle, OC obliqueness, and ALID using SD-OCT in patients with POAG. Then, we investigated correlations between the parameters, the correlation with axial length (AL), and spatial correspondence with glaucomatous ONH damage.

2. Methods

2.1. Participants

For this cross-sectional observational study, patients with OAG (with myopia less than −0.5 diopters (D)) who visited Samsung Medical Center (Seoul, Korea) for their first ophthalmic examination between January 2015 and March 2017 were reviewed, and patients who met the inclusion and exclusion criteria were included. This study was approved by the Institutional Review Board (IRB)/Ethics Committee of Samsung Medical Center and followed the tenets of the Declaration of Helsinki.

The inclusion criteria were as follows: (1) patients diagnosed with OAG at least in one eye after a comprehensive ophthalmic examination; (2) patients with myopia less than −0.5 D in eyes with OAG; and (3) patients with ONH with visible EOBT on OCT examination in eyes with OAG. Patients or eyes satisfying the following criteria were not included: (1) eyes with media opacities, such as a corneal or vitreous opacity or moderate to severe cataract; (2) patients who had systemic or ocular diseases that could affect VF test results; (3) eyes with a high degree of myopia with AL > 28 mm accompanied by myopic degeneration or retinal schisis around the ONH; and (4) eyes with a VF MD of −12 dB or less, for which the glaucomatous VF pattern would be difficult to determine. If the patient had OAG in both eyes, only the eye with less-severe MD was included in the analysis.

Each participant underwent a comprehensive ophthalmic examination, including slit-lamp biomicroscopy, Goldmann applanation tonometry (GAT), manifest refraction, gonioscopic examination, dilated stereoscopic examination of the ONH, color and red-free fundus photography (TRC-50DX; Topcon Medical System, Inc., Oakland, NJ, USA), automated perimetry using a central 30–2 Humphrey Field Analyzer (HFA, model 640; Humphrey Instruments, Inc., San Leandro, CA, USA) with the Swedish interactive threshold algorithm standard, AL measurement (IOL Master; Carl Zeiss Meditec, Jena, Germany), ultrasound pachymetry (Tomey SP-3000; Tomey Ltd., Nagoya, Japan), and SD-OCT examination (Heidelberg Engineering, Heidelberg, Germany). The extent of the VF defect was measured using the mean deviation (MD), pattern standard deviation (PSD), and visual field index (VFI). Reliable VF analysis was defined as a false-negative rate < 15%, a false-positive rate < 15%, and a fixation loss of <20%. IOPs were measured at the first and second visits without IOP-lowering medications. Average IOP values were used in the analysis.

OAG was diagnosed based on the following criteria: (1) the presence of glaucomatous optic disc changes, such as increased cupping (vertical cup-to-disc ratio > 0.7), diffuse or focal neuroretinal rim thinning, disc hemorrhage, or RNFL defects; (2) an open angle on gonioscopic examination with no identifiable causes of secondary glaucoma; and (3) glaucomatous VF defects positive by more than one reliable test for at least two of the following criteria: (1) a cluster of three points with a probability less than 5% on the pattern deviation map in at least one hemifield, including at least one point with a probability less than 1% or a cluster of two points with a probability less than 1%; (2) a glaucoma hemifield test result outside the normal limits; or (3) a PSD of 95% outside the normal limits.

2.2. Imaging of Optic Nerve Head Using SD-OCT

For imaging of the deep structure of the ONH, spectral-domain OCT (SD-OCT; Heidelberg Engineering) with the enhanced depth-imaging (EDI) mode was used. Details of the methods were given previously [7]. Briefly, 48 radial B-scan images (interval of 3.75°) centered on the optic disc were acquired using the EDI mode. Each scan included an average of 20 OCT frames. Magnification errors were corrected using a formula provided by the manufacturer based on results of autorefraction keratometry and focus setting during image acquisition. To measure the parameters of the deep ONH, every other section among the 48 scans (24 radial EDI scans in total) was selected and the scaling was adjusted to 1:1 µm in the software. If the scan section contained a poor-quality OCT image that did not provide interpretable information regarding the BMO or border tissue due to the presence of preluminar tissue or overlying vessels, the next image was used. If more than three of the twenty-four radial scans were unrecognizable, the eye was excluded from the analysis.

The presence of EOBT on OCT images was assessed by two investigators (HN and JCH) in a masked fashion. Disagreement between the investigators was resolved by a third adjudicator (CK).

2.3. Measurement of the Extent and Angular Location of Deep ONH Parameters Using SD-OCT

In a previous study, we defined several parameters representing deep ONH structures on OCT images, such as EOBT length, ONH tilt angle, and optic canal (OC) obliqueness [7]. As previously described, EOBT length was defined as the length between the two end points of the EOBT tissue and ONH tilt angle was defined as the angle between the BMO plane and the optic canal plane. The BMO plane was defined as the line connecting the two BMOs, nasal and temporal. The optic canal plane was defined as the line connecting the nasal BMO and the innermost margin of the EOBT. OC obliqueness was defined as the angle formed by a vertical line and the EOBT [7]. Anterior lamina cribrosa insertion (ALI) was also defined as previously described as the intersection of the scleral canal wall and the anterior surface of the lamina cribrosa in each of the 24 radial scans [12]. ALI depth (ALID) was defined as the distance from the anterior scleral canal opening (ASCO) to the ALI. The maximal value of each parameter among all scanned sections measured was defined as the maximum deep ONH parameter.

The angular location of the maximum deep ONH parameters was measured using the infrared (IR) scanning laser ophthalmoscopy (SLO) image provided by SD-OCT. The line connecting the center of the BMO and fovea was defined as the fovea–BMO (FoBMO) axis. In case the IR photo did not contain the fovea, we set the position of the fovea after aligning the IR and red-free photos using Photoshop CS5 (Adobe System, San Jose, CA, USA). The angular location was defined as the angle between the location of each maximum deep ONH parameter and the FoBMO axis. If the angular location of each parameter was below the FoBMO axis, the location was assigned a positive value. Otherwise, the location of each parameter was assigned a negative value. A schematic diagram of these parameters is provided in the authors' previous work [6,7] (Figure 1).

The extent and angular location of all parameters described above were assessed by two investigators (HN and JCH), and the average values of the two investigators were used in the final analysis.

2.4. Determination of Dominant VF Defect Locations

We divided the VF defect patterns based on the dominant VF defect location (superior vs. inferior dominant). To determine the location of the dominant VF defect, we calculated the average values in pattern deviation plots at the superior and inferior hemifield, respectively (26 points in each hemifield). When one hemifield had a greater absolute value than the other, we regarded it as a dominant VF defect location.

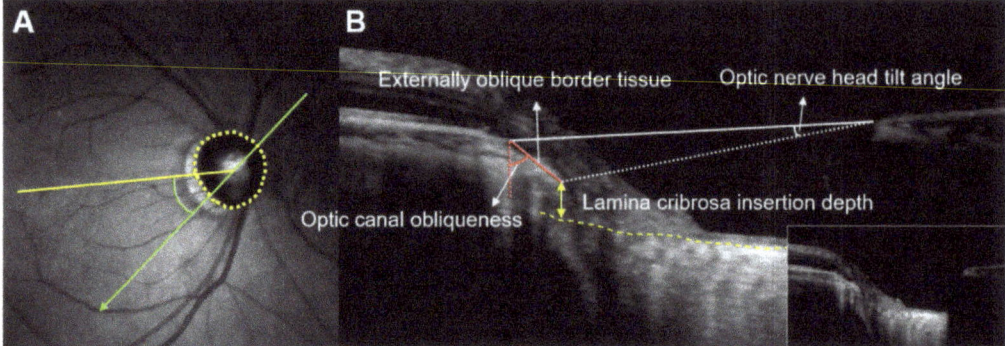

Figure 1. Measurement of the extent and location of the deep ONH parameters EOBT length, ONH tilt angle, OC obliqueness, and ALID. (**A**) BMOs (yellow dots) were marked and the FoBMO axis (yellow line), which is the line connecting the center of the BMO and fovea, was used as the reference line. The locations of maximum deep ONH parameters were measured as angles (green) from the FoBMO axis. When the directions were located below the FoBMO axis, they were assigned positive values. (**B**) Methods for measuring EOBT length, ONH tilt angle, OC obliqueness, and ALID are displayed.

2.5. Statistical Analysis

The intraobserver (two consecutive measurements by HN) and interobserver (measured by HN and JCH) reproducibility of measurements of the OCT parameters were assessed by calculating the intraclass correlation coefficients (ICCs). SD-OCT images of 20 randomly selected patients were used for this analysis. To compare the mean values of continuous variables between the two subgroups, the Mann–Whitney U test was used. A Chi-square test or Fisher's exact test was performed for comparison of categorical variables. Correlations between the parameters and AL and correlations among the parameters were evaluated by Pearson's correlation analysis, and the correlation coefficient (R) was calculated. The Brown–Forsythe test was performed to assess the equality of distribution of the parameters. An AL of 25 mm was arbitrarily set as a cutoff for comparison between the two subgroups according to AL. A logistic regression analysis was performed to confirm the factors associated with the location of the dominant VF defect. A p-value < 0.05 was considered statistically significant. Statistical analyses were performed using IBM SPSS software version 24.0 (IBM Corp., Armonk, NY, USA) and R statistical package version 3.5.3 (R Foundation for Statistical Computing, Vienna, Austria).

3. Results

A total of 139 eyes were analyzed from 139 enrolled patients. Among these eyes, 21 (15.1%) were excluded because of the poor quality of OCT images that did not allow for clear visualization of deep ONH structures such as the BMO or EOBT. Eight eyes with unreliable VF tests, six eyes of advanced glaucoma with VF MD < -12 dB, and four highly myopic eyes with AL > 28 were also excluded from the analysis. In total, 100 eyes from 100 patients were included in the analysis. Intraobserver and interobserver ICCs showed good agreement for the assessment of the extent and the angular location of all four parameters (Table S1). Baseline characteristics of the subjects are described in Table 1.

3.1. Spatial Correspondence between Deep ONH Structures and VF Defects

When the eyes were divided into two groups according to the location of the predominant VF defect, there were 68 (68.0%) eyes in the superior dominant group and 32 (32.0%) eyes in the inferior dominant group. Baseline characteristics, such as age, IOP, AL, CCT, and MD, did not show significant differences between the two groups. The maximum deep ONH parameters, such as EOBT length, ONH tilt angle, OC obliqueness, and ALID, did not differ between the two groups in terms of their extent. However, all the maximum deep ONH parameters except for ALID were significantly inferiorly located in the superior dominant VF group compared with the inferior dominant VF defect group ($p = 0.008$ for maximum EOBT length; $p = 0.008$ for maximum ONH tilt angle; $p = 0.001$ for maximum OC obliqueness; $p = 0.150$ for maximum ALID) (Table 1). A logistic regression analysis also showed that the angular locations of all the deep ONH parameters except for ALID were significantly associated with the inferiorly located dominant VF defect (Table S2). When the angular locations were divided by binary values of positive and negative directions relative to the FoBMO axis, the binary values of the locations of all maximum deep ONH parameters were significantly associated with the dominant location of the VF defect ($p = 0.026$ for the maximum EOBT length location; $p = 0.035$ for the maximum ONH tilt angle location; $p = 0.001$ for the maximum OC obliqueness location; $p = 0.028$ for the maximum ALID location) (Table 1).

Table 1. Baseline characteristics and deep optic nerve head parameters of the patients depending on the dominant VF involvement.

	Total ($n = 100$)	Superior Dominant VF Defect ($n = 68$)	Inferior Dominant VF Defect ($n = 32$)	p Value
Age, years	50.7 ± 11.7	49.4 ± 12.2	53.5 ± 10.4	0.102 *
IOP, mmHg	16.8 ± 3.1	16.8 ± 2.6	16.7 ± 3.9	0.921 *
AL, mm	25.4 ± 1.4	25.4 ± 1.5	25.5 ± 1.2	0.699 *
CCT, μm	538.8 ± 35.0	541.2 ± 36.4	533.7 ± 31.9	0.319 *
MD, dB	−3.9 ± 2.9	−4.1 ± 2.8	−3.4 ± 3.0	0.262 *
Deep ONH parameters				
Extent				
Maximum EOBT length, μm	445.0 ± 203.2	456.4 ± 213.2	420.8 ± 181.0	0.417 *
Maximum ONH tilt angle, °	10.6 ± 4.2	10.6 ± 4.2	10.6 ± 4.3	0.962 *
Maximum OC obliqueness, °	52.4 ± 16.0	51.2 ± 16.3	54.7 ± 15.4	0.309 *
Maximum ALID, μm	573.0 ± 119.1	579.4 ± 119.1	559.5 ± 119.8	0.440 *
Angular location, °				
Maximum EOBT location	16.9 ± 34.9	23.2 ± 34.0	3.5 ± 33.5	**0.008** *
Maximum ONH tilt angle location	17.7 ± 33.2	23.7 ± 33.3	5.0 ± 29.8	**0.008** *
Maximum OC obliqueness location	20.0 ± 34.0	27.4 ± 31.0	4.2 ± 35.3	**0.001** *
Maximum ALID location	38.6 ± 27.6	41.4 ± 25.9	32.8 ± 30.5	0.150 *
Inferior dominant location, n (%)				
Maximum EOBT location	71 (71.0)	53 (77.9)	18 (56.3)	**0.026** †
Maximum ONH tilt angle location	73 (73.0)	54 (79.4)	19 (59.4)	**0.035** †
Maximum OC obliqueness location	74 (74.0)	57 (83.8)	17 (53.1)	**0.001** †
Maximum ALID location	91 (91.0)	65 (95.6)	26 (81.3)	**0.028** †

VF, visual field; IOP, intraocular pressure; AL, axial length; CCT, central corneal thickness; MD, mean deviation; ONH, optic nerve head; EOBT, externally oblique border tissue; OC, optic canal; ALID, anterior lamina cribrosa insertion depth; °: degree. Values are mean ± SD or frequency (%); p values < 0.05 are shown in bold; * Independent t-test; † χ^2 test or Fisher's exact test for comparison between superior dominant VF defects and inferior dominant VF defects.

3.2. Extent and Location of Deep ONH Parameters According to AL

When we analyzed the correlation between the deep ONH parameters, significant correlations were observed between all parameters except ALID in both aspects of the extent and angular location (Table 2).

Next, we analyzed the correlation between the AL and the extent of deep ONH parameters. The extent of all deep ONH parameters except ALID were significantly positively correlated with AL (R = 0.52, $p < 0.001$ for the maximum EOBT length; R = 0.28, $p = 0.005$ for the maximum ONH tilt angle; R = 0.43, $p < 0.001$ for the maximum OC oblique-ness; R = −0.19, $p = 0.061$ for the maximum ALID) (Figure 2).

Table 2. Correlations among the extent and location of the deep ONH parameters.

Parameters, Extent	Maximum ONH Tilt Angle	Maximum OC Obliqueness	Maximum ALID
Maximum EOBT			
Pearson's coefficient	0.707	0.577	−0.050
p value *	<0.001	<0.001	0.619
Maximum ONH tilt angle			
Pearson's coefficient		0.255	0.149
p value *		0.011	0.140
Maximum OC Obliqueness			
Pearson's coefficient			−0.172
p value *			0.087
Parameters, Location	**Maximum ONH Tilt Angle Location**	**Maximum OC Obliqueness Location**	**Maximum ALID Location**
Maximum EOBT location			
Pearson's coefficient	0.883	0.819	0.290
p value *	<0.001	<0.001	0.003
Maximum ONH tilt angle location			
Pearson's coefficient		0.803	0.159
p value *		<0.001	0.114
Maximum OC Obliqueness location			
Pearson's coefficient			0.243
p value *			0.015

ONH, optic nerve head; EOBT, externally oblique border tissue; OC, optic canal; ALID, anterior lamina cribrosa insertion depth. p values < 0.05 are shown in bold; * Pearson's correlation.

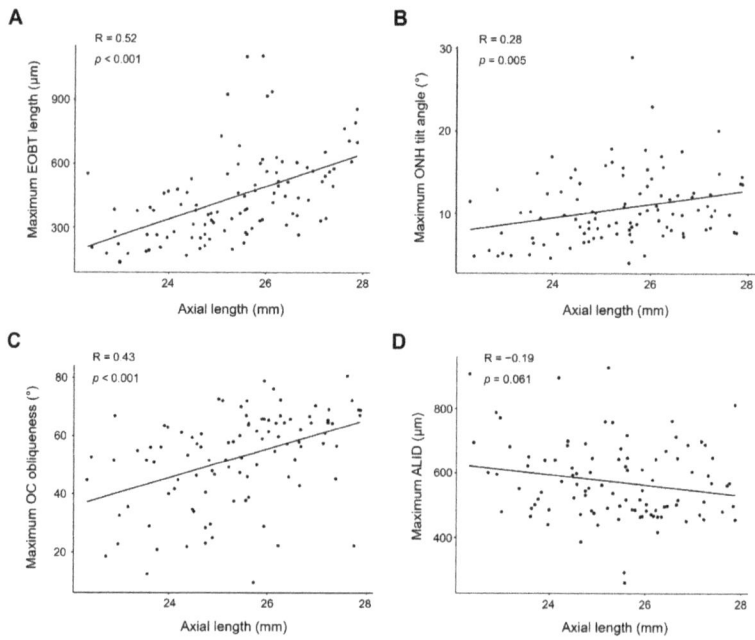

Figure 2. Pearson's correlation plots showing correlations between AL and maximal EOBT length (**A**), maximal ONH tilt angle (**B**), maximal OC obliqueness (**C**), and ALID (**D**). All parameters except ALID showed significant correlations with AL.

The angular locations of the parameters are shown in Figure 3. The angular locations of the deep ONH parameters were mainly positioned in the inferotemporal region of the ONH. When the AL was divided into two groups (AL ≥ 25 mm and AL < 25 mm), in eyes with AL ≥ 25 mm, the maximum EOBT location, maximum ONH tilt angle location, and maximum OC obliqueness location were located more superiorly (temporally) than in eyes with AL < 25 mm, while the maximum ALID location was not significantly different between the two groups ($p = 0.047$ for the maximum EOBT length; $p = 0.020$ for the maximum ONH tilt angle; $p = 0.013$ for the maximum OC obliqueness; $p = 0.806$ for the maximum ALID). In addition, eyes with AL ≥ 25 mm showed significantly narrower distributions in the maximum EOBT location, maximum ONH tilt angle location, and maximum OC obliqueness location than those with AL < 25 mm, while the maximum ALID did not ($p = 0.007$ for the maximum EOBT length; $p = 0.049$ for the maximum ONH tilt angle; $p = 0.002$ for the maximum OC obliqueness; $p = 0.067$ for the maximum ALID).

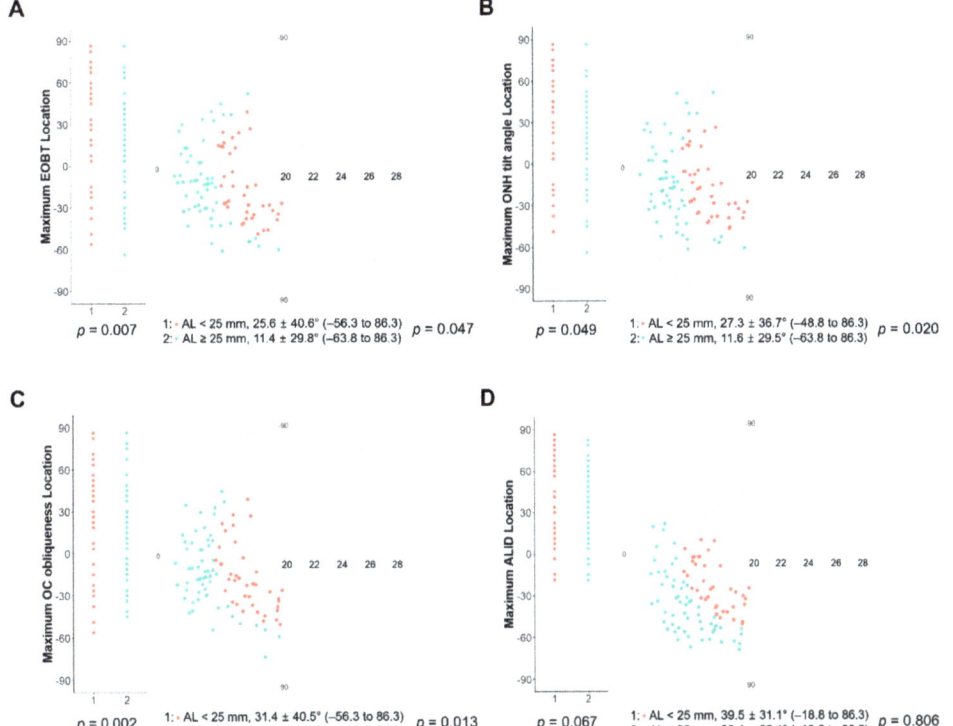

Figure 3. Frequency distribution of the location of each deep ONH parameter with the maximal value (maximal EOBT length (**A**), maximal ONH tilt angle (**B**), maximal OC obliqueness (**C**), and ALID (**D**)) according to the meridian clock. The eyes were divided into two groups with a cutoff of 25 mm. In eyes with AL ≥ 25 mm, all the maximum deep ONH parameters except ALID were significantly located temporally compared with the eyes with AL < 25 mm. All of the deep ONH parameters with their maximal values were placed in the inferotemporal direction. In eyes with AL ≥ 25 mm, all the parameters except ALID showed narrower distributions than in eyes with AL < 25 mm.

3.3. Relationship between RNFL Thickness and Location of Deep ONH Parameters

We divided the deep ONH parameters into 'superior' and 'inferior' groups according to the position of their maximum values. When we compared the RNFL thickness at the superior, temporal, inferior, and nasal positions between the two groups of each deep ONH parameter, the inferior RNFL thickness was significantly lower in inferiorly located groups with the parameters of EOBT location, ONH tilt location, and OC obliqueness location compared with superiorly located groups. On the other hand, there was no significant difference in the inferior RNFL thickness according to the location of the maximum ALID (Table 3).

Table 3. Comparisons of RNFL thickness according to the location of the deep ONH parameters.

	Inferior Maximum EOBT Location, n = 71	Superior Maximum EOBT Location, n = 29	p Value
RNFL thickness, μm			
Superior	93.5 ± 16.8 (58 to 138)	95.8 ± 18.8 (64 to 145)	0.555 *
Temporal	64.1 ± 12.5 (37 to 97)	64.9 ± 11.0 (41 to 81)	0.761 *
Inferior	77.8 ± 15.0 (47 to 117)	92.7 ± 17.2 (65 to 129)	<0.001 *
Nasal	63.1 ± 8.9 (43 to 87)	64.4 ± 9.2 (49 to 84)	0.508 *
	Inferior Maximum ONH Tilt Location, n = 73	Superior Maximum ONH Tilt Location, n = 27	p Value
RNFL thickness, μm			
Superior	94.6 ± 16.9 (58 to 138)	93.1 ± 18.8 (64 to 145)	0.720 *
Temporal	64.5 ± 12.2 (37 to 97)	63.9 ± 11.8 (41 to 89)	0.829 *
Inferior	79.4 ± 15.7 (47 to 129)	89.5 ± 18.5 (55 to 125)	**0.008 ***
Nasal	62.7 ± 8.8 (43 to 87)	65.5 ± 9.3 (49 to 84)	0.168 *
	Inferior Maximum OC Obliqueness Location, n = 74	Superior Maximum OC Obliqueness Location, n = 26	p Value
RNFL thickness, μm			
Superior	94.3 ± 17.1 (58 to 145)	93.8 ± 18.4 (64 to 129)	0.910 *
Temporal	64.2 ± 12.5 (37 to 97)	64.6 ± 10.7 (41 to 81)	0.885 *
Inferior	79.0 ± 14.5 (47 to 117)	90.1 ± 19.6 (55 to 129)	**0.002 ***
Nasal	63.7 ± 9.2 (43 to 87)	62.7 ± 8.5 (49 to 83)	0.623 *
	Inferior Maximum ALID location, n = 91	Superior Maximum ALID location, n = 9	p Value
RNFL thickness, μm			
Superior	94.7 ± 17.7 (58 to 145)	89.2 ± 13.0 (71 to 115)	0.323 *
Temporal	64.3 ± 12.3 (37 to 97)	64.9 ± 9.0 (53 to 78)	0.763 *
Inferior	81.5 ± 17.3 (47 to 129)	88.1 ± 14.1 (73 to 120)	0.250 *
Nasal	63.3 ± 9.1 (43 to 87)	65.0 ± 7.0 (57 to 76)	0.531 *

ONH, optic nerve head; EOBT, externally oblique border tissue; OC, optic canal; ALID, anterior lamina cribrosa insertion depth; RNFL, retinal nerve fiber layer. Values are mean ± SD (range); p values < 0.05 are shown in bold; * Independent t-test or Mann–Whitney U test.

4. Discussion

In this study, we analyzed the characteristics of four deep ONH parameters measured by SD-OCT in patients with POAG in terms of correlations between the parameters, correlations with AL, and spatial correspondence with the glaucomatous ONH damage. As a result, we found that EOBT length, ONH tilt angle, and OC obliqueness, which are known to be regionally correlated with PPA, were correlated with each other and with AL, whereas ALID showed less correlation with other parameters and AL. In addition, the location where these three inter-related parameters had maximum values corresponded well to the predominant region of the glaucomatous ONH damage, while the location where ALI was the deepest corresponded less. These results indicate that each of the parameters representing the features of deep ONH may have varying degrees of association with myopia or the location of the glaucomatous damage, which should be taken into account when we interpret the myopic or glaucomatous ONH change.

In this study, four parameters were investigated as parameters characterizing the deep ONH: EOBT length, ONH tilt angle, OC obliqueness, and ALID. Of these, as previously reported, the extent of EOBT length, ONH tilt angle, and OC obliqueness, which were associated with the presence of PPA, were strongly correlated with the AL [7]. The location of their maximum values was positioned temporally as the AL elongated. In addition to these three parameters, we analyzed ALID in this study. ALI is the part of the wall of the scleral canal in contact with the anterior surface of the LC, and its depth (ALID) can represent how much the LC is deformed posteriorly [17]. ALID has been reported to be located deeply in superior and inferior parts of the optic disc of healthy controls, and another study showed that ONHs of patients with POAG had a deeper ALID than those of healthy controls [12–14]. Therefore, ALID has been considered to be a factor related to the development of glaucomatous ONH change.

The interesting finding of this study was that, compared with the other three parameters, ALID had less correlation with the other parameters and with AL. We interpreted the reason for such a difference between the parameters as follows. When the AL is elongated and glaucomatous ONH changes occur at the same time, the ONH undergoes both passive changes and active remodeling. Among the four parameters we analyzed in this study, EOBT length, ONH tilt angle, and OC obliqueness are thought to be parameters representing the passive changes that occur as the AL increases based on findings that they show a strong correlation with AL [7]. On the other hand, ALID is a factor related to the active remodeling of the ONH occurring at the level of the LC [12,17], and it may not be directly related to the changes in AL. In other words, unlike the other three parameters, ALID can change even after the myopic AL elongation process stops.

In the analysis of the relationship between the positional characteristics of four ONH parameters and the predominant region of the glaucomatous ONH damage, contrary to our expectations, the AL-related factors EOBT length, ONH tilt angle, and OC obliqueness corresponded more to the location of glaucomatous ONH damage compared with the LC-related factor ALID. If the deepening of ALI is a phenomenon that reflects the glaucomatous change in the LC, ALID would seem to correlate better with the location of glaucomatous damage, but this was not the case in this study. This may be related to the fact that most patients (95%) included in this study had early stage normal tension glaucoma with a mild VF defect (MD −3.9 dB). Disc cupping due to elevated IOP may deepen ALI as the LC is excavated posteriorly, but disc cupping in eyes with NTG more involves focal prelaminar and neuroretinal rim thinning than lamina deformation, especially in early stage glaucoma [12,18,19]. In addition, even if the LC depth increases as glaucoma progresses, this phenomenon may occur in a diffuse manner rather than a localized manner, and the ALID will have a less localized value to correlate with glaucomatous damage. We think that parameters such as BMO-MRW representing the prelamina or neuroretinal rim can be correlated better in terms of the location of the glaucomatous ONH damage in eyes with NTG [20]. Analyzing more patients separately from eyes with NTG and POAG in the future will help to determine whether the topographical relationship between ALID and glaucomatous ONH damage is affected by IOP or the severity of glaucoma.

This study has several limitations. First, this study was a cross-sectional study, so it is not possible to establish causal relationships. In other words, the issues of whether parameters related to AL affect the location of the glaucomatous damage and whether changes in the ONH parameters and glaucomatous damage occur together due to other unknown factors remain unresolved. Similarly, the ALID can be deepened as the LC excavates backward as glaucoma progresses; however, on the other hand, an ONH with a deeper ALID may be more prone to glaucoma. Second, although the positions of each ONH parameter were measured precisely by angle, the location of glaucomatous damage in the ONH was inferred by comparing the superior and inferior regions of the VFD or RNFL thickness. If the thinnest location of the BMO-MRW is measured by angle in the future, it will provide a more detailed correlation analysis between the ONH parameters and the location of ONH damage. Finally, this study included a single disease group with a limited sample size. Further studies are needed to examine the differences between the parameters analyzed in this study, including the longitudinal changes, with a larger number of patients and healthy controls.

In conclusion, we found that among the deep ONH parameters, EOBT length, ONH tilt angle, and OC obliqueness were strongly correlated with AL and the location of the glaucomatous ONH damage whereas the LC-related parameter ALID was correlated with neither AL nor the region with glaucomatous ONH damage in eyes of patients with POAG. These findings suggest that AL-related ONH parameters and LC-related ONH parameters may have different influences on the localization of glaucomatous ONH damage. Further studies are needed to determine how these differences affect the development of glaucomatous ONH damage.

Supplementary Materials: The following supporting information can be downloaded at: https://www.mdpi.com/article/10.3390/jcm11051320/s1, Table S1: Intra- and inter-observer reproducibility in measurement of parameters; Table S2: Factors associated with an inferiorly located dominant VF defect.

Author Contributions: Conceptualization, J.-C.H. and C.K.; Data curation, H.N.; Formal analysis, H.N.; Funding acquisition, D.-Y.P. and J.-C.H.; Investigation, D.-Y.P. and J.-C.H.; Methodology, D.-Y.P. and J.-C.H.; Resources, J.-C.H. and C.K.; Supervision, J.-C.H. and C.K.; Validation, J.-C.H.; Writing—original draft, D.-Y.P. and H.N.; Writing—review and editing, D.-Y.P. and J.-C.H. All authors have read and agreed to the published version of the manuscript.

Funding: This work was supported by a 2020 Yeungnam University Research Grant and the Basic Science Research Program through the National Research Foundation of Korea (NRF) funded by the Ministry of Education (2017R1D1A1B03034834). The funders had no role in the study design, the data collection and analysis, the decision to publish, or the preparation of the manuscript.

Institutional Review Board Statement: The study was conducted in accordance with the Declaration of Helsinki, and approved by the Institutional Review Board of Samsung Medical Center (IRB no. 2019-06-066).

Informed Consent Statement: Informed consent was waived due to the nature of the retrospective study.

Data Availability Statement: The data presented in this study are available from the authors upon reasonable request. The data are not publicly available due to privacy and ethical issue.

Conflicts of Interest: The authors declare no conflict of interest.

References

1. Burgoyne, C.F.; Downs, J.C.; Bellezza, A.J.; Suh, J.K.F.; Hart, R.T. The optic nerve head as a biomechanical structure: A new paradigm for understanding the role of IOP-related stress and strain in the pathophysiology of glaucomatous optic nerve head damage. *Prog. Retin. Eye Res.* **2005**, *24*, 39–73. [CrossRef]
2. Bellezza, A.J.; Hart, R.T.; Burgoyne, C.F. The optic nerve head as a biomechanical structure: Initial finite element modeling. *Investig. Ophthalmol. Vis. Sci.* **2000**, *41*, 2991–3000.
3. Downs, J.C.; Girkin, C.A. Lamina cribrosa in glaucoma. *Curr. Opin. Ophthalmol.* **2017**, *28*, 113–119. [CrossRef] [PubMed]
4. Cho, B.J.; Park, K.H. Topographic correlation between beta-zone parapapillary atrophy and retinal nerve fiber layer defect. *Ophthalmology* **2013**, *120*, 528–534. [CrossRef]
5. Choi, J.A.; Park, H.Y.L.; Shin, H.Y.; Park, C.K. Optic disc tilt direction determines the location of initial glaucomatous damage. *Investig. Ophthalmol. Vis. Sci.* **2014**, *55*, 4991–4998. [CrossRef]
6. Han, J.C.; Choi, J.H.; Park, D.Y.; Lee, E.J.; Kee, C. Deep optic nerve head morphology is associated with pattern of glaucomatous visual field defect in open-angle glaucoma. *Investig. Ophthalmol. Vis. Sci.* **2018**, *59*, 3842–3851. [CrossRef]
7. Han, J.C.; Lee, E.J.; Kim, S.B.; Kee, C. The characteristics of deep optic nerve head morphology in myopic normal tension glaucoma. *Investig. Ophthalmol. Vis. Sci.* **2017**, *58*, 2695–2704. [CrossRef]
8. Reis, A.S.C.; O'Leary, N.; Yang, H.L.; Sharpe, G.P.; Nicolela, M.T.; Burgoyne, C.F.; Chauhan, B.C. Influence of clinically invisible, but optical coherence tomography detected, optic disc margin anatomy on neuroretinal rim evaluation. *Investig. Ophthalmol. Vis. Sci.* **2012**, *53*, 1852–1860. [CrossRef] [PubMed]
9. Reis, A.S.C.; Sharpe, G.P.; Yang, H.L.; Nicolela, M.T.; Burgoyne, C.F.; Chauhan, B.C. Optic disc margin anatomy in patients with glaucoma and normal controls with spectral domain optical coherence tomography. *Ophthalmology* **2012**, *119*, 738–747. [CrossRef] [PubMed]
10. Hosseini, H.; Nassiri, N.; Azarbod, P.; Giaconi, J.; Chou, T.; Caprioli, J.; Nouri-Mahdavi, K. Measurement of the optic disc vertical tilt angle with spectral-domain optical coherence tomography and influencing factors. *Am. J. Ophthalmol.* **2013**, *156*, 737–744. [CrossRef] [PubMed]
11. Strouthidis, N.G.; Grimm, J.; Williams, G.A.; Cull, G.A.; Wilson, D.J.; Burgoyne, C.F. A comparison of optic nerve head morphology viewed by spectral domain optical coherence tomography and by serial histology. *Investig. Ophthalmol. Vis. Sci.* **2010**, *51*, 1464–1474. [CrossRef] [PubMed]

12. Lee, K.M.; Kim, T.W.; Weinreb, R.N.; Lee, E.J.; Girard, M.J.; Mari, J.M. Anterior lamina cribrosa insertion in primary open-Angle glaucoma patients and healthy subjects. *PLoS ONE* **2014**, *9*, e114935. [CrossRef] [PubMed]
13. Park, S.C.; Kiumehr, S.; Teng, C.C.; Tello, C.; Liehmann, J.M.; Ritch, R. Horizontal central ridge of the lamina cribrosa and regional differences in laminar insertion in healthy subjects. *Investig. Ophthalmol. Vis. Sci.* **2012**, *53*, 1610–1616. [CrossRef] [PubMed]
14. Kim, Y.W.; Jeoung, J.W.; Kim, D.W.; Girard, M.J.; Mari, J.M.; Park, K.H.; Kim, D.M. Clinical assessment of lamina cribrosa curvature in eyes with primary open-Angle glaucoma. *PLoS ONE* **2016**, *11*, e0150260. [CrossRef] [PubMed]
15. Kim, Y.W.; Kim, D.W.; Jeoung, J.W.; Kim, D.M.; Park, K.H. Peripheral lamina cribrosa depth in primary open-angle glaucoma: A swept-source optical coherence tomography study of lamina cribrosa. *Eye* **2015**, *29*, 1368–1374. [CrossRef] [PubMed]
16. Sawada, Y.; Hangai, M.; Murata, K.; Ishikawa, M.; Yoshitomi, T. Lamina cribrosa depth variation measured by spectral-Domain optical coherence tomography within and between four glaucomatous optic disc phenotypes. *Investig. Ophthalmol. Vis. Sci.* **2015**, *56*, 5777–5784. [CrossRef] [PubMed]
17. Yang, H.L.; Williams, G.; Downs, J.C.; Sigal, I.A.; Roberts, M.D.; Thompson, H.; Burgoyne, C.F. Posterior (outward) migration of the lamina cribrosa and early cupping in monkey experimental glaucoma. *Investig. Ophthalmol. Vis. Sci.* **2011**, *52*, 7109–7121. [CrossRef] [PubMed]
18. Li, R.H.; Wang, X.; Wei, Y.H.; Fang, Y.; Tian, T.; Li, M.; Cai, Y.; Pan, Y. Structure-Function relationship between Bruch's membrane opening-Minimum rim width and perimetry in open-Angle glaucoma subtypes. *Graefes Arch. Clin. Exp. Ophthalmol.* **2020**, *258*, 595–605. [CrossRef] [PubMed]
19. Kim, Y.W.; Jeoung, J.W.; Girard, M.J.A.; Mari, J.M.; Park, K.H. Positional and curvature difference of lamina cribrosa according to the baseline intraocular pressure in primary open-Angle glaucoma: A swept-Source optical coherence tomography (ss-oct) study. *PLoS ONE* **2016**, *11*, e0162182. [CrossRef] [PubMed]
20. Gmeiner, J.M.D.; Schrems, W.A.; Mardin, C.Y.; Laemmer, R.; Kruse, F.E. Schrems-Hoesl LM. Comparison of bruch's membrane opening minimum rim width and peripapillary retinal nerve fiber layer thickness in early glaucoma assessment. *Investig. Ophthalmol. Vis. Sci.* **2016**, *57*, 575–584. [CrossRef] [PubMed]

Review

Optical Coherence Tomography Findings in Rhegmatogenous Retinal Detachment: A Systematic Review

Carla Danese [1] and Paolo Lanzetta [1,2,*]

[1] Department of Medicine—Ophthalmology, University of Udine, 33100 Udine, Italy
[2] Istituto Europeo di Microchirurgia Oculare (IEMO), 33100 Udine, Italy
* Correspondence: paolo.lanzetta@uniud.it; Tel.: +39-0432559907

Abstract: Rhegmatogenous retinal detachment is a sight-threatening condition that may lead to blindness if left untreated. Surgical treatments may vary and are tailored to a single patient. Anatomical and functional results may vary, due to factors that are currently under study. Optical coherence tomography (OCT) allows a detailed visualization of the retinal structure. Some studies have been performed using OCT on eyes with retinal detachment. We performed a review on the subject. Several data have been obtained using different OCT applications. Some alterations may represent potential biomarkers since they are associated with visual and anatomical prognoses. Increased knowledge on the subject may be helpful to choose among different surgical strategies and endotamponades. More research on the topic is needed.

Keywords: OCT; optical coherence tomography; retinal detachment; rhegmatogenous retinal detachment; angiography; en face; adaptive optics; biomarkers

1. Introduction

Retinal detachment is defined as the separation of the neurosensory retina from the underlying retinal pigment epithelium (RPE). In its rhegmatogenous form, liquefied vitreous detaches the retina by passing through a retinal tear or hole. Its incidence is around 1 in 10,000 persons per year [1]. According to the macular involvement, it may be classified as "macula on" or "macula off" retinal detachment. Especially when it is of recent onset and without macular involvement, it is considered a surgical emergency. Potential risks of delayed surgery are a progression of the detached retina, development of proliferative vitreoretinopathy, and worse functional outcomes if the macula becomes involved [2]. It may lead to blindness of the affected eye unless surgical treatment is promptly performed. There is no ideal strategy for its treatment. The currently available options are scleral buckling, pars plana vitrectomy, and pneumatic retinopexy. Each one has characteristic advantages for certain patients. After vitrectomy, a tamponade with gas or silicone oil is required [3]. In some cases, visual results may be unsatisfying. In order to better understand factors affecting postoperative prognosis, several studies have been conducted correlating optical coherence tomography (OCT) findings with clinical outcomes [4]. Spectral-domain OCT (SD-OCT) and swept-source OCT (SS-OCT) are both types of Fourier domain OCT. Nowadays, they have a high sensitivity, providing high imaging speed, improved image contrast, full volumetric tissue information, and high resolution in the three dimensions [5]. OCT usually refers to B-scan imaging, derived from sagittal and transverse sections. C-scan, or en face OCT, is an application of SD-OCT, producing frontal sections of retinal layers [6]. Three-dimensional images are obtained with serial horizontal or vertical B-scan images, which are reconstructed in a three-dimensional "cube" [7]. OCT angiography (OCT-A) is a novel development, allowing visualization of the retinal vascularization without a contrast agent [5]. Recently, instruments using adaptive optics have been combined with SS-OCT imaging (AO-OCT). Adaptive optics produce a two-dimensional areal image of the retina with a cellular resolution. Therefore, this multimodal retina imaging system may add cellular resolution to images obtained with SS-OCT [8].

This review aims to be an update of the knowledge on the subject so far, taking into account SD-OCT, SS-OCT, OCT-A, three-dimensional OCT (3D-OCT), and AO-OCT.

Although some authors have performed OCT studies specifically focused on the postoperative period in order to study surgical complications, such as macular hole formation, these findings will be only briefly touched on the present review [9,10].

2. Materials and Methods

Articles published in PubMed, without restriction on the year of publication and published until July 2022, were considered. Appropriate keywords were used in order to retrieve research articles on rhegmatogenous retinal detachment and OCT. Only articles in English wereincluded. Research works conducted with time-domain OCT were not included.

Tables 1–5 report the included publications, divided according to the type of study and OCT examination.

Table 1. Spectral-domain and swept-source OCT.

Authors	Year	Study	No. of Eyes
Lai et al.	2010	Retrospective	37
Stopa et al.	2011	Prospective	25
Dell'Omo et al.	2012	Retrospective	33
Huang et al.	2013	Retrospective	58
Nagpal et al.	2014	Prospective	30
Terauchi et al.	2015	Retrospective	49
Srydar et al.	2015	Case report	2
Tee et al.	2016	Retrospective	61
Purtskhvanidze et al.	2017	Retrospective	20
Yang et al.	2018	Case report	1
Raczynska et al.	2018	Prospective	57
Poulsen et al.	2019	Prospective	84
Noda et al.	2019	Retrospective	42
Borowicz et al.	2019	Prospective	62
Yeo et al.	2020	Retrospective	114
Mané et al.	2021	Retrospective	85
Ozsaygili et al.	2021	Retrospective	86
Felfeli et al.	2021	Retrospective	406
Klaas et al.	2021	Retrospective	102
Kumar et al.	2021	Case control	39
Muni et al.	2021	RCT	150
Zgolli et al.	2021	Prospective	90
Uemura et al.	2021	Retrospective	11
Guan et al.	2021	Retrospective	49
Baudin et al.	2021	Prospective	115
Iwase et al.	2021	Retrospective	69
Chatziralli et al.	2021	Prospective	86
Gharbiya et al.	2012	Retrospective	35
Bansal et al.	2021	Prospective	15
Hostovsky et al.	2021	Retrospective	44
Lee et al.	2021	Retrospective	30
Lee et al.	2022	RCT	83
Horozoglu et al.	2022	Retrospective	20

RCT: randomized clinical trial.

Table 2. OCT angiography.

Authors	Year	Study	No. of Eyes
Hong et al.	2020	Retrospective	31
Chatziralli et al.	2020	Prospective	103
Xu et al.	2020	Retrospective	71
Roohipoor et al.	2020	Prospective	45
Nam et al.	2021	Retrospective	34
Lee et al.	2021	Retrospective	30

Table 3. En face OCT.

Authors	Year	Study	No. of Eyes
Fukuyama et al.	2019	Retrospective	33
Comet et al.	2021	Case report	2
Matoba et al.	2021	Retrospective	64

Table 4. Three-dimensional OCT.

Authors	Year	Study	No. of Eyes
Hisatomi et al.	2018	Retrospective	68

Table 5. Adaptive optics OCT.

Authors	Year	Study	No. of eyes
Reumueller et al.	2020	Prospective	5

3. Results

3.1. Spectral-Domain OCT and Swept-Source OCT

Studies conducted on macula-off retinal detachment showed that the baseline visual acuity and time to surgical repair are among the best predictors of vision outcomes [11,12]. The number of detached quadrants and the stage of proliferative vitreoretinopathy are also related to poor postoperative anatomical results and poor visual prognosis [11–13]. In addition, the integrity of the ellipsoid zone and the external limiting membrane is useful to predict postoperative visual acuity [12,14–17]. However, Sridhar and colleagues reported that two patients with macula-off retinal detachment experienced a postoperative improvement in visual acuity secondary to ellipsoid zone restoration [18]. Changes in the thickness of the outer nuclear layer may also predict the postoperative visual outcome [19]. A lower mean preoperative central retinal thickness is associated with a good visual prognosis [20].

Terauchi and colleagues found that the thickness of the inner segments of the photoreceptors was significantly thinner in the early postoperative period. They also showed that the thickness of the inner and outer segments of the photoreceptors in an early postoperative period may be a good indicator of the final visual acuity [21].

Some authors found a correlation between outer retinal folds and postoperative metamorphopsia. They also showed abrupt changes in the reflectivity of the ellipsoid zone, associated with folds [22]. Nagpal and colleagues found that outer retinal corrugation was associated with a poor postoperative visual outcome. Therefore, it may be an important predictor of visual outcome [17].

Poulsen and colleagues demonstrated that in eyes with macula-off retinal detachment, a detached macula with a near-normal appearance had a better visual prognosis than a detached macula with a disrupted intraretinal appearance [23].

Some authors observed that the percentage of eyes with integrity of the photoreceptor layer increased progressively over time after surgery for macula-off retinal detachment. A delayed surgery was associated with a higher risk of layer disruption, and it was therefore associated with a worse visual prognosis. Cystoid macular edema and epiretinal membranes were associated with a lower postoperative visual acuity [24].

Iwase and colleagues studied intraretinal cystoid cavities in macula-off retinal detachment. They found that they were associated with the anterior protrusion of the macula. While their presence was associated with worse preoperative visual function and morphology, it did not affect postoperative outcomes [25].

OCT allows the recognition of whitish outer retinal spots, occasionally appearing in the detached retina as hyperreflective foci in the ellipsoid or interdigitation layers [26].

SD-OCT permits the detection of microscopic macular changes in macula-off retinal detachment. Zgolli and colleagues measured the height of the subretinal fluid, finding that a greater level of macular detachment was correlated with lower preoperative and postoperative visual acuity and with the formation of cavitations in the external nuclear layer [13]. Other authors, on the other hand, found no statistically significant correlation between the height of macula-off retinal detachment and the final visual acuity. They observed that the presence of a macular hole was the only preoperative variable with a significant correlation with postoperative visual acuity [27].

Outer retinal undulation is a debated potential biomarker. It is thought to be caused by a disparity in the amount of edema between the inner and outer retina. This is likely caused by more severe damage in the outer retina than in the inner retina. Yeo and colleagues did not find a significant influence of outer retinal undulation on visual outcomes in patients with macula-off retinal detachment. Performing SS-OCT, they also showed that outer retinal undulation was associated with younger age and better preoperative visual acuity. Most importantly, patients with a recent retinal detachment had a higher incidence of outer retinal undulation, which may therefore be used to determine retinal detachment duration in patients with an unknown duration of symptoms [14].

Research has been conducted in order to identify factors associated with postoperative metamorphopsia following successful vitrectomy for retinal detachment. Using SS-OCT, Kumar and colleagues found that the preoperative extent of the detachment, postoperative foveal contour, and the continuity of the ellipsoid zone are significantly associated with the occurrence of postoperative metamorphopsia [28].

Mané et al. conducted a retrospective study using SD-OCT. They observed that preoperative OCT examination detected a shallow macular detachment extending beyond the fovea in patients diagnosed with fovea-splitting retinal detachment by clinical examination with a non-contact lens. These patients were considered to have macula-off from an anatomical point of view, but their postoperative prognosis was closer to macula-on. The authors assumed that the favorable postoperative functional outcome in these eyes was due to a shallow macular detachment with moderate preoperative visual loss and a short duration of the detachment, allowing the restoration of the ellipsoid zone and external limiting membrane [29].

Klaas and colleagues used SD-OCT to define a more precise classification of rhegmatogenous retinal detachment according to the state of the macula and the fovea. They also showed that the grade of retinal detachment and the extent of the cystoid macular edema were good preoperative biomarkers to predict functional recovery in eyes with detached fovea [30].

Bansal et al. monitored retinal reattachment with SS-OCT after pneumatic retinopexy, identifying five specific stages. Stage 1 is characterized by a rapid reduction in the height of the detachment, leading to an improvement in the metabolic transport between the retina and the RPE and dehydration of the inner and outer retina. The subsequent reduction in cystoid macular edema and the improvement in hydration folds and outer retinal corrugations define stage 2. In stage 3, the retina makes contact with the RPE. The subsequent rapid deturgescence of the inner and the outer segments of the photoreceptors defines stage 4. Stage 5 is characterized by an improvement in the integrity of the outer retina, involving the external limiting membrane and the ellipsoid zone, and eventual recovery of the foveal bulge. The authors also observed that in eyes with acute retinal detachment and symptom occurrence lasting less than 24 h, the outer retina may still be intact, therefore achieving a quicker recovery of the foveal bulge [31].

When performing SD-OCT on eyes that underwent a pars plana vitrectomy for macula-off retinal detachment, Ozsaygili and colleagues observed that different endotamponades may have different effects on the thickness of the retinal layers. No significant difference was observed in the eyes after gas tamponade. On the other hand, significant changes, especially in the ganglion cells layer and in the outer nuclear layer, were seen in the eyes when silicone oil was used; they also had a worse visual recovery. The difference in the thickness of the ganglion cells layer showed the strongest correlation with worse visual outcomes [32]. These results confirmed a similar finding from other authors, who found that a reduction in the thickness of the ganglion cell layer and inner plexiform layer after tamponade with silicone oil, with an unclear mechanism [33]. The thickness of the ganglion cells layer and inner plexiform layer may be a predictive factor for the final visual acuity, according to Raczynska and colleagues [34]. Lee et al. found that silicone oil tamponade may cause a temporary thinning of the parafoveal inner retina, which recovered after silicone oil removal. However, the thinning of the peripapillary nerve fiber layer remained unchanged after removal. These changes were likely due to the mechanical pressure of the endotamponade on the retina [35].

Horozoglu et al. found that the long-term use of heavy silicone oil for the treatment of retinal detachment resulted in a good anatomical reattachment of the retina with good ellipsoid zone continuity and foveal thickness. However, extended use of heavy silicone oil increased the rate of epiretinal membrane formation [36].

There is still no consensus regarding the best surgical strategy to treat retinal detachment. The advantages of one technique over the other are still debated. Although OCT studies may provide useful information on the most indicated surgical approach, there is still limited evidence to draw any substantial conclusion [37].

It has been suggested that postoperative discontinuity of the ellipsoid zone and of the external limiting membrane and the development of outer retinal folds, may be influenced by the surgical technique [38,39]. Some authors found that outer retinal folds were associated with significantly worse visual acuity. In addition, there was a negative correlation between the closest distance of an outer retinal fold from the fovea and vertical metamorphopsia [39].

Stopa and colleagues found that the functional outcome of eyes affected by retinal detachment complicated by proliferative vitreoretinopathy might be influenced by an abnormal macular status, which can be found in the majority of these eyes [40].

The persistent subfoveolar fluid following surgery for macula-off retinal detachment has been studied by Tee et al. They found that the fluid was almost always present in eyes with retinal detachment secondary to atrophic round holes or dialyses, while it was present in one third of eyes with a detachment secondary to tractional tears. The fluid may persist for up to one year. It slowly resolves with time, but in some cases it is associated with the development of progressive foveal photoreceptor atrophy and loss of visual acuity [41].

Borowicz and colleagues found that macular changes shown through OCT examination occurred postoperatively both in macula-on and macula-off eyes. Specifically, they identified epiretinal membranes, macular edema, subretinal fluid, and increased central retinal thickness [42].

3.2. OCT Angiography

Some authors have performed OCT-A after rhegmatogenous retinal detachment in order to investigate visual prognostic factors with vessel density (VD) measurements. Hong and colleagues found that the postoperative state of the outer retinal layer was associated with the subfoveal choriocapillaris VD, which correlated well with visual outcomes. An intact outer retina was associated with a normal VD of the choriocapillaris, while patients with outer retinal defects presented a significantly lower choriocapillaris VD [43].

After successful pars plana vitrectomy for macula-off retinal detachment, Chatziralli et al. found an enlargement of the foveal avascular zone (FAZ), accompanied by a significant decrease in VD in both superficial and deep capillary plexuses. A significant thinning of inner retinal layers was also observed, corresponding to the areas of decreased VD [44].

In a study by Xu and colleagues, the superficial FAZ was found to be normal, while the deep FAZ was enlarged postoperatively. Moreover, in eyes with rhegmatogenous retinal detachment and choroidal detachment, the deep FAZ continued to increase in size in the postoperative period. In this group of patients, there was a significant negative correlation between the deep FAZ area and visual acuity [45].

Some authors confirmed that the FAZ area increased and VD decreased when compared to normal eyes. The parafoveal VD progressively increased in the postoperative period, but it did not reach a normal status. However, these alterations did not have a correlation with visual outcomes. They also found that eyes with a thinner preoperative foveal sensory thickness presented a lower VD in the superficial capillary plexus postoperatively. The VD of the superficial capillary plexus was lower in eyes treated with pars plana vitrectomy than in eyes treated with scleral buckling [46].

Roohipoor and colleagues performed OCT-A on eyes with silicone oil tamponade following vitrectomy for macula-off retinal detachment. They found a significantly lower VD of the parafoveal superficial capillary layer and the total retina, compared to a normal eye. The parafoveal VD progressively increased postoperatively, but it did not return to normal. The VD of the deep capillary plexus and the choroidal flow were less than normal in silicone oil-filled eyes, but the difference did not reach statistical significance. In eyes with silicone oil tamponade, the FAZ was not affected [47]. Other authors found that the macular VD and FAZ were not affected by silicone oil [35].

3.3. En Face OCT

Some authors observed in some cases that en face OCT may represent a useful imaging technique in order to monitor outer retinal folds occurring postoperatively after vitrectomy. It is indeed well known that outer retinal folds are less likely to cause metamorphopsia and they spontaneously resolve after some months in the majority of the cases. En face OCT is useful since it may provide several pieces of structural information, especially on the outer retina [48,49].

En face OCT is also more sensitive than B-scan OCT for detecting epiretinal membrane formation after vitrectomy for the treatment of retinal detachment. Studies performed using en face OCT for detecting epiretinal membranes also showed that they have a marginal impact on postoperative visual acuity [50].

3.4. Three-Dimensional OCT

Hisatomi and colleagues used three-dimensional OCT (3D-OCT) to study the retinal changes after vitrectomy with the internal limiting membrane (ILM) peeling for the treatment of macula-on and macula-off rhegmatogenous retinal detachment. The observed changes were: thinning of the ILM peeling area, dissociation of the outer nerve fiber layer, dimple sign, temporal macular thinning, and forceps-related retinal thinning. These developed in the first two postoperative months and remained stable thereafter. Proliferative changes such as epiretinal membrane and proliferative vitreoretinopathy were not noted as a consequence of ILM peeling, suggesting that this maneuver may decrease the occurrence of this complication [51]. However, there is no extensive literature on the subject and this finding needs to be confirmed by further studies.

3.5. Adaptive Optics OCT

It has been suggested that post-surgical receptor regeneration may play a role in determining visual prognosis after retinal detachment. However, traditional OCT technology is not adequate to identify and track the evolution of single cone photoreceptors. Adaptive optics (AO) have been recently introduced to enhance ophthalmic imaging, analyzing single photoreceptors in vivo [4]. Some authors have tried to study photoreceptors using a fundus camera integrated with AO. In their studies, they found that cone density was reduced following retinal detachment, even if it improved after surgery. However, since fundus cameras provide two-dimensional images, information on all the retinal layers was captured, leading to artifacts and reduced visualization of single cones [52–54]. The combination of AO with OCT instead allows for increased lateral resolution, acquiring information for each individual retinal layer [55].

Reumueller et al. have conducted a prospective study on patients undergoing vitrectomy with gas tamponade for macula-off retinal detachment. They performed SD-OCT as well as AO-OCT with follow up times of 6 and 56 weeks after surgery. Even if cone morphology improved 6 weeks after surgery, significant distortion of the cone mosaic was still present after one year. This finding was correlated to reduced retinal sensitivity through microperimetry. Even if the visual acuity was satisfying, the regular mosaic of the cones appeared to be completely lost [4]. Distortion of cones may also explain the micrometamorphopsia reported by some patients despite macular reattachment after surgery in the absence of a secondary epiretinal membrane.

Table 6 summarizes possible biomarkers which have emerged from different studies.

Table 6. Potential biomarkers.

Type of OCT	Potential Biomarkers
SD-OCT and SS-OCT	Integrity of ellipsoid zone Integrity of external limiting membrane Thickness of the outer retinal layers Central retinal thickness Thickness and integrity of the inner and outer segments of the photoreceptors Outer retinal folds and undulations Integrity of the detached macula Macular edema Epiretinal membranes Hyper-reflective foci in the ellipsoid zone Height of subretinal fluid Macular hole Postoperative foveal contour Thickness of the ganglion cells layer Thickness of the outer nuclear layer Thickness of the inner plexiform layer Thickness of the peripapillary nerve fiber layer Persistence of subfoveolar fluid
OCT-A	Subfoveal choriocapillaris vessel density Dimensions of the foveal avascular zone Vessel density of the superficial and capillary plexuses Choroidal flow
En face OCT	Outer retinal folds Epiretinal membranes
Adaptive optics OCT	Cone morphology

OCT: optical coherence tomography; SD-OCT: spectral-domain OCT; SS-OCT: swept-source OCT; OCT-A: OCT angiography.

4. Discussion

Rhegmatogenous retinal detachment is a potential cause of permanent vision loss. Its treatment requires surgical intervention, which aims to reattach the retina closing the breaks and releasing vitreoretinal tractions. Pneumatic retinopexy, scleral buckling, and vitrectomy are efficacious techniques with high success rates [56–59]. However, anatomical and functional postoperative success is affected by several factors.

OCT imaging enables the detection of structural changes which are not always evident in clinical examination. Therefore, several studies have been performed in order to obtain a better understanding of rhegmatogenous retinal detachment, and to identify possible biomarkers which may influence the prognosis [60,61].

In the literature, there are limited data on the subject. Most importantly, the majority of studies are retrospective in nature and only a few RCTs are available. Currently, a meta-analysis on the subject cannot be performed. The present narrative review sums up the different and sometimes conflicting evidence from the available studies to date. More research is needed in order to define the best practice pattern for the management of retinal detachment and its prognosis.

Actual knowledge on the physiology of retinal reattachment has improved thanks to studies using SS-OCT. This enhances the understanding of certain anatomic abnormalities occurring after retinal reattachments, such as outer retinal folds, outer retinal corrugations, and residual subfoveal fluid blebs [31].

Studies on OCT are not only useful to find new predictors of visual prognoses but also to improve the classification of rhegmatogenous retinal detachment. Traditionally, rhegmatogenous retinal detachment is classified according to the presence/absence of proliferative vitreoretinopathy and the status of the macula (macula-on/macula-off). In some cases of foveal-splitting retinal detachment diagnosed with clinical examination, SD-OCT allows the identification of a complete macular detachment, which was, however, associated with a better visual prognosis than a macula-off detachment. It may be useful to classify these cases as macula-on/off retinal detachment, in order to better stratify the visual prognosis [29].

Among the potential biomarkers predicting functional recovery, the grade of detachment and the extent of cystoid macular edema seems promising in eyes with a detached fovea, as well as the integrity of the ellipsoid zone [14,30]. The extent of the detachment, the postoperative foveal contour, the integrity of the ellipsoid zone and of the external limiting membrane, and the presence of outer retinal folds, seem to be predictors of visual prognoses and metamorphopsia following a successful vitrectomy [12,15–17,22,28,48,49]. In addition, the thickness of the inner and outer segments of the photoreceptors, and thickness changes in the outer nuclear layer, may be predictors of the final visual outcome [19,21]. Lower preoperative central retinal thickness is associated with a good visual prognosis [12,20]. Irregularity in the reflectivity of the ellipsoid zone may be associated with outer retinal folds. These alterations may represent subtle damage to the photoreceptors [22]. Outer retinal undulation may have a role in assessing the duration of retinal detachment, but it does not seem to be related to the visual prognosis [14]. Recovery of the integrity of the ellipsoid zone may be associated with postoperative improvement in visual acuity [18]. Persistent subfoveal fluid resolves spontaneously in the majority of cases, but it may also be rarely associated with progressive foveal photoreceptor atrophy and loss of visual acuity. It occurs more frequently when the macula-off retinal detachment is secondary to atrophic round holes or dialysis [41]. The quantity of macular subretinal fluid may also be considered a biomarker since it is correlated with low visual acuity and cavitations of the external nuclear layer [13]. On the other hand, other studies failed to find a significant correlation between the height of the retinal detachment and the visual outcome. The preoperative presence of a macular hole, instead, significantly affects postoperative visual acuity [27]. Intraretinal cystoid cavities do not seem to impair postoperative anatomical and functional outcomes [25].

OCT-A studies may also help to identify biomarkers useful for predicting functional and anatomical visual prognoses. OCT-A findings have suggested a potential relationship between outer retinal restoration, the VD of the choriocapillaris, and visual prognosis in macula-off retinal detachment after a vitrectomy [43]. In these patients, an enlargement of the FAZ with reduced VD of the superficial and deep capillary plexuses have been observed, together with inner retinal layer thinning [44]. The enlarged area of the deep FAZ continues to increase in eyes with retinal detachment and choroidal detachment, suggesting that choroidal lesions may have an acute pathological effect on ischemia of the deep retinal capillary network. Therefore, early intervention on retinal and choroidal ischemia may improve the structural recovery of the retina and the visual prognosis. Moreover, the extent of the deep FAZ may be used to predict postoperative visual acuity [45]. On the other hand, some authors have also found no correlation between FAZ, VD, and visual prognosis. The finding that eyes treated with vitrectomy have a lower VD than eyes treated with scleral buckling suggests that vitrectomy may potentially damage the microvascular structure of the vessels [46]. However, further studies are needed.

The timing of intervention for the treatment of retinal detachment is also a debated issue. High-risk indicators may facilitate the identification of eyes that benefit more than others from urgent surgery [62]. The evidence that a disrupted intraretinal appearance of the detached macula may be associated with a worse visual prognosis may aid in the selection of patients who may potentially benefit from early surgery [23]. The integrity of the photoreceptor layer seems to improve postoperatively over time. A longer time period before surgery is associated with a worse status of the photoreceptors, and it is subsequently associated with a worse visual outcome. This highlights the importance of early intervention, even in macula-off retinal detachment [24].

Studies on AO-OCT, though conducted on small samples, have highlighted that retinal reattachment after surgery does not correspond to a restoration of the outer segments of the photoreceptors, which remain considerably misaligned even after a quite long follow-up time. Structural damage to the photoreceptors prevents normal coupling of light, causing distorted and attenuated signals [4].

Postoperative photoreceptor integrity may represent a predictor of better postoperative functional outcomes. Discontinuity of the outer retinal layers and development of outer retinal folds, which are also associated with vertical metamorphopsia if close to the fovea, seem to be associated with worse visual outcomes. The surgical technique used to treat the retinal detachment may play a role in the genesis of these alterations, as suggested by some recently published studies [38,39]. However, no large RCTs are available and there is still limited data on the topic, insufficient to suggest a preferred surgical strategy. Further research on the subject should be encouraged in order to identify those OCT findings that may be relevant and crucial for choosing the most appropriate surgical technique.

It has been suggested that an abnormal macular status in the postoperative period may lead to a poor visual outcome [40]. Morphological OCT changes in the macular region seem to affect both macula-on and macula-off detachments [42]. Further studies are needed in order to clarify the role of ILM peeling, especially regarding the formation of epiretinal membranes and proliferative vitreoretinopathy in the postoperative period [51]. At the same time, studies performed with en face OCT for the detection of postoperative epiretinal membranes concluded that they are usually not severe and they have only a marginal impact on postoperative visual acuity [50].

OCT findings are useful to choose among the different endotamponades available since it is known that silicone oil, but not gases, is associated with retinal thinning. The inner retinal layers are affected: mainly the ganglion cell layer and the inner plexiform layer. Their thickness may be a predictive factor to assess the final visual acuity [34]. The parafoveal inner retinal thickness may return to normal after silicone oil removal, while the peripapillary nerve fiber layer thinning remains constant. A mechanical effect caused by the pressure of silicone oil on the retina, especially in the prone position, may be assumed [35]. The mechanism of action and the effects on visual outcome are still unclear, therefore it may be advisable to use silicone oil only in complicated cases. Moreover, monitoring of retinal thinning using SD-OCT may support the decision to remove silicone oil with the correct timing in order to minimize the potential thinning effect on the retina [32,33]. Extended use of heavy silicone oil is associated with an increased risk of ERM formation [36]. It is likely that the retina is more susceptible to damage from silicone oil than the choroid since silicone oil makes contact only with the retina. OCT-A may show a reduced VD of the superficial capillary plexus only, although no alterations of FAZ and VD may be observed [35,46].

5. Conclusions

In conclusion, OCT provides a more detailed knowledge of the retinal structure and of its alterations. At present, there is no gold standard for the treatment of rhegmatogenous retinal detachment, and the treatment strategy needs to be tailored to each patient. Detailed information on the preoperative retina status is useful in order to improve diagnostic accuracy and identify the prognosis. Some OCT patterns may be defined as biomarkers, predictive of anatomical and functional prognoses. OCT may be also useful in defining the retinal alterations subsequent to different endotamponades, although the evidence is still limited. In this narrative review, we have taken into consideration all of the OCT techniques available at present, since each of them may contribute to increasing the knowledge and understanding of the disease. The limit of the studies analyzed is that they are mostly retrospective in nature. Differences in patients and retinal detachment characteristics are also present, as well as disparities in surgical techniques. At present, a detailed meta-analysis on the subject cannot be conducted and there is no strong evidence supporting the choice of a surgical technique based on OCT findings. Larger prospective studies should be encouraged.

Author Contributions: Conceptualization: P.L.; methodology: C.D.; validation: P.L. and C.D.; formal analysis: P.L. and C.D.; investigation: C.D.; resources: C.D.; data curation: P.L. and C.D.; writing—original draft preparation: C.D.; writing—review and editing: P.L. and C.D.; visualization: P.L. and C.D.; supervision: P.L.; project administration: P.L. All authors have read and agreed to the published version of the manuscript.

Funding: This research received no external funding.

Institutional Review Board Statement: Not applicable.

Informed Consent Statement: Not applicable.

Data Availability Statement: The data presented in in this study are openly available in PubMed.

Conflicts of Interest: Carla Danese is consultant for Bayer, outside the submitted work. Paolo Lanzetta is consultant for Aerie, Apellis, Bayer, Biogen, Centervue, Novartis, Roche, outside the submitted work.

References

1. Feltgen, N.; Walter, P. Rhegmatogenous retinal detachment—An ophthalmologic emergency. *Dtsch. Arztebl. Int.* **2014**, *111*, 12–22. [CrossRef]
2. Callizo, J.; Pfeiffer, S.; Lahme, E.; van Oterendorp, C.; Khattab, M.; Bemme, S.; Kulanga, M.; Hoerauf, H.; Feltgen, N. Risk of progression in macula-on rhegmatogenous retinal detachment. *Graefes Arch. Clin. Exp. Ophthalmol.* **2017**, *255*, 1559–1564. [CrossRef]
3. Kunikata, H.; Abe, T.; Nakazawa, T. Historical, Current and Future Approaches to Surgery for Rhegmatogenous Retinal Detachment. *Tohoku J. Exp. Med.* **2019**, *248*, 159–168. [CrossRef]
4. Reumueller, A.; Wassermann, L.; Salas, M.; Karantonis, M.G.; Sacu, S.; Georgopoulos, M.; Drexler, W.; Pircher, M.; Pollreisz, A.; Schmidt-Erfurth, U. Morphologic and Functional Assessment of Photoreceptors after Macula-Off Retinal Detachment With Adaptive-Optics OCT and Microperimetry. *Am. J. Ophthalmol.* **2020**, *214*, 72–85. [CrossRef] [PubMed]
5. de Boer, J.F.; Leitgeb, R.; Wojtkowski, M. Twenty-five years of optical coherence tomography: The paradigm shift in sensitivity and speed provided by Fourier domain OCT [Invited]. *Biomed. Opt. Express.* **2017**, *8*, 3248–3280. [CrossRef]
6. Wolff, B.; Matet, A.; Vasseur, V.; Sahel, J.A.; Mauget-Faÿsse, M. En Face OCT Imaging for the Diagnosis of Outer Retinal Tubulations in Age-Related Macular Degeneration. *J. Ophthalmol.* **2012**, *2012*, 542417. [CrossRef]
7. Ishikawa, H.; Kim, J.; Friberg, T.R.; Wollstein, G.; Kagemann, L.; Gabriele, M.L.; Townsend, K.A.; Sung, K.R.; Duker, J.S.; Fujimoto, J.G.; et al. Three-dimensional optical coherence tomography (3D-OCT) image enhancement with segmentation-free contour modeling C-mode. *Investig. Ophthalmol. Vis. Sci.* **2009**, *50*, 1344–1349. [CrossRef]
8. Azimipour, M.; Jonnal, R.S.; Werner, J.S.; Zawadzki, R.J. Coextensive synchronized SLO-OCT with adaptive optics for human retinal imaging. *Opt. Lett.* **2019**, *44*, 4219–4222. [CrossRef] [PubMed]
9. Uemura, A.; Arimura, N.; Yamakiri, K.; Fujiwara, K.; Furue, E.; Sakamoto, T. Macular holes following vitrectomy for rhegmatogenous retinal detachment: Epiretinal proliferation and spontaneous closure of macular holes. *Graefes Arch. Clin. Exp. Ophthalmol.* **2021**, *259*, 2235–2241. [CrossRef] [PubMed]
10. Yang, H.Y.; Yang, C.S. Development of a full thickness macular hole after vitrectomy for rhegmatogenous retinal detachment: A sequential study via optical coherence tomography. *BMC Ophthalmol.* **2018**, *18*, 265. [CrossRef] [PubMed]

11. Felfeli, T.; Murtaza, F.; Abueh, B.; Mandelcorn, M.S.; Wong, D.D.; Mandelcorn, E.D. Clinical Significance of Macula-Off Rhegmatogenous Retinal Detachment Preoperative Features on Optical Coherence Tomography. *Ophthalmic Surg. Lasers Imaging Retina* **2021**, *52*, S23–S29. [CrossRef]
12. Chatziralli, I.; Chatzirallis, A.; Kazantzis, D.; Dimitriou, E.; Machairoudia, G.; Theodossiadis, G.; Parikakis, E.; Theodossiadis, P. Predictive Factors for Long-Term Postoperative Visual Outcome in Patients with Macula-Off Rhegmatogenous Retinal Detachment Treated with Vitrectomy. *Ophthalmologica* **2021**, *244*, 213–217. [CrossRef]
13. Zgolli, H.; Mabrouk, S.; Khayrallah, O.; Fekih, O.; Zeghal, I.; Nacef, L. Prognostic factors for visual recovery in idiopathic rhegmatogenous retinal detachment: A prospective study of 90 patients. *Tunis. Med.* **2021**, *99*, 972–979. [PubMed]
14. Yeo, Y.D.; Kim, Y.C. Significance of outer retinal undulation on preoperative optical coherence tomography in rhegmatogenous retinal detachment. *Sci. Rep.* **2020**, *10*, 15747. [CrossRef] [PubMed]
15. Noda, H.; Kimura, S.; Morizane, Y.; Toshima, S.; Hosokawa, M.M.; Shiode, Y.; Doi, S.; Takahashi, K.; Hosogi, M.; Fujiwara, A.; et al. RELATIONSHIP BETWEEN PREOPERATIVE FOVEAL MICROSTRUCTURE AND VISUAL ACUITY IN MACULA-OFF RHEGMATOGENOUS RETINAL DETACHMENT: Imaging Analysis By Swept Source Optical Coherence Tomography. *Retina* **2020**, *40*, 1873–1880. [CrossRef]
16. Lai, W.W.; Leung, G.Y.; Chan, C.W.; Yeung, I.Y.; Wong, D. Simultaneous spectral domain OCT and fundus autofluorescence imaging of the macula and microperimetric correspondence after successful repair of rhegmatogenous retinal detachment. *Br. J. Ophthalmol.* **2010**, *94*, 311–318. [CrossRef] [PubMed]
17. Nagpal, M.; Shakya, K.; Mehrotra, N.; Kothari, K.; Bhatt, K.; Mehta, R.; Shukla, C. Morphometric analysis of fovea with spectral-domain optical coherence tomography and visual outcome postsurgery for retinal detachment. *Indian J. Ophthalmol.* **2014**, *62*, 846–850. [CrossRef]
18. Sridhar, J.; Flynn, H.W., Jr.; Fisher, Y. Inner segment ellipsoid layer restoration after macula-off rhegmatogenous retinal detachment. *Ophthalmic Surg. Lasers Imaging Retina* **2015**, *46*, 103–106. [CrossRef] [PubMed]
19. Gharbiya, M.; Grandinetti, F.; Scavella, V.; Cecere, M.; Esposito, M.; Segnalini, A.; Gabrieli, C.B. Correlation between spectral-domain optical coherence tomography findings and visual outcome after primary rhegmatogenous retinal detachment repair. *Retina* **2012**, *32*, 43–53. [CrossRef]
20. Guan, I.; Gupta, M.P.; Papakostas, T.; Wu, A.; Nadelmann, J.; D'Amico, D.J.; Kiss, S.; Orlin, A. Role of optical coherence tomography for predicting postoperative visual outcomes after repair of macula-off rhegmatogenous retinal detachment. *Retina* **2021**, *41*, 2017–2025. [CrossRef]
21. Terauchi, G.; Shinoda, K.; Matsumoto, C.S.; Watanabe, E.; Matsumoto, H.; Mizota, A. Recovery of photoreceptor inner and outer segment layer thickness after reattachment of rhegmatogenous retinal detachment. *Br. J. Ophthalmol.* **2015**, *99*, 1323–1327. [CrossRef]
22. Dell'Omo, R.; Mura, M.; Lesnik Oberstein, S.Y.; Bijl, H.; Tan, H.S. Early simultaneous fundus autofluorescence and optical coherence tomography features after pars plana vitrectomy for primary rhegmatogenous retinal detachment. *Retina* **2012**, *32*, 719–728. [CrossRef]
23. Poulsen, C.D.; Petersen, M.P.; Green, A.; Peto, T.; Grauslund, J. Fundus autofluorescence and spectral domain optical coherence tomography as predictors for long-term functional outcome in rhegmatogenous retinal detachment. *Graefes Arch. Clin. Exp. Ophthalmol.* **2019**, *257*, 715–723. [CrossRef]
24. Baudin, F.; Deschasse, C.; Gabrielle, P.H.; Berrod, J.P.; Le Mer, Y.; Arndt, C.; Tadayoni, R.; Delyfer, M.N.; Weber, M.; Gaucher, D.; et al. Functional and anatomical outcomes after successful repair of macula-off retinal detachment: A 12-month follow-up of the DOREFA study. *Acta Ophthalmol.* **2021**, *99*, e1190–e1197. [CrossRef]
25. Iwase, T.; Tomita, R.; Ra, E.; Iwase, C.; Terasaki, H. Investigation of causative factors for unusual shape of macula in eyes with macula-off rhegmatogenous retinal detachment. *Jpn. J. Ophthalmol.* **2021**, *65*, 363–371. [CrossRef]
26. Russell, J.F. Whitish Outer Retinal Spots in Retinal Detachment: Longitudinal Follow-up, Multimodal Imaging, and Clinical Utility. *Ophthalmol. Retina* **2022**, *6*, 469–477. [CrossRef]
27. Hostovsky, A.; Trussart, R.; AlAli, A.; Kertes, P.J.; Eng, K.T. Pre-operative optical coherence tomography findings in macula-off retinal detachments and visual outcome. *Eye* **2021**, *35*, 3285–3291. [CrossRef]
28. Kumar, V.; Naik, A.; Kumawat, D.; Sundar, D.; Chawla, R.; Chandra, P.; Kumar, A. Multimodal imaging of eyes with metamorphopsia after vitrectomy for rhegmatogenous retinal detachment. *Indian J. Ophthalmol.* **2021**, *69*, 2757–2765. [CrossRef]
29. Mané, V.; Chehaibou, I.; Lehmann, M.; Philippakis, E.; Rothschild, P.R.; Bousquet, E.; Tadayoni, R. Preoperative Optical Coherence Tomography Findings of Foveal-Splitting Rhegmatogenous Retinal Detachment. *Ophthalmologica* **2021**, *244*, 127–132. [CrossRef]
30. Klaas, J.E.; Rechl, P.; Feucht, N.; Siedlecki, J.; Friedrich, J.; Lohmann, C.P.; Maier, M. Functional recovery after macula involving retinal detachment and its correlation with preoperative biomarkers in optical coherence tomography. *Graefes Arch. Clin. Exp. Ophthalmol.* **2021**, *259*, 2521–2531. [CrossRef]
31. Bansal, A.; Lee, W.W.; Felfeli, T.; Muni, R.H. Real-Time In Vivo Assessment of Retinal Reattachment in Humans Using Swept-Source Optical Coherence Tomography. *Am. J. Ophthalmol.* **2021**, *227*, 265–274. [CrossRef]
32. Ozsaygili, C.; Bayram, N. Effects of different tamponade materials on macular segmentation after retinal detachment repair. *Jpn. J. Ophthalmol.* **2021**, *65*, 227–236. [CrossRef] [PubMed]

33. Purtskhvanidze, K.; Hillenkamp, J.; Tode, J.; Junge, O.; Hedderich, J.; Roider, J.; Treumer, F. Thinning of Inner Retinal Layers after Vitrectomy with Silicone Oil versus Gas Endotamponade in Eyes with Macula-Off Retinal Detachment. *Ophthalmologica* **2017**, *238*, 124–132. [CrossRef] [PubMed]
34. Raczyńska, D.; Mitrosz, K.; Raczyńska, K.; Glasner, L. The Influence of Silicone Oil on the Ganglion Cell Complex After Pars Plana Vitrectomy for Rhegmatogenous Retinal Detachment. *Curr. Pharm. Des.* **2018**, *24*, 3476–3493. [CrossRef]
35. Lee, J.; Cho, H.; Kang, M.; Hong, R.; Seong, M.; Shin, Y. Retinal Changes before and after Silicone Oil Removal in Eyes with Rhegmatogenous Retinal Detachment Using Swept-Source Optical Coherence Tomography. *J. Clin. Med.* **2021**, *10*, 5436. [CrossRef]
36. Horozoglu, F.; Sener, H.; Polat, O.A.; Sever, O.; Potoglu, B.; Celik, E.; Turkoglu, E.B.; Evereklioglu, C. Evaluation of long-term outcomes associated with extended heavy-silicone oil use for the treatment of inferior retinal detachment. *Sci. Rep.* **2022**, *12*, 11636. [CrossRef]
37. Huang, C.; Fu, T.; Zhang, T.; Wu, X.; Ji, Q.; Tan, R. Scleral buckling versus vitrectomy for macula-off rhegmatogenous retinal detachment as accessed with spectral-domain optical coherence tomography: A retrospective observational case series. *BMC Ophthalmol.* **2013**, *13*, 12. [CrossRef]
38. Muni, R.H.; Felfeli, T.; Sadda, S.R.; Juncal, V.R.; Francisconi, C.L.; Nittala, M.G.; Lindenberg, S.; Gunnemann, F.; Berger, A.R.; Wong, D.T.; et al. Postoperative Photoreceptor Integrity Following Pneumatic Retinopexy vs Pars Plana Vitrectomy for Retinal Detachment Repair: A Post Hoc Optical Coherence Tomography Analysis From the Pneumatic Retinopexy Versus Vitrectomy for the Management of Primary Rhegmatogenous Retinal Detachment Outcomes Randomized Trial. *J. AMA Ophthalmol.* **2021**, *139*, 620–627. [CrossRef]
39. Lee, W.W.; Bansal, A.; Sadda, S.R.; Sarraf, D.; Berger, A.R.; Wong, D.T.; Kertes, P.J.; Kohly, R.P.; Hillier, R.J.; Muni, R.H. Outer Retinal Folds after Pars Plana Vitrectomy vs. Pneumatic Retinopexy for Retinal Detachment Repair: Post hoc analysis from PIVOT. *Ophthalmol. Retina* **2022**, *6*, 234–242. [CrossRef]
40. Stopa, M.; Kociecki, J. Anatomy and function of the macula in patients after retinectomy for retinal detachment complicated by proliferative vitreoretinopathy. *Eur. J. Ophthalmol.* **2011**, *21*, 468–472. [CrossRef]
41. Tee, J.J.; Veckeneer, M.; Laidlaw, D.A. Persistent subfoveolar fluid following retinal detachment surgery: An SD-OCT guided study on the incidence, aetiological associations, and natural history. *Eye* **2016**, *30*, 481–487. [CrossRef]
42. Borowicz, D.; Nowomiejska, K.; Nowakowska, D.; Brzozowska, A.; Toro, M.D.; Avitabile, T.; Jünemann, A.G.; Rejdak, R. Functional and morphological results of treatment of macula-on and macula-off rhegmatogenous retinal detachment with pars plana vitrectomy and sulfur hexafluoride gas tamponade. *BMC Ophthalmol.* **2019**, *19*, 118. [CrossRef]
43. Hong, E.H.; Cho, H.; Kim, D.R.; Kang, M.H.; Shin, Y.U.; Seong, M. Changes in Retinal Vessel and Retinal Layer Thickness After Vitrectomy in Retinal Detachment via Swept-Source OCT Angiography. *Investig. Ophthalmol. Vis. Sci.* **2020**, *61*, 35. [CrossRef]
44. Chatziralli, I.; Theodossiadis, G.; Parikakis, E.; Chatzirallis, A.; Dimitriou, E.; Theodossiadis, P. Inner retinal layers' alterations and microvasculature changes after vitrectomy for rhegmatogenous retinal detachment. *Int. Ophthalmol.* **2020**, *40*, 3349–3356. [CrossRef]
45. Xu, C.; Wu, J.; Feng, C. Changes in the postoperative foveal avascular zone in patients with rhegmatogenous retinal detachment associated with choroidal detachment. *Int. Ophthalmol.* **2020**, *40*, 2535–2543. [CrossRef]
46. Nam, S.H.; Kim, K.; Kim, E.S.; Kim, D.G.; Yu, S.Y. Longitudinal Microvascular Changes on Optical Coherence Tomographic Angiography after Macula-Off Rhegmatogenous Retinal Detachment Repair Surgery. *Ophthalmologica* **2021**, *244*, 34–41. [CrossRef]
47. Roohipoor, R.; Tayebi, F.; Riazi-Esfahani, H.; Khodabandeh, A.; Karkhaneh, R.; Davoudi, S.; Khurshid, G.S.; Momenaei, B.; Ebrahimiadib, N.; Modjtahedi, B.S. Optical coherence tomography angiography changes in macula-off rhegmatogenous retinal detachments repaired with silicone oil. *Int. Ophthalmol.* **2020**, *40*, 3295–3302. [CrossRef]
48. Comet, A.; Ramtohul, P.; Stolowy, N.; Gascon, P.; Denis, D.; David, T. Role of en face OCT in following outer retinal folds after rhegmatogenous retinal detachment. *J. Fr. Ophtalmol.* **2021**, *44*, e479–e481. [CrossRef]
49. Fukuyama, H.; Yagiri, H.; Araki, T.; Iwami, H.; Yoshida, Y.; Ishikawa, H.; Kimura, N.; Kakusho, K.; Okadome, T.; Gomi, F. Quantitative assessment of outer retinal folds on enface optical coherence tomography after vitrectomy for rhegmatogenous retinal detachment. *Sci. Rep.* **2019**, *9*, 2327. [CrossRef]
50. Matoba, R.; Kanzaki, Y.; Doi, S.; Kanzaki, S.; Kimura, S.; Hosokawa, M.M.; Shiode, Y.; Takahashi, K.; Morizane, Y. Assessment of epiretinal membrane formation using en face optical coherence tomography after rhegmatogenous retinal detachment repair. *Graefes Arch. Clin. Exp. Ophthalmol.* **2021**, *259*, 2503–2512. [CrossRef]
51. Hisatomi, T.; Tachibana, T.; Notomi, S.; Koyanagi, Y.; Murakami, Y.; Takeda, A.; Ikeda, Y.; Yoshida, S.; Enaida, H.; Murata, T.; et al. Internal limiting membrane peeling-dependent retinal structural changes after vitrectomy in rhegmatogenous retinal detachment. *Retina* **2018**, *38*, 471–479. [CrossRef] [PubMed]
52. Ra, E.; Ito, Y.; Kawano, K.; Iwase, T.; Kaneko, H.; Ueno, S.; Yasuda, S.; Kataoka, K.; Terasaki, H. Regeneration of Photoreceptor Outer Segments after Scleral Buckling Surgery for Rhegmatogenous Retinal Detachment. *Am. J. Ophthalmol.* **2017**, *177*, 17–26. [CrossRef]
53. Saleh, M.; Debellemanière, G.; Meillat, M.; Tumahai, P.; Garnier, M.B.; Flores, M.; Schwartz, C.; Delbosc, B. Quantification of cone loss after surgery for retinal detachment involving the macula using adaptive optics. *Br. J. Ophthalmol.* **2014**, *98*, 1343–1348. [CrossRef]
54. Potic, J.; Bergin, C.; Giacuzzo, C.; Daruich, A.; Pournaras, J.A.; Kowalczuk, L.; Behar-Cohen, F.; Konstantinidis, L. Changes in visual acuity and photoreceptor density using adaptive optics after retinal detachment repair. *Retina* **2020**, *40*, 376–386. [CrossRef]

55. Zawadzki, R.J.; Choi, S.S.; Jones, S.M.; Oliver, S.S.; Werner, J.S. Adaptive optics-optical coherence tomography: Optimizing visualization of microscopic retinal structures in three dimensions. *J. Opt. Soc. Am. A Opt. Image Sci. Vis.* **2007**, *24*, 1373–1383. [CrossRef]
56. Han, D.P.; Mohsin, N.C.; Guse, C.E.; Hartz, A.; Tarkanian, C.N. Comparison of pneumatic retinopexy and scleral buckling in the management of primary rhegmatogenous retinal detachment. Southern Wisconsin Pneumatic Retinopexy Study Group. *Am. J. Ophthalmol.* **1998**, *126*, 658–668. [CrossRef]
57. Heimann, H.; Bartz-Schmidt, K.U.; Bornfeld, N.; Weiss, C.; Hilgers, R.D.; Foerster, M.H. Scleral buckling versus primary vitrectomy in rhegmatogenous retinal detachment: A prospective randomized multicenter clinical study. *Ophthalmology* **2007**, *114*, 2142–2154. [CrossRef]
58. Campo, R.V.; Sipperley, J.O.; Sneed, S.R.; Park, D.W.; Dugel, P.U.; Jacobsen, J.; Flindall, R.J. Pars plana vitrectomy without scleral buckle for pseudophakic retinal detachments. *Ophthalmology* **1999**, *106*, 1811–1816. [CrossRef]
59. Soni, C.; Hainsworth, D.P.; Almony, A. Surgical management of rhegmatogenous retinal detachment: A meta-analysis of randomized controlled trials. *Ophthalmology* **2013**, *120*, 1440–1447. [CrossRef]
60. Fercher, A.F.; Hitzenberger, C.K.; Drexler, W.; Kamp, G.; Sattmann, H. In vivo optical coherence tomography. *Am. J. Ophthalmol.* **1993**, *116*, 113–114. [CrossRef]
61. Swanson, E.A.; Izatt, J.A.; Hee, M.R.; Huang, D.; Lin, C.P.; Schuman, J.S.; Puliafito, C.A.; Fujimoto, J.G. In vivo retinal imaging by optical coherence tomography. *Opt. Lett.* **1993**, *18*, 1864–1866. [CrossRef] [PubMed]
62. Mahmoudi, S.; Almony, A. Macula-Sparing Rhegmatogenous Retinal Detachment: Is Emergent Surgery Necessary? *J. Ophthalmic Vis. Res.* **2016**, *11*, 100–107. [CrossRef]

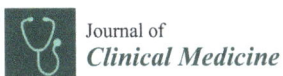

Review

Advances in Optical Coherence Tomography Imaging Technology and Techniques for Choroidal and Retinal Disorders

Joshua Ong [1], Arman Zarnegar [1], Giulia Corradetti [2,3], Sumit Randhir Singh [4] and Jay Chhablani [1,*]

1. Department of Ophthalmology, University of Pittsburgh School of Medicine, Pittsburgh, PA 15213, USA
2. Department of Ophthalmology, Doheny Eye Institute, Los Angeles, CA 90095, USA
3. Stein Eye Institute, David Geffen School of Medicine at the University of California, Los Angeles, CA 90033, USA
4. Nilima Sinha Medical College & Hospital, Rampur 852113, India
* Correspondence: jay.chhablani@gmail.com

Abstract: Optical coherence tomography (OCT) imaging has played a pivotal role in the field of retina. This light-based, non-invasive imaging modality provides high-quality, cross-sectional analysis of the retina and has revolutionized the diagnosis and management of retinal and choroid diseases. Since its introduction in the early 1990s, OCT technology has continued to advance to provide quicker acquisition times and higher resolution. In this manuscript, we discuss some of the most recent advances in OCT technology and techniques for choroidal and retinal diseases. The emerging innovations discussed include wide-field OCT, adaptive optics OCT, polarization sensitive OCT, full-field OCT, hand-held OCT, intraoperative OCT, at-home OCT, and more. The applications of these rising OCT systems and techniques will allow for a closer monitoring of chorioretinal diseases and treatment response, more robust analysis in basic science research, and further insights into surgical management. In addition, these innovations to optimize visualization of the choroid and retina offer a promising future for advancing our understanding of the pathophysiology of chorioretinal diseases.

Keywords: optical coherence tomography; retina; choroid; advances; technology

1. Introduction

Optical coherence tomography (OCT) is an imaging modality that has revolutionized the field of ophthalmology. As a non-invasive imaging technique, OCT utilizes light and light interference to capture high resolution, cross-sectional tomographic information of biological tissue such as the retina and choroid at the micron level. This technology was first introduced in 1991 [1] and has been rapidly adopted into clinical practice in retina. Diagnostic evaluation in retinal and choroidal diseases are often conducted with OCT, including neovascular age-related macular degeneration (AMD) [2], central serous chorioretinopathy (CSCR) [3], vascular retinal disorders [4], and other vitreoretinal disorders [5]. OCT biomarkers have also been instrumental in further understanding and monitoring chorioretinal disease status; these biomarkers include central macular thickness, subretinal/intraretinal fluid, neurosensory detachment height, subfoveal choroid thickness, choroidal vessel diameter, and choroidal vascularity index [6–8]. More recently, in the attempt to optimize the design of early interventional clinical trials for non-neovascular AMD, a number of structural OCT biomarkers, such as intraretinal hyperreflective foci, subretinal drusenoid deposits, drusen with hyporeflective core, high central drusen volume, have been described as high-risk for AMD progression to late stages [9–12].

Time-domain OCT (TD-OCT) was the first OCT system introduced to the world of clinical ophthalmology [13,14]. Compared to current systems, TD-OCT had a relatively slow scanning speed of 400 axial scans (A-scans)/second. Rapid advances allowed for increased axial

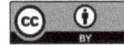

resolution and scanning speed to optimize evaluation of the retina and choroid. For example, spectral-domain (SD) OCT and swept-source (SS) OCT were developed after TD-OCT and have acquisition times ranging from 27,000 A-scans/second to 100,000 A-scans/second. Axial resolution also increased, from around 10 μm with TD-OCT to 2 μm with SD-OCT and SS-OCT [13].

The advances in OCT technology have strengthened the ability to detect and diagnose for retinal disorders, often leading to earlier interventions and preservation of vision. OCT and OCT angiography (OCTA) of the retina have also been found to visualize and quantify the structure and the microvasculature of the retina. Moreover, enhanced penetration provides details of choroidal vasculature not previously seen with TD-OCT. Researchers have visualized sites of penetration of short posterior ciliary arteries and in eyes with thin choroid (i.e., especially highly myopic eyes) even the scleral vessels, posterior episcleral tissue, and Tenon's layer can be delineated [15]. In addition, their applications are not limited to the retina field. In fact, OCT and OCTA imaging have been revolutionary in the field of glaucoma and neuro-ophthalmology by helping with early diagnosis of neurodegenerative diseases, including Alzheimer's disease and possibly preclinical Alzheimer's [16]. Thus, advances in OCT technology are promising in various fields of ophthalmology and neurology for earlier detection of the diseases, which may potentially improve the design of early interventional clinical trials. Given the wide application and evolving OCTA technology, including all OCTA advances is out of the scope of this article. In this paper, we review advances in OCT technology and techniques including wide-field OCT, visible light OCT, adaptive optics OCT, polarization-sensitive OCT, high-resolution OCT, intraoperative OCT, and handheld OCT. The emerging innovations made in this imaging modality will help advance several critical aspects in retinal care including imaging acquisition times, field of view, portability/accessibility, and intraoperative management.

2. Recent Advances in OCT Technology and Techniques

In this section and the following sections, we discuss the recent advances in OCT technology and techniques. Many of these techniques help to address current limitations to this clinically useful imaging modality. We organize these advances into three categories: (1) emerging advancements for clinical use, (2) advancements at the basic science/research level, and (3) recent advancements in currently available technology (Table 1). As these advances continue to progress in the future, these technologies will likely become more integrated and applied in the clinical setting.

Table 1. Advances in optical coherence tomography (OCT) imaging technology and techniques. Advances are categorized into emerging advances for clinical use, advances for basic science/research, and recent advances in available technology.

Advances in OCT	Summary of Primary Advancement	References
Emerging Advances for Clinical Use		
Visible-Light (Vis) OCT	Utilizes visible light illumination for OCT as opposed to commonly used near-infrared (NIR) light to capture fine details of the retina	[17,18]
Adaptive Optics (AO) OCT	Wavefront correcting component and computational controller software to compensate for aberrations and quality degradation, increasing the quality of OCT images.	[19,20]
Polarization Sensitive (PS) OCT	Measures and quantifies the polarization and depolarization of tissue for precision, high-quality imaging of retinal pigment epithelium layers	[21,22]
High-Resolution OCT (High-Res OCT)	Broadened bandwidth of the OCT light source to improve axial resolution and capture clearer details of the retinal microstructures and microvasculature.	[23,24]

Table 1. *Cont.*

Advances in OCT	Summary of Primary Advancement	References
Advances for Basic Science/Research		
Full-Field (FF) and Dynamic Full-Field (DFF) OCT	Acquires images with charge coupled device cameras in 2D enface orientation at different depths for high resolution images at the cellular level.	[25,26]
Recent Advances in Available Technology		
Wide-field (WF) and Ultrawide-field (UWF) OCT	Increased field of view to 40–55 degrees with wide-field OCT and up to 200 degrees with ultrawide-field OCT	[27,28]
Hand-Held and Intraoperative OCT (iOCT)	Hand-held OCT is portable OCT technology that is particularly useful for infants and bed ridden patients. Intraoperative OCT (microscope integrated) allows for image guidance and real-time feedback during ophthalmic surgery.	[29,30]
At-Home OCT	At-home, self-imaging OCT that allows for more frequent imaging and good agreement when compared to in-clinic OCT for more precise management of retinal diseases.	[31,32]

3. Visible Light OCT (Vis-OCT)

Visible light OCT (vis-OCT) utilizes visible light for OCT illumination, rather than near-infrared (NIR) light, to capture images [33]. This technique allows for improved resolution of biological features of the retina due to shorter illumination wavelengths [33]. Zhang et al. recently reported the utilization of vis-OCT to quantify subcellular reflectivity contributions to the outermost retinal hyperreflective bands (Figure 1) [18]. Vis-OCT was first described by Povazay et al. [17]. Using a sub-15fs Ti:sapphire laser and photonic crystal fibers, this group demonstrated light emission in the range of 535 nm to 700 nm of the electromagnetic spectrum that improved axial resolution to <2 microns. This was achieved with a smaller bandwidth compared to current OCT illumination methods such as NIR. While most OCT devices currently utilize light in the NIR range because of its tissue penetration and reduced cost, there has been increasing interest in using vis-OCT [17]. Primary uses of vis-OCT are currently in blood vessel oximetry and imaging of healthy eyes [34,35].

Vis-OCT systems predominantly rely on supercontinuum lasers, which intrinsically generate relative intensity noise that restricts their clinical utility. Relative intensity noise can be attenuated by lengthening the camera's exposure time, which subjects patients to excess light thus increasing their eye movements and hindering quality image acquisition. Rubinoff et al. proposed a balanced-detection vis-OCT model that uses two spectrometers to reduce relative intensity noise and tested it in a phantom retina and in vivo in human patients [36]. Results from their study indicated there may be a reduced need for exposing patients to excess light when employing balanced detection. The study results are unique as their method demonstrates more significant levels of relative intensity noise reduction than in previous setups.

Speckle noise, which is often caused by the scattering of light waves, can negatively impact image interpretation in vis-OCT. Multi-volume image registration and modulation of B-scans have been suggested to reduce speckle noise [37,38]. The resultant improvement in vis-OCT image quality enhanced the visualization of neurons throughout all layers of rat retina. It allows vis-OCT to rival the capabilities of NIR AO-OCT. In particular, vis-OCT can now image structures such as the inner plexiform layer, the retinal pigment epithelium, and Bruch's membrane [18,39]. Limitations to vis-OCT include depth-dependent dispersion limiting image quality. Zhang et al. demonstrated that water wavenumber calibration eliminates additional resampling steps and corrects dispersion [40].

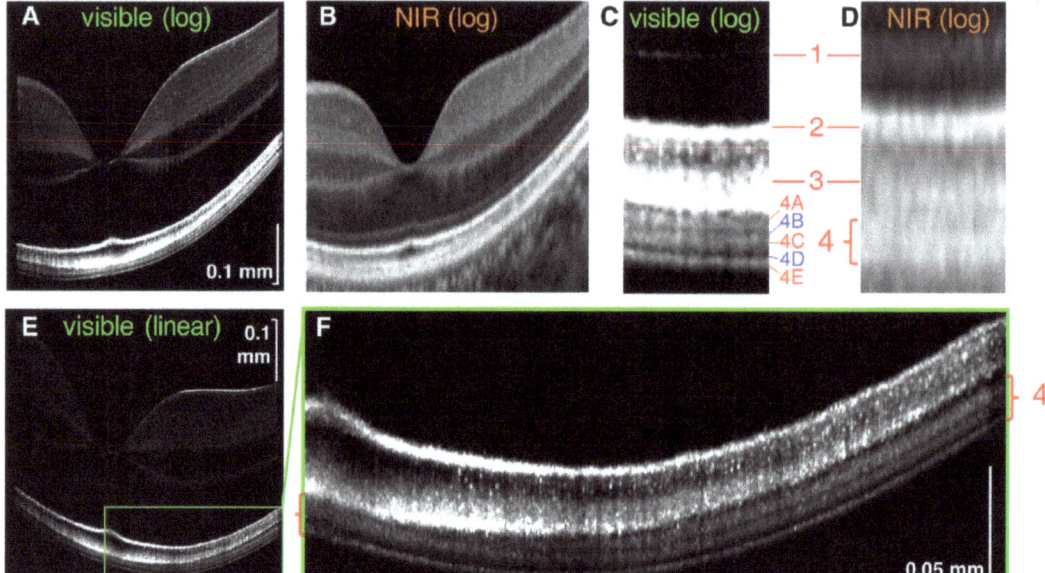

Figure 1. Visible light OCT (vis-OCT) imaging. Side-by-side comparison of vis-OCT (**A**) and commercial NIR-based OCT (**B**). (**C**) Magnified vis-OCT that shows outer retinal bands 1–4, with segmented hyperreflective bands and hyporeflective zones in outer retinal band 4, compared to magnified commercial NIR-based OCT (**D**). (**E,F**) Vis-OCT (linear scale). Reprinted with permission from Zhang et al. [18]. Visible Light Optical Coherence Tomography (OCT) Quantifies Subcellular Contributions to Outer Retinal Band 4. *Transl. Vis Sci. Technol.* 2021; 10(3): 30. with license permissions obtained from Creative Commons; Creative Commons Attribution 4.0 International License (CC BY 4.0, https://creativecommons.org/licenses/by/4.0/legalcode accessed on 1 August 2022).

4. Adaptive Optics (AO) in OCT (AO-OCT)

AO was initially developed to reduce dynamic wave-front errors in astronomical imaging [41]. It has since been found to quantify and eliminate high-order monochromatic aberrations from light passing through ocular tissues such as the cornea and lens. These aberrations cause poor lateral resolution in ophthalmic imaging and previously limited the clinical applications of various ophthalmic imaging systems [42,43]. AO systems are composed of a wavefront sensor (generally a Shack-Hartmann wavefront sensor) that measures distortions, and a wavefront corrector (typically a deformable mirror) that alters its shape to cancel out aberrations, and a controller that connects these elements (Figure 2) [44,45].

Arguably the most impactful feature of AO in ophthalmology is that it permits the imaging of individual cells, such as photoreceptors, in vivo [42,46,47]. AO has a lateral resolution of 2 microns, a considerable improvement from the ~15-micron lateral resolution of OCT [48]. Initially, AO was used with en-face imaging modalities to demonstrate individual rods and cones in 2D. When combined with OCT, AO allows for 3D imaging and the resolution of structures such as photoreceptors and the retinal pigment epithelium. Efforts have been made to increase the FOV of AO-OCT systems in imaging these cells, increasing the area from ~1 degree to 4 degrees × 4 degrees (Figure 3) [49].

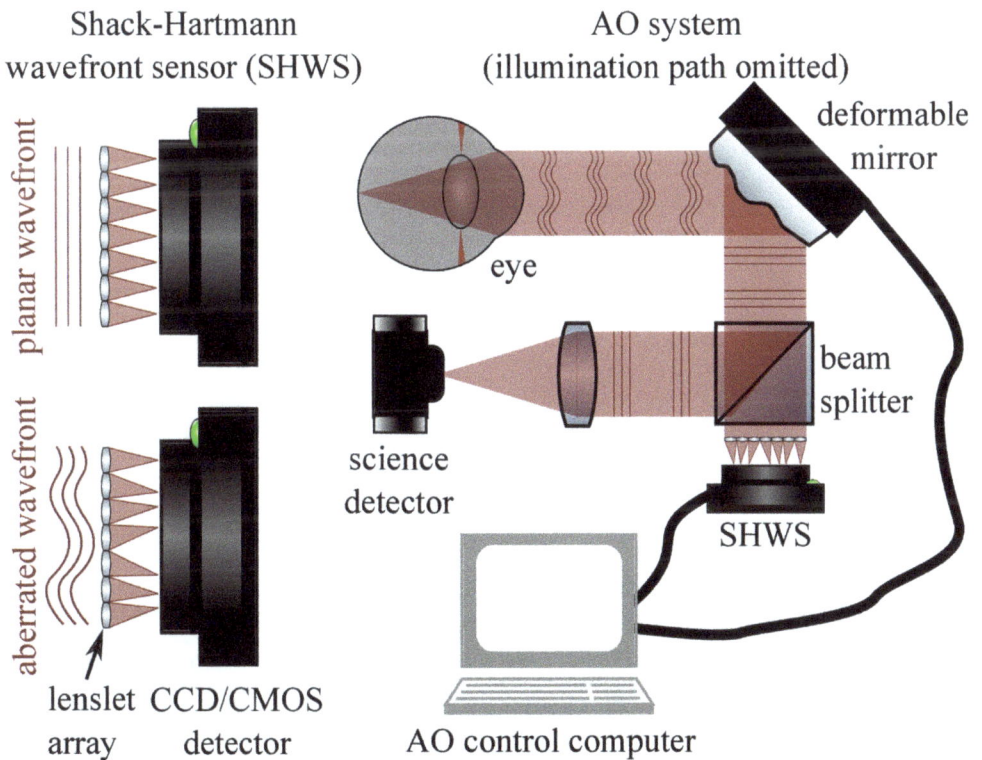

Figure 2. Adaptive optics technology system with Shack–Harmann wavefront sensor (SHWS) and deformable mirror schematic. SHWS utilizes a small lenslet array and samples a wavefront; displacements due to aberrations can drive a corrector (e.g., deformable mirror). This technology can help to visualize individual cells in the human retina [42,45]. Reprinted with permission from Jonnal et al. [45]. A Review of Adaptive Optics Optical Coherence Tomography: Technical Advances, Scientific Applications, and the Future. *Invest Ophthalmol. Vis Sci.* 2016; 57(9): OCT51-68 with license permissions obtained from Creative Commons; Creative Commons Attribution-Non-Commercial-No Derivatives 4.0 International (CC BY-NC-ND 4.0, https://creativecommons.org/licenses/by-nc-nd/4.0/legalcode (accessed on 1 August 2022)).

Computational AO (CAO) reduces aberrations by modifying the phase of OCT data in the spectral domain and has been studied with much fervor in recent years. While image quality tends to be sacrificed with CAO, it was designed to reduce the need for costly hardware by correcting distortions after data collection [44,51]. The primary CAO modality today is interferometric synthetic aperture microscopy (ISAM), a computational imaging technique that enhances depth-independent resolution [52]. ISAM requires limited movement from the patient for optimal imaging quality. A stretched-pulse mode-locked laser light source was tested to increase the A-scan rate and combat the adverse effects of eye movement [53]. Boppart et al. established the first model of CAO in polarization-sensitive OCT (PS-OCT), which corrects low-order aberrations in ex vivo human tissues [54]. There have also been proposed advances in improving CAO aberration correction capabilities and image quality [55]. CAO may streamline image collection workflows and promote cost-savings in the clinic, though with loss of image quality.

Sensorless AO (SAO) is another alternative to hardware-based AO-OCT that relies on the images' properties rather than a wavefront sensor to ultimately measure and correct aberrations [56]. SAO optimization methods and algorithms include Zernike Mode Hill

Climbing [57], stochastic parallel gradient descent [58,59], deep reinforcement learning [60], and others. SAO features have been tested to some extent in CAO models as well [58,61]. Since its description 15 years ago, AO-OCT is still not commonly used in ophthalmology clinics due to certain limitations. High magnification images are prone to motion artifacts and require constant fixation [62]. This becomes increasingly difficult in eyes with AMD-related geographic atrophy, retinal dystrophy such as cone dystrophy. Moreover, poor mydriasis, or presence of any media opacity significantly affect the quality of the images [62]. Other concerns are related to the very high acquisition cost, lack of commercial interest, need for trained manpower, and availability of ample space to house AO-OCT. Despite these limitations, researchers and clinicians can identify and broaden the clinical utility of AO-OCT in AMD, diabetic retinopathy, inherited retinal dystrophies, and other specialties such as glaucoma.

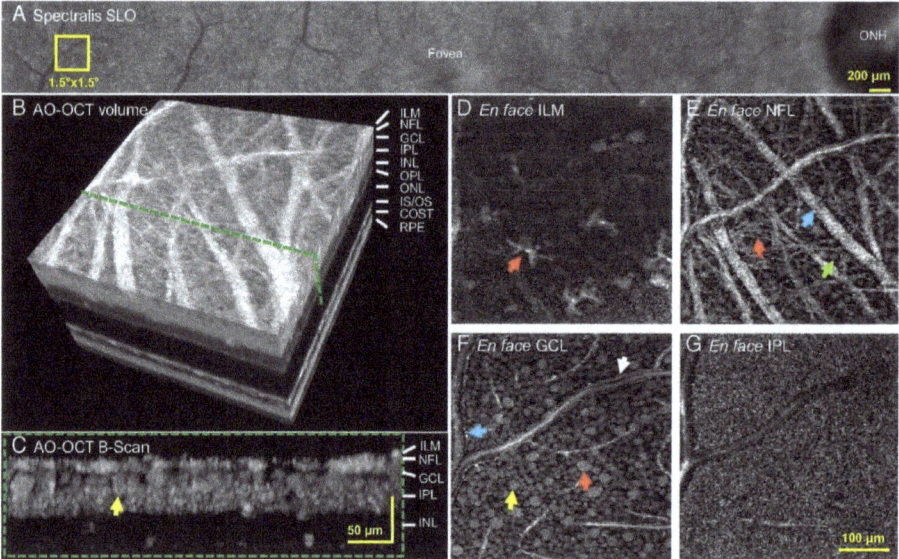

Figure 3. Adaptive optics (AO) OCT showcasing cellular structures of the retina. Yellow 1.5 × 1.5 box in (**A**) (Spectralis scanning laser ophthalmoscope) showcases location imaged by AO-OCT. (**B**) 3D AO-OCT with layers and green dotted line showcases the cross-section of the retina in (**C**) with yellow arrow highlighting ganglion cell layer soma. (**D–G**) Different layers of the retina (internal limiting membrane, nerve fiber layer, ganglion cell layer, and inner plexiform layer). (**D**) Red arrow shows astrocyte/microglial cells. (**E**) Blue arrow shows nerve fiber webs. (**F**) Red arrow shows large soma, yellow arrow shows ganglion cell layer soma, blue and white arrows show edges of vessel walls. (**G**) Synaptic connections in the internal plexiform layer. Reprinted with permission from Liu et al. [50]. Imaging and quantifying ganglion cells and other transparent neurons in the living human retina. *Proc. Natl. Acad. Sci. USA* 2017; 114(48): 12803-8 with license permissions obtained from Creative Commons; Creative Commons Attribution-Non-Commercial-No Derivatives 4.0 International (CC BY-NC-ND 4.0, https://creativecommons.org/licenses/by-nc-nd/4.0/legalcode (accessed on 1 August 2022)).

5. Polarization-Sensitive (PS) OCT

First demonstrated in 1992, PS-OCT functions by analyzing the polarization state of backscattered light and measuring birefringence in the tissue sample. Different tissues can change the polarization state of the OCT light source [63]. Initial PS-OCT schemes were based on TD-OCT. However, PS is now employed in both SS-OCT and SD-OCT to image various ocular structures such as the macula and peripheral retina [21,64,65]. A challenge in recognizing AMD early is detecting drusen; PS-OCT can be used to segment the RPE and identify drusen [66]. In many fiber-based PS-OCT setups, the laser light is initially polarized, then the optical fiber is fixed to prevent changes in the polarization state. Any changes to the optical fiber after that would affect the polarization state of the light source. A variation of SS-based PS-OCT was tested that uses a depolarizer and a polarizer to achieve a model independent of the input polarization, albeit with a drop in sensitivity and considerable loss of input light [67]. Another technique minimizes changes in the polarization state of the incident light beam by using a common-path interferometer in conjunction with polarization-maintaining fibers to promote stability of the optical fiber [68].

Adaptations of PS-OCT include polarization-sensitive quantitative OCT (PS-QOCT). QOCT provides dispersion-cancellation and identifies the refractive index of a media, and when combined with PS, offers improved resolution compared to traditional methods [69,70]. In a recent study, Sukharenko et al. demonstrated imaging and characterization of a birefringent material using PS-QOCT, which may have future applications in imaging biological tissues [71].

PS-OCT carries many promising applications in both basic and clinical ophthalmic research, particularly in automated segmentation of retinal structures such as RPE [66]. Similarly, geographic atrophy commonly seen in the dry form of AMD can be segmented using PS-OCT [21]. Fibrotic tissues, which contain collagen, are particularly birefringent and are thus imaged well by PS-OCT. Schütze et al. demonstrated that PS-OCT was useful for the evaluation of RPE lesions in choroidal neovascularization in eyes with neovascular AMD (Figure 4) [72]. Retinal fibrosis growth in the setting of neovascular AMD can be tracked using PS-OCT and segmentation algorithms [73].

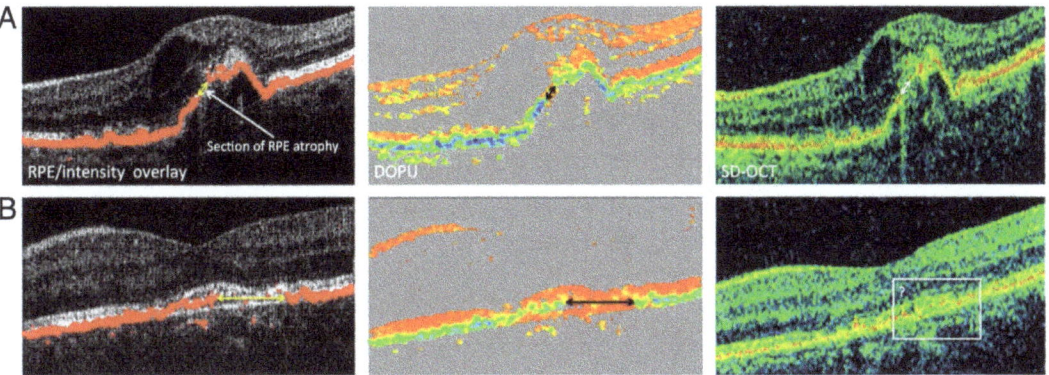

Figure 4. Polarization-sensitive optical coherence tomography (PS-OCT). (**A**) Three-figure panel showcases a comparison of PS-OCT (**top middle**) and SD-OCT (**top right**) where both modalities are able to identify retinal pigment epithelium atrophy. (**B**) Three-figure panel showcases a comparison of PS-OCT (**bottom middle**) and SD-OCT (bottom right) where PS-OCT can more clearly identify the retinal pigment epithelium atrophy. Reprinted with permission from Schütze, C et al. Polarisation-sensitive OCT is useful for evaluating retinal pigment epithelial lesions in patients with neovascular AMD. *British Journal of Ophthalmology* 2016; 100: 371–377 with license permissions obtained from Creative Commons; Attribution-NonCommercial 4.0 International (CC BY-NC 4.0, https://creativecommons.org/licenses/by-nc/4.0/legalcode (accessed on 1 August 2022)).

6. High-Resolution OCT (High-Res OCT)

One of Heidelberg Engineering's recent developments is the introduction of high-resolution OCT (High-Res OCT). High-Res OCT increases the bandwidth of the OCT light source which allows for an increase in optical axial resolution [23]. High-Res OCT is capable of 3 μm axial resolution, allowing for capturing clearer images of the small vasculature, including the choriocapillaris [23,24]. The choriocapillaris has been found to play a role in many retinal diseases, thus more detailed visualization of this microvasculature will likely advance understanding of its dysfunction in these diseases [74]. Spaide and Lally reported the utilization of High-Res OCT to evaluate a patient with multiple evanescent white dot syndrome (MEWDS) [24]. Their investigation with this OCT imaging of up to 3 μm axial resolution suggested that the interdigitation zone (IZ) showed persistent abnormalities in this patient with MEWDS rather than the ellipsoid zone (EZ), the primary zone of involvement noted in previous MEWDS studies [24]. The utilization of this advancement in OCT imaging may help to provide additional insight into the microstructures and microvasculature of the retina in chorioretinal diseases.

7. Full-Field OCT (FFOCT) and Dynamic FFOCT (D-FFOCT)

Full-field OCT (FFOCT) captures 2D enface scans of ocular tissue at different depths. These can be used to reconstruct 3D volumetric images with resolutions of up to 1 micron. The setup most commonly relies on incoherent illumination and a Linnik interferometer, with two microscope objectives in the reference and sample arms. FFOCT possesses clinical value as an optical microscopy tool because it can capture subcellular structures for tissue examination in a non-invasive, efficient manner. Its current utilization has bolstered basic science research in cellular-resolution analysis. Current research has employed FFOCT to visualize detailed aspects of the human retinal ganglion cell axons [25] (Figure 5).

A derivative of FFOCT has been described that similarly provides visualization of dynamic structures at the microscopic level. In D-FFOCT, backscattered light from subcellular structures in motion can be measured in a time-dependent fashion that potentiates live or time-lapse imaging [75]. Like FFOCT, D-FFOCT primarily utilizes incoherent light and a Linnik interferometer, though without a reference arm [76]. When used in conjunction with fluorescence microscopy, histological techniques, or multimodal setups, highly specific structures can be marked, identified, and examined in situ. A full-field form of confocal microscopy, structured illumination microscopy, has been used with dynamic and static FFOCT methods [77].

A recently described application of D-FFOCT is in the 3D imaging of retinal organoids (ROs). Derived from human-induced pluripotent stem cells, ROs are tissues that form 3D structures such as the developmental optical vesicle and optic cups and, ultimately, the retina. The design and implementation of ROs have been ground-breaking in ophthalmologic research because it closely mimics the structure and functionality of the human retina. Areas of study that benefit from using ROs include retinal transplantation [78,79], drug delivery, optic nerve diseases [80], and others.

Scholler et al. introduced a novel method of label-free imaging of retinal organoids using D-FFOCT and used it to monitor the temporal development of ROs with a temporal resolution of 20 ms [81]. The authors showed that the metabolic activity of cells could be determined and used to differentiate cells, such as those undergoing apoptosis and rapidly dividing. Validated by multimodal imaging that overlayed fluorescence with D-FFOCT images, the success of this method suggests an imaging system that can identify specific without the need for exogenous dyes or antibodies is on the horizon. Groux et al. recently presented findings from an experiment in which porcine RPE cells and human-induced pluripotent stem cell-derived RPE were captured with live D-FFOCT imaging before and after exposure to toxic stress [82]. The authors explored the dynamics of intracellular organelles during wound healing and showcased a semi-automatic segmentation-based software (SAVE Profiler) that segmented the RPE wound and determined its dimensions. Their results indicate that D-FFOCT and the SAVE Profiler may have applications in diseases of the RPE, such as age-related macular degeneration.

In summary, FF-OCT offers 2D en face imaging of ex vivo tissues with resolution that is quickly approaching that seen in histological sample preparation. Its in vivo use is made difficult due to motion artifact. The study of ROs has potential to model human retinal in health and disease, and D-FFOCT now offers a means of imaging individual cells in situ to follow retinal development.

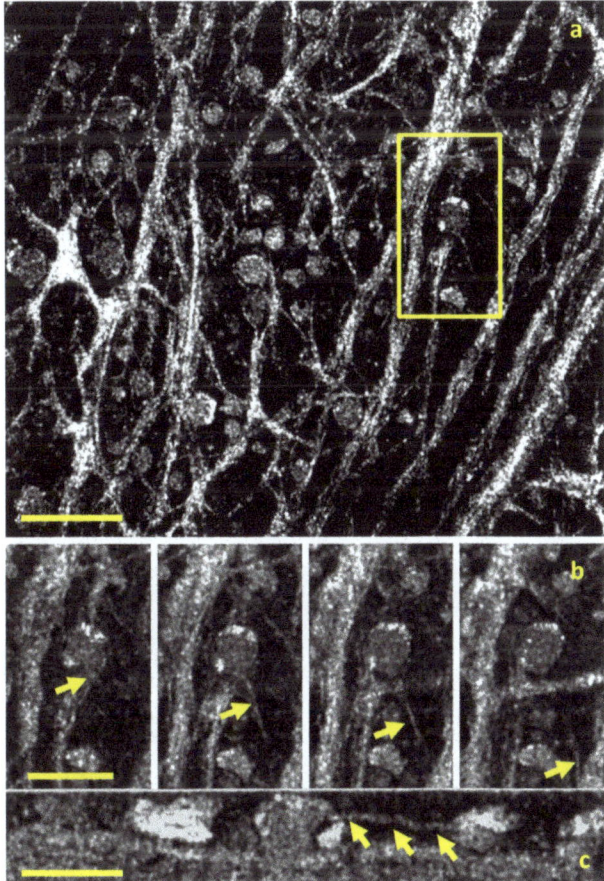

Figure 5. Full-field optical coherence tomography (FF-OCT) imaging the human retina. (**a**) The en face view of the human nerve fiber layer (scale bar is 500 μm). (**b**) A four-panel image of a 2 μm thick axon (yellow arrow) moving away from a ganglion cell soma. (**c**) A cross-section the same cell in (**b**) along the length of the axon (scale bar is 50 μm). Reprinted with permission from Grieve et al. [25]. Appearance of the Retina With Full-Field Optical Coherence Tomography. Invest. Ophthalmol. Vis. Sci. 2016; 57(9): OCT96–OCT104 with license permissions obtained from Creative Commons; Creative Commons Attribution-NonCommercial-NoDerivatives 4.0 International (CC BY-NC-ND 4.0, https://creativecommons.org/licenses/by-nc-nd/4.0/legalcode (accessed on 1 August 2022)).

8. Wide-Field and Ultrawide-Field OCT (WF-OCT and UWF-OCT)

Although a powerful ocular imaging tool, OCT imaging is often limited with a relatively narrow field of view (FOV). The FOV is usually constrained to around 20 degrees × 20 degrees [83]. Fundus cameras such as the Pomerantzeff equator-plus camera [84] and ultrawide-field scanning laser ophthalmoscopy (SLO) [85] addressed the issue of narrow FOV but only produced 2D scans. To address this gap in imaging capability, wide-field OCT technology (WF-OCT) with FOV around 40–55 degrees and ultrawide-field OCT (UWF-OCT) with FOV up to 200 degrees in a volumetric scan were developed (Figure 6) [28,86]. SS-OCT with a higher imaging speed (100,000 A scans/s) also has an advantage of enhanced depth scan range which is essential to image the curved contour of the peripheral retina [87]. Early WF-OCTs were based upon an InGaAs diode array that enabled a higher readout rate and a FOV of 38 degrees [27]. The initial UWF-OCT system described by

Klein et al. [88] is based upon ultrahigh speed swept source (SS) OCT that employs a 1050 nm Fourier domain mode locked laser. It can produce 1900 × 1900 A-scans with a 70–degree FOV within three to six seconds. In 2018, Gresores et al. demonstrated that a prototype multimodal system that combined ultrawide-field SLO and OCT could provide similar visualization of retinal structures to standalone OCT yet allowed for observation of additional lesions outside the OCT scanning field [89]. At present, commercially available WF OCT machines include the NIDEK Mirante® (NIDEK Co. Ltd., Gamagori, Japan) high definition SLO/OCT model which includes an adapter that allows for 163 degree UWF imaging [90,91]. Another system is Heidelberg Engineering's Spectralis® OCT (Heidelberg Engineering, Heidelberg, Germany) which utilizes a similar multimodal SD-OCT with confocal scanning laser ophthalmoscope to generate a FOV of up to 55 degrees. This system can be combined with the Ocular Staurenghi 230 SLO Retina Lens to produce a FOV of 150 degrees [92]. The Optos' Silverstone® (Optos PLC, Dunfermline, UK) integrates scanning laser ophthalmoscope and UWF imaging with SS-OCT for a 200-degree single-capture image in less than 0.5 s [93,94]. Another Optos OCT device, the Optos' Monaco® (Optos PLC, Dunfermline, UK), integrates UWF imaging with SD-OCT for a 200-degree single-capture image in less than 0.5 s [95]. Integration of these advances to capture the peripheral retina allows for peripheral OCT of retinal diseases including retinal tears, retinal holes, retinoschisis, retinal tuft, lattice degeneration, CSCR, choroidal nevi, and choroidal lesions (Figure 7) [96].

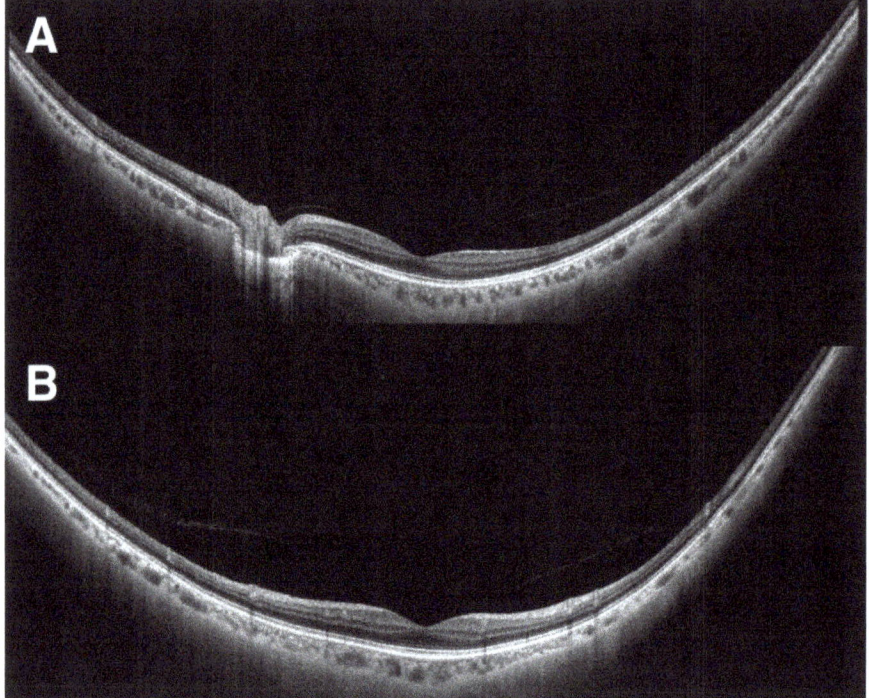

Figure 6. Ultrawide-field optical coherence tomography (UWF-OCT) Image. (**A**) Horizonal scan image (23 mm in length). (**B**) showcases vertical scan (20 mm in length). Reprinted with permission from Takahashi et al. [28]. Ultra-Widefield Optical Coherence Tomographic Imaging of Posterior Vitreous in Eyes With High Myopia. *Am J Ophthalmol.* 2019;206:102-12. with license permissions obtained from Elsevier and Copyright Clearance Center.

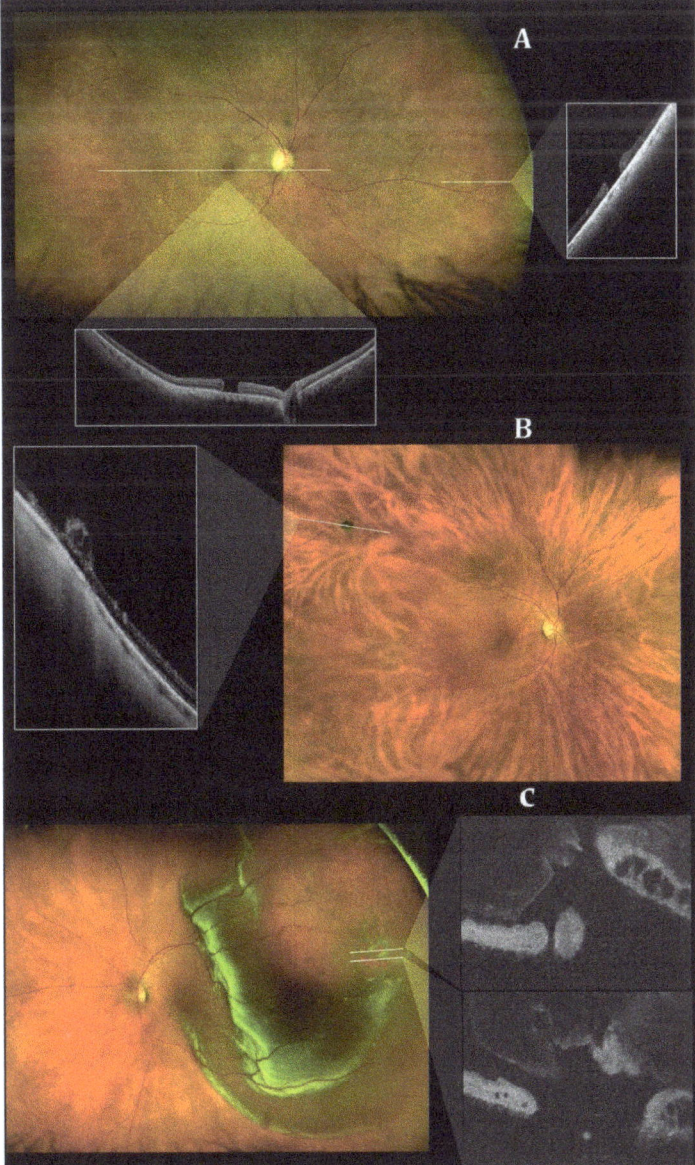

Figure 7. Integrated scanning laser ophthalmoscope and ultra-widefield imaging for peripheral optical coherence tomography with Optos' Silverstone swept-source optical coherence tomography (Optos PLC, Dunfermline, UK). (**A**) A peripheral atrophic retinal hole (right rectangle) and macular hole (lower rectangle). (**B**) A cystic retinal tuft in the peripheral retina. (**C**) A retinal detachment in the peripheral retina. Reprinted with permission from Sodhi et al. [96]. Feasibility of peripheral OCT imaging using a novel integrated SLO ultra-widefield imaging swept-source OCT device. Int Ophthalmol 2021; 41(8): 2805-15 with license permissions obtained from Creative Commons; Creative Commons Attribution 4.0 International License (CC BY 4.0, https://creativecommons.org/licenses/by/4.0/legalcode (accessed on 1 August 2022)).

Experimental methods of widening the FOV of OCT include extended field imaging (EFI). Described by Uji et al. [97], EFI utilizes swept-source OCT with a +20.00-diopter lens between the eye and the OCT probe to increase the FOV to nearly 60 or 70 degrees. This offers a simple way to achieve wider FOV for imaging the periphery. A recent study swapped the +20.00-diopter lens for a +90.00-diopter double aspheric noncontact slit-lamp lens in a swept-source OCT system. This method was dubbed "innovative wide-field" OCT. In the study, innovative wide-field OCT was compared to standard 12 mm OCT in imaging the retina in 50 eyes of 25 patients with proliferative diabetic retinopathy. Innovative wide-field technology increased the scan length by a factor of 1.65 ± 0.67; however, this setup had more rim and edge artifacts and poorer image quality compared to standard OCT [98].

Mori et al. described a technique that combines multiple SD-OCT scans of the posterior vitreous cortex and vitreoretinal interface into a montage of images that mimics WF-OCT [99]. The montage can be achieved by obtaining multiple scans with the subject focusing on different targets, then combining the images via image editing software. This methodology has been adopted to increase scan sizes in OCT angiography (OCTA) as well. Though it improves the visualization of microvasculature in the peripheral retina, montaging is susceptible to distortions, low-OCT-signaling, reduced sampling density, and other artifacts negatively impacting its clinical utility [100].

WF-OCT provides additional information compared to the routine 6–9 mm scans in conditions such as DR, CSCR, polypoidal choroidal vasculopathy (PCV), peripapillary choroidal neovascular membrane (CNVM) or uveitic entities. Anatomical details of peripheral retinal changes such as ischemic areas in DR, retinal vein occlusions, or site of retinal breaks, peripheral retinal detachment, retinoschisis and choroidal lesions (melanoma, nevus, hemangioma, choroidal metastasis) can be easily obtained.

Artificial intelligence (AI) has played an increasingly important role in optimizing delivery of care and research in ophthalmology [101]. As such, this powerful technology has been applied to WF SS-OCT imaging for retinal diseases. Deep learning (DL), especially convolutional neural networks (CNN), have been implicated in studying age-related macular degeneration (AMD) progression. A prominent challenge in utilizing AI in understanding retinal disease is a general paucity of 3-dimensional (3D), volumetric scan data. A novel deep learning technique, SLIVER-net, can be trained on a dataset of 2-dimensional (2D) scans to predict AMD biomarkers (intraretinal hyperreflective foci, subretinal drusenoid deposits, and hyporeflective drusen cores) and risk factors in 3D volumes via transfer learning [102]. Zhang et. al. used deep-learning to automatically detect and quantify geographic atrophy in patients with AMD in 2D B-scans with success [103]. In this study, models were generated to identify features such as RPE loss that are used to grade geographic atrophy. As this technology continues to become further validated, the pairing of AI with OCT will likely help clinicians to monitor retinal diseases even more closely.

Wide field imaging techniques including WF-OCT are prone to certain challenges. Optical aberrations increase with increase in FOV manifesting as increased noise to signal ratio [104]. Pupillary and ciliary shadowing related artifacts further reduce the image quality. Increased peripheral retinal curvature and inter-individual variation in retinal curvature and the need for very high A scan rate (>1 million A scan per second) are other variables which need to be addressed to obtain analyzable dense wide-field OCT scans. To summarize, WF-OCT and ultrawide-field OCT provide the clinicians with high quality, non-invasive, in-vivo tomographic details of chorioretinal layers and aid in the management of these chorioretinal disorders.

9. Hand-Held and Intraoperative OCT (iOCT)

Although a powerful imaging technology, commercially available OCTs are relatively large and typically table-mounted and with limited portability [105]. Hand-Held OCT technology has been developed to address these limitations and serve as an efficient and diagnostic point-of-care imaging tool [106]. One of the key utilizations noted for hand-held OCT is to help remove barriers to care for OCT imaging in the infant and young child population [107–109]. As commercial OCT systems are typically not designed for infants; the use of a portable OCT can help address this limitation in this OCT for identifying vision-threatening diseases in this patient population. In addition hand-held OCT can also address limitations for imaging bedridden patients [110]. Hand-Held OCT usually have two components: a lighter, hand-held piece, and a bulkier, base unit which contains the light source, reference arm, spectrometer, and computer with its display. An overall reduction in size of base unit, its constituents and transferring the interferometer to handpiece led to significant reduction in cost. Low-cost OCT therefore can be available at market prices of approximately 5000–7000 USD i.e., a reduction of >70% compared to the commercially available OCT devices [105,111]. Several challenges for a handheld OCT system include operator variability, hand movement, and manual alignment [112].

Widefield technology has also been integrated into handheld OCT imaging, as well as OCTA, increasing the field of view of this useful, portable technique [29]. Continued clinical validation is needed for this promising technology, and its development has served as a powerful catalyst for OCT utilization during vitreoretinal surgery [113].

As a powerful imaging tool in the clinic, OCT imaging has been explored to provide additional visualization for ophthalmic surgeries [114]. Intraoperative OCT (iOCT) allows for surgeons to utilize microscope-integrated, OCT imaging in real-time for feedback and image guidance in the operating room (Figure 8) [115].

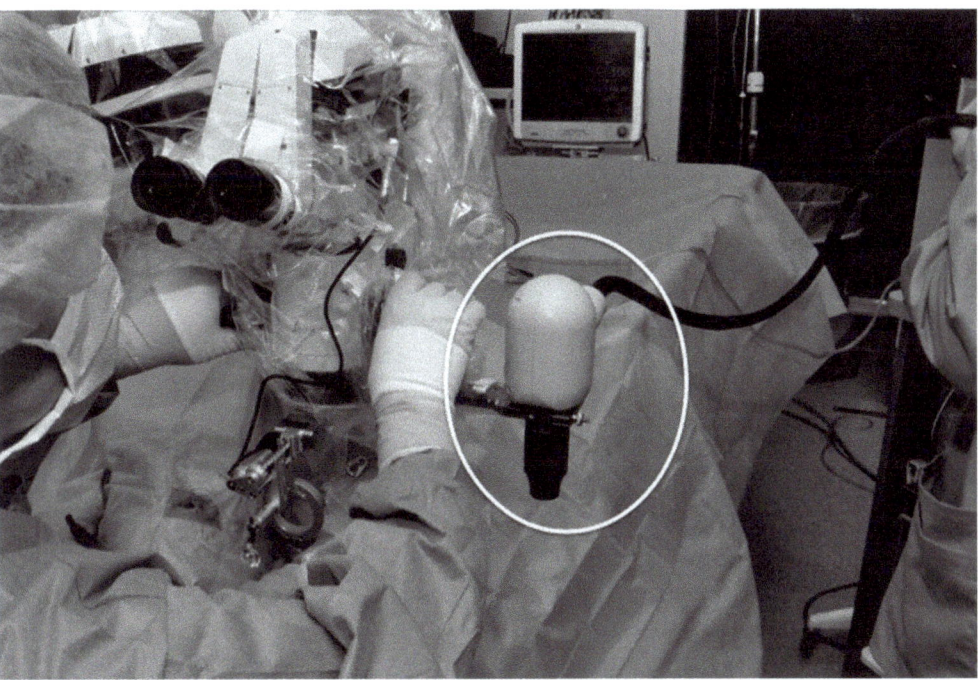

Figure 8. Intraoperative OCT with portable mounted microscope (circled) by Ehlers et al. [115]. Reprinted with permission from Ehlers et al. The Prospective Intraoperative and Perioperative Ophthalmic ImagiNg with Optical CoherEncE TomogRaphy (PIONEER) Study: 2-year results. *Am J Ophthalmol.* 2014 Nov; 158(5): 999–1007 with license permissions obtained from Elsevier and Copyright Clearance Center.

The Prospective Intraoperative and Perioperative Ophthalmic ImagiNg with Optical CoherEncE TomogRaphy (PIONEER) and Determination of Feasibility of Intraoperative Spectral Domain Microscope Combined/Integrated OCT Visualization During En Face

Retinal and Ophthalmic Surgery (DISCOVER) studies were started to investigate the utility of iOCT in various ophthalmic surgeries [115,116]. These studies included both anterior and posterior segment surgeries for preoperative diagnoses including epiretinal membrane, retinal detachment (Figure 9), vitreous hemorrhage, and vitreomacular traction [115]. Surgeries with iOCT included fluocinolone intravitreal implant and pars plana vitrectomy [115,116]. The DISCOVER study also included pars plana vitrectomy with combined iOCT and Ngenuity's digital heads-up, 3-dimensional visualization system (Ngenuity, Alcon, Fort Worth, TX, USA) [117]. This digital integration with iOCT allowed for the surgeon to view an overlay of the OCT data on top of the surgical field on a 4K high-definition monitor. The digital system allowed for the surgeons to review OCT data without turning away from the surgical field, and the surgeons reported excellent image visualization and contrast [117].

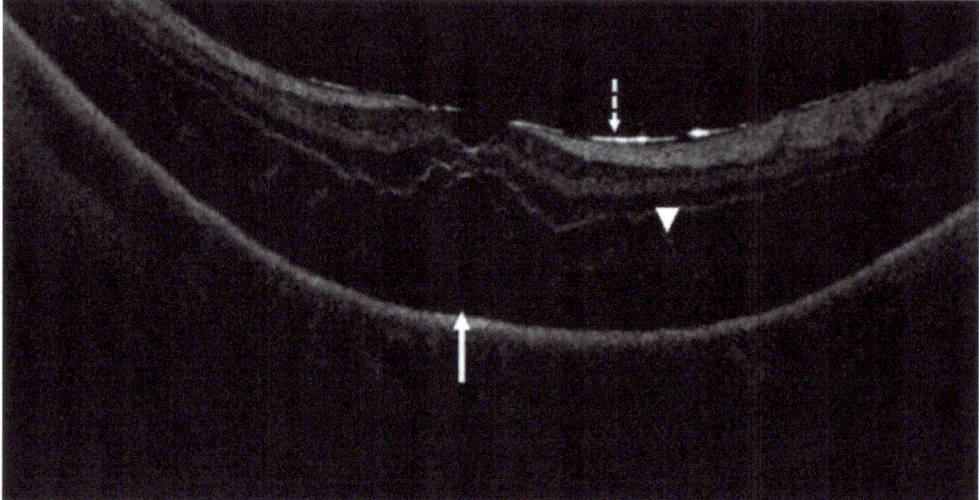

Figure 9. Retinal detachment visualized by intraoperative OCT. Dashed arrow shows hyperreflective retina and perfluorocarbon liquid interface, arrowhead shows outer retinal corrugations, and solid arrow shows persistent subretinal fluid. Reprinted with permission from Ehlers et al. [115]. The Prospective Intraoperative and Perioperative Ophthalmic ImagiNg with Optical CoherEncE Tomog-Raphy (PIONEER) Study: 2-year results. *Am J Ophthalmol.* 2014 Nov; 158(5): 999–1007 with license permissions obtained from Elsevier and Copyright Clearance Center.

Various systems have been developed and iOCT continues to be an area of high interest for optimizing surgical retinal care. Multiple iOCT options including hand-held portable probe, microscope mounted, and microscope integrated are available at present [118]. Microscope-integrated design helps to visualize the real-time vitreoretinal interface interaction with surgical instruments and corresponding changes intraoperatively. For instance, surgeons can assess intraoperative macular hole closure or identify remnants of epiretinal membrane during membrane peel. iOCT may also obviate the need to use dye staining during macular surgeries. iOCT may also facilitate the therapeutic delivery of drugs e.g., tissue plasminogen activator [119] or placement of electrodes array for subretinal implants [120]. Further research must be conducted to evaluate the widespread impact that iOCT has on vitreoretinal surgery [30].

10. At-Home OCT

Given the nature of certain retinal diseases (e.g., neovascular AMD), frequent monitoring via clinic visits and OCT imaging is required to ensure proper management [31]. These visits can often be burdensome, especially for the elderly population [121]. Notal

Vision Home OCT, an at-home SD-OCT, allows for daily self-imaging for patients at risk for worsening retinal disease. Studies that have evaluated this at-home, self-imaging OCT technology have reported good agreement on retina biomarkers with scans from in-clinic OCT [31,32,121]. Liu et al. reported a prospective, longitudinal study with 15 participants with this technology and observed a mean daily self-imaging rate of 80% (or 5.7 scans per week) [121]. The consistent, near-daily monitoring of retinal and choroidal diseases may allow for precise treatment planning. Artificial intelligence has also been developed with the Notal OCT Analyzer to automate the identification of intra- and subretinal fluid [31,122]. While this technology will continue to undergo testing and further research prior to widespread adoption, the ability to have OCT scans done near-daily at home may help to prevent vision loss for many in the future.

11. Conclusions

OCT technology continues to progress to address certain limitations observed in the current standards of care for choroidal and retinal diseases. In addition, these advances will help to advance basic science research and our understanding of the pathophysiology of chorioretinal diseases. As evidenced by technologies such as ultrawide-field OCT, these applications can help to detect and monitor retinal diseases with OCT capabilities at the periphery. As observed with full-field OCT, this innovation allows for analysis up to the individual human retinal ganglion cell axon. As seen with OCT advances in currently available technologies, such as intraoperative OCT, these innovations allow for further insight into the surgical management of chorioretinal disorders. At-home OCT demonstrates the ability to bring this powerful technology to the homes of at-risk individuals for a new frontier of retinal monitoring. As future research continues to develop, the goal is for emerging, clinically validated OCT technology to become more widely adopted. These technologies represent a promising future in optimizing the understanding, diagnosis, monitoring, and management of diseases in retina.

Author Contributions: Conceptualization, J.O., S.R.S. and J.C.; writing—original draft preparation, J.O., A.Z., G.C., S.R.S. and J.C.; writing—review and editing, J.O., A.Z., G.C., S.R.S. and J.C. All authors have read and agreed to the published version of the manuscript.

Funding: This paper received no external funding.

Conflicts of Interest: The authors declare no conflict of interest.

References

1. Huang, D.; Swanson, E.A.; Lin, C.P.; Schuman, J.S.; Stinson, W.G.; Chang, W.; Hee, M.R.; Flotte, T.; Gregory, K.; Puliafito, C.A.; et al. Optical coherence tomography. *Science* **1991**, *254*, 1178–1181. [CrossRef]
2. Stahl, A. The Diagnosis and Treatment of Age-Related Macular Degeneration. *Dtsch Arztebl Int.* **2020**, *117*, 513–520. [CrossRef]
3. Semeraro, F.; Morescalchi, F.; Russo, A.; Gambicorti, E.; Pilotto, A.; Parmeggiani, F.; Bartollino, S.; Costagliola, C. Central Serous Chorioretinopathy: Pathogenesis and Management. *Clin. Ophthalmol.* **2019**, *13*, 2341–2352. [CrossRef]
4. Boned-Murillo, A.; Albertos-Arranz, H.; Diaz-Barreda, M.D.; Orduna-Hospital, E.; Sánchez-Cano, A.; Ferreras, A.; Cuenca, N.; Pinilla, I. Optical Coherence Tomography Angiography in Diabetic Patients: A Systematic Review. *Biomedicines* **2021**, *10*, 88. [CrossRef]
5. Majumdar, S.; Tripathy, K. Macular Hole. In *StatPearls*; StatPearls: Treasure Island, FL, USA, 2022.
6. Metrangolo, C.; Donati, S.; Mazzola, M.; Fontanel, L.; Messina, W.; D'Alterio, G.; Rubino, M.; Radice, P.; Premi, E.; Azzolini, C. OCT Biomarkers in Neovascular Age-Related Macular Degeneration: A Narrative Review. *J. Ophthalmol.* **2021**, *2021*, 9994098. [CrossRef]
7. Dhurandhar, D.S.; Singh, S.R.; Sahoo, N.K.; Goud, A.; Lupidi, M.; Chhablani, J. Identifying central serous chorioretinopathy biomarkers in coexisting diabetic retinopathy: A multimodal imaging study. *Br. J. Ophthalmol.* **2020**, *104*, 904–909. [CrossRef]
8. Sahoo, N.K.; Ong, J.; Selvam, A.; Maltsev, D.; Sacconi, R.; Venkatesh, R.; Reddy, N.G.; Madan, S.; Tombolini, B.; Lima, L.H.; et al. Longitudinal follow-up and outcome analysis in central serous chorioretinopathy. *Eye* **2022**, 1–7. [CrossRef]
9. Corradetti, G.; Corvi, F.; Nittala, M.G.; Nassisi, M.; Alagorie, A.R.; Scharf, J.; Lee, M.Y.; Sadda, S.R.; Sarraf, D. Natural history of incomplete retinal pigment epithelial and outer retinal atrophy in age-related macular degeneration. *Can. J. Ophthalmol.* **2021**, *56*, 325–334. [CrossRef]

10. Nassisi, M.; Fan, W.; Shi, Y.; Lei, J.; Borrelli, E.; Ip, M.; Sadda, S.R. Quantity of Intraretinal Hyperreflective Foci in Patients With Intermediate Age-Related Macular Degeneration Correlates With 1-Year Progression. *Investig. Ophthalmol. Vis. Sci.* **2018**, *59*, 3431–3439. [CrossRef]
11. Lei, J.; Balasubramanian, S.; Abdelfattah, N.S.; Nittala, M.G.; Sadda, S.R. Proposal of a simple optical coherence tomography-based scoring system for progression of age-related macular degeneration. *Graefes Arch. Clin. Exp. Ophthalmol.* **2017**, *255*, 1551–1558. [CrossRef]
12. Nassisi, M.; Lei, J.; Abdelfattah, N.S.; Karamat, A.; Balasubramanian, S.; Fan, W.; Uji, A.; Marion, K.M.; Baker, K.; Huang, X.; et al. OCT Risk Factors for Development of Late Age-Related Macular Degeneration in the Fellow Eyes of Patients Enrolled in the HARBOR Study. *Ophthalmology* **2019**, *126*, 1667–1674. [CrossRef]
13. Gabriele, M.L.; Wollstein, G.; Ishikawa, H.; Kagemann, L.; Xu, J.; Folio, L.S.; Schuman, J.S. Optical coherence tomography: History, current status, and laboratory work. *Investig. Ophthalmol. Vis. Sci.* **2011**, *52*, 2425–2436. [CrossRef]
14. Aumann, S.; Donner, S.; Fischer, J.; Muller, F. Optical Coherence Tomography (OCT): Principle and Technical Realization. In *High Resolution Imaging in Microscopy and Ophthalmology: New Frontiers in Biomedical Optics*; Bille, J.F., Ed.; Springer Nature: Cham, Switzerland, 2019; pp. 59–85.
15. Ohno-Matsui, K.; Fang, Y.; Morohoshi, K.; Jonas, J.B. Optical Coherence Tomographic Imaging of Posterior Episclera and Tenon's Capsule. *Investig. Ophthalmol. Vis. Sci.* **2017**, *58*, 3389–3394. [CrossRef]
16. Zhang, Y.; Wang, Y.; Shi, C.; Shen, M.; Lu, F. Advances in retina imaging as potential biomarkers for early diagnosis of Alzheimer's disease. *Transl. Neurodegen.* **2021**, *10*, 6. [CrossRef]
17. Povazay, B.; Bizheva, K.; Unterhuber, A.; Hermann, B.; Sattmann, H.; Fercher, A.F.; Drexler, W.; Apolonski, A.; Wadsworth, W.J.; Knight, J.C.; et al. Submicrometer axial resolution optical coherence tomography. *Opt. Lett.* **2002**, *27*, 1800–1802. [CrossRef]
18. Zhang, T.; Kho, A.M.; Yiu, G.; Srinivasan, V.J. Visible Light Optical Coherence Tomography (OCT) Quantifies Subcellular Contributions to Outer Retinal Band 4. *Transl. Vis. Sci. Technol.* **2021**, *10*, 30. [CrossRef]
19. Miller, D.T.; Kocaoglu, O.P.; Wang, Q.; Lee, S. Adaptive optics and the eye (super resolution OCT). *Eye* **2011**, *25*, 321–330. [CrossRef]
20. Zawadzki, R.J.; Jones, S.M.; Olivier, S.S.; Zhao, M.; Bower, B.A.; Izatt, J.A.; Choi, S.; Laut, S.; Werner, J.S. Adaptive-optics optical coherence tomography for high-resolution and high-speed 3D retinal in vivo imaging. *Opt. Express* **2005**, *13*, 8532–8546. [CrossRef]
21. Sayegh, R.G.; Zotter, S.; Roberts, P.K.; Kandula, M.M.; Sacu, S.; Kreil, D.P.; Baumann, B.; Pircher, M.; Hitzenberger, C.K.; Schmidt-Erfurth, U. Polarization-Sensitive Optical Coherence Tomography and Conventional Retinal Imaging Strategies in Assessing Foveal Integrity in Geographic Atrophy. *Investig. Ophthalmol. Vis. Sci.* **2015**, *56*, 5246–5255. [CrossRef]
22. De Boer, J.F.; Hitzenberger, C.K.; Yasuno, Y. Polarization sensitive optical coherence tomography—A review [Invited]. *Biomed. Opt. Express* **2017**, *8*, 1838–1873. [CrossRef]
23. Imaging that Enlightens. Deeper insights into retinal structures with High-Resolution OCT. *Ophthalmologist.* 2020. Available online: https://theophthalmologist.com/subspecialties/imaging-that-enlightens (accessed on 1 August 2022).
24. Spaide, R.F.; Lally, D.R. High Resolution Spectral Domain Optical Coherence Tomography of Multiple Evanescent White Dot Syndrome. *Retin. Cases Brief Rep.* **2021**. [CrossRef]
25. Grieve, K.; Thouvenin, O.; Sengupta, A.; Borderie, V.M.; Paques, M. Appearance of the Retina With Full-Field Optical Coherence Tomography. *Investig. Ophthalmol. Vis. Sci.* **2016**, *57*, OCT96–OCT104. [CrossRef]
26. Mece, P.; Scholler, J.; Groux, K.; Boccara, C. High-resolution in-vivo human retinal imaging using full-field OCT with optical stabilization of axial motion. *Biomed. Opt. Express* **2020**, *11*, 492–504. [CrossRef]
27. Povazay, B.; Hermann, B.; Hofer, B.; Kajić, V.; Simpson, E.; Bridgford, T.; Drexler, W. Wide-field optical coherence tomography of the choroid in vivo. *Investig. Ophthalmol. Vis. Sci.* **2009**, *50*, 1856–1863. [CrossRef]
28. Takahashi, H.; Tanaka, N.; Shinohara, K.; Yokoi, T.; Yoshida, T.; Uramoto, K.; Ohno-Matsui, K. Ultra-Widefield Optical Coherence Tomographic Imaging of Posterior Vitreous in Eyes With High Myopia. *Am. J. Ophthalmol.* **2019**, *206*, 102–112. [CrossRef]
29. Ni, S.; Wei, X.; Ng, R.; Ostmo, S.; Chiang, M.F.; Huang, D.; Jia, Y.; Campbell, J.P.; Jian, Y. High-speed and widefield handheld swept-source OCT angiography with a VCSEL light source. *Biomed. Opt. Express* **2021**, *12*, 3553–3570. [CrossRef]
30. Ehlers, J.P.; Tao, Y.K.; Srivastava, S.K. The value of intraoperative optical coherence tomography imaging in vitreoretinal surgery. *Curr. Opin. Ophthalmol.* **2014**, *25*, 221–227. [CrossRef]
31. Nahen, K.; Benyamini, G.; Loewenstein, A. Evaluation of a Self-Imaging SD-OCT System for Remote Monitoring of Patients with Neovascular Age Related Macular Degeneration. *Klin. Mon. Für Augenheilkd.* **2020**, *237*, 1410–1418. [CrossRef]
32. Kim, J.E.; Tomkins-Netzer, O.; Elman, M.J.; Lally, D.R.; Goldstein, M.; Goldenberg, D.; Shulman, S.; Benyamini, G.; Loewenstein, A. Evaluation of a self-imaging SD-OCT system designed for remote home monitoring. *BMC Ophthalmol.* **2022**, *22*, 261. [CrossRef]
33. Shu, X.; Beckmann, L.; Zhang, H. Visible-light optical coherence tomography: A review. *J. Biomed Opt.* **2017**, *22*, 1–14. [CrossRef]
34. Yi, J.; Wei, Q.; Liu, W.; Backman, V.; Zhang, H.F. Visibl.le-light optical coherence tomography for retinal oximetry. *Opt. Lett.* **2013**, *38*, 1796–1798. [CrossRef]
35. Yi, J.; Liu, W.; Chen, S.; Backman, V.; Sheibani, N.; Sorenson, C.M.; Fawzi, A.A.; Linsenmeier, R.A.; Zhang, H.F. Visible light optical coherence tomography measures retinal oxygen metabolic response to systemic oxygenation. *Light Sci. Appl.* **2015**, *4*, e334. [CrossRef]

36. Rubinoff, I.; Miller, D.A.; Kuranov, R.; Wang, Y.; Fang, R.; Volpe, N.J.; Zhang, H.F. High-speed balanced-detection visible-light optical coherence tomography in the human retina using subpixel spectrometer calibration. *IEEE Trans. Med. Imaging* **2022**. [CrossRef]
37. Rubinoff, I.; Beckmann, L.; Wang, Y.; Fawzi, A.A.; Liu, X.; Tauber, J.; Jones, K.; Ishikawa, H.; Schuman, J.S.; Kuranov, R.; et al. Speckle reduction in visible-light optical coherence tomography using scan modulation. *Neurophotonics* **2019**, *6*, 041107. [CrossRef]
38. Pi, S.; Hormel, T.T.; Wei, X.; Cepurna, W.; Morrison, J.C.; Jia, Y. Imaging retinal structures at cellular-level resolution by visible-light optical coherence tomography. *Opt. Lett.* **2020**, *45*, 2107–2110. [CrossRef]
39. Zhang, T.; Kho, A.M.; Srinivasan, V.J. Morphometry of Inner Plexiform Layer (IPL) Stratification in the Human Retina With Visible Light Optical Coherence Tomography. *Front. Cell Neuro Sci.* **2021**, *15*, 655096. [CrossRef]
40. Zhang, T.; Kho, A.M.; Srinivasan, V.J. Water wavenumber calibration for visible light optical coherence tomography. *J. Biomed. Opt.* **2020**, *25*, 090501. [CrossRef]
41. Babcock, H.W. The possibility of compensating astronomical seeing. In *Publications of the Astronomical Society of the Pacific*, 386th ed.; The Astronomical Society of the Pacific: San Francisco, WI, USA, 1953; Volume 65, pp. 229–236.
42. Liang, J.; Williams, D.R.; Miller, D.T. Supernormal vision and high-resolution retinal imaging through adaptive optics. *J. Opt. Soc. Am. A Opt. Image Sci. Vis.* **1997**, *14*, 2884–2892. [CrossRef]
43. Roorda, A.; Romero-Borja, F.; Donnelly Iii, W.; Queener, H.; Hebert, T.; Campbell, M. Adaptive optics scanning laser ophthalmoscopy. *Opt. Express* **2002**, *10*, 405–412. [CrossRef]
44. Akyol, E.; Hagag, A.M.; Sivaprasad, S.; Lotery, A.J. Adaptive optics: Principles and applications in ophthalmology. *Eye* **2021**, *35*, 244–264. [CrossRef]
45. Jonnal, R.S.; Kocaoglu, O.P.; Zawadzki, R.J.; Liu, Z.; Miller, D.T.; Werner, J.S. A Review of Adaptive Optics Optical Coherence Tomography: Technical Advances, Scientific Applications, and the Future. *Investig. Ophthalmol. Vis. Sci.* **2016**, *57*, OCT51-68. [CrossRef]
46. Roorda, A.; Williams, D.R. The arrangement of the three cone classes in the living human eye. *Nature* **1999**, *397*, 520–522. [CrossRef]
47. Kadomoto, S.; Muraoka, Y.; Uji, A.; Ooto, S.; Kawai, K.; Ishikura, M.; Nishigori, N.; Akagi, T.; Tsujikawa, A. Human Foveal Cone and Müller Cells Examined by Adaptive Optics Optical Coherence Tomography. *Transl. Vis. Sci. Technol.* **2021**, *10*, 17. [CrossRef]
48. Fernández, E.; Drexler, W. Influence of ocular chromatic aberration and pupil size on transverse resolution in ophthalmic adaptive optics optical coherence tomography. *Opt. Express* **2005**, *13*, 8184–8197. [CrossRef]
49. Shirazi, M.F.; Brunner, E.; Laslandes, M.; Pollreisz, A.; Hitzenberger, C.K.; Pircher, M. Visualizing human photoreceptor and retinal pigment epithelium cell mosaics in a single volume scan over an extended field of view with adaptive optics optical coherence tomography. *Biomed. Opt. Express* **2020**, *11*, 4520–4535. [CrossRef]
50. Liu, Z.; Kurokawa, K.; Zhang, F.; Lee, J.J.; Miller, D.T. Imaging and quantifying ganglion cells and other transparent neurons in the living human retina. *Proc. Natl. Acad. Sci. USA* **2017**, *114*, 12803–12808. [CrossRef]
51. Adie, S.G.; Graf, B.W.; Ahmad, A.; Carney, P.S.; Boppart, S.A. Computational adaptive optics for broadband optical interferometric tomography of biological tissue. *Proc. Natl. Acad. Sci. USA* **2012**, *109*, 7175–7180. [CrossRef]
52. Ralston, T.S.; Marks, D.L.; Carney, P.S.; Boppart, S.A. Interferometric synthetic aperture microscopy. *Nat. Phys.* **2007**, *3*, 129–134. [CrossRef]
53. Lee, B.; Lee, J.; Jeong, S.; Kang, W.; Oh, W.-Y. Video-rate computational adaptive optics optical coherence tomography with a stretched-pulse mode-locked laser. In *European Conference on Biomedical Optics*; Optical Society of America: Washington, DC, USA, 2021.
54. Wang, J.; Chaney, E.J.; Aksamitiene, E.; Marjanovic, M.; Boppart, S.A. Computational adaptive optics for polarization-sensitive optical coherence tomography. *Opt. Lett.* **2021**, *46*, 2071–2074. [CrossRef]
55. Ruiz-Lopera, S.; Restrepo, R.; Cuartas-Vélez, C.; Bouma, B.E.; Uribe-Patarroyo, N. Computational adaptive optics in phase-unstable optical coherence tomography. *Opt. Lett.* **2020**, *45*, 5982–5985. [CrossRef]
56. Liu, L.; Wu, Z.; Qi, M.; Li, Y.; Zhang, M.; Liao, D.; Gao, P. Application of Adaptive Optics in Ophthalmology. *Photonics* **2022**, *9*, 288. [CrossRef]
57. Camino, A.; Ng, R.; Huang, J.; Guo, Y.; Ni, S.; Jia, Y.; Huang, D.; Jian, Y. Depth-resolved optimization of a real-time sensorless adaptive optics optical coherence tomography. *Opt. Lett.* **2020**, *45*, 2612–2615. [CrossRef]
58. Zhu, D.; Wang, R.; Žurauskas, M.; Pande, P.; Bi, J.; Yuan, Q.; Wang, L.; Gao, Z.; Boppart, S.A. Automated fast computational adaptive optics for optical coherence tomography based on a stochastic parallel gradient descent algorithm. *Opt. Express* **2020**, *28*, 23306–23319. [CrossRef]
59. Hofer, H.; Sredar, N.; Queener, H.; Li, C.; Porter, J. Wavefront sensorless adaptive optics ophthalmoscopy in the human eye. *Opt. Express* **2011**, *19*, 14160–14171. [CrossRef]
60. Durech, E.; Newberry, W.; Franke, J.; Sarunic, M.V. Wavefront sensor-less adaptive optics using deep reinforcement learning. *Biomed. Opt. Express* **2021**, *12*, 5423–5438. [CrossRef]
61. Iyer, R.R.; Sorrells, J.E.; Yang, L.; Chaney, E.J.; Spillman, D.R.; Tibble, B.E.; Renteria, C.A.; Tu, H.; Žurauskas, M.; Marjanovic, M.; et al. Label-free metabolic and structural profiling of dynamic biological samples using multimodal optical microscopy with sensorless adaptive optics. *Sci. Rep.* **2022**, *12*, 3438. [CrossRef]
62. Pircher, M.; Zawadzki, R.J. Review of adaptive optics OCT (AO-OCT): Principles and applications for retinal imaging [Invited]. *Biomed. Opt. Express* **2017**, *8*, 2536–2562. [CrossRef]

63. Hee, M.R.; Huang, D.; Swanson, E.A.; Fujimoto, J.G. Polarization-sensitive low-coherence reflectometer for birefringence characterization and ranging. *JOSA B* **1992**, *9*, 903–908. [CrossRef]
64. Pircher, M.; Hitzenberger, C.K.; Schmidt-Erfurth, U. Polarization sensitive optical coherence tomography in the human eye. *Prog. Retin. Eye Res.* **2011**, *30*, 431–451. [CrossRef]
65. Ueno, Y.; Mori, H.; Kikuchi, K.; Yamanari, M.; Oshika, T. Visualization of Anterior Chamber Angle Structures With Scattering- and Polarization-Sensitive Anterior Segment Optical Coherence Tomography. *Transl. Vis. Sci. Technol.* **2021**, *10*, 29. [CrossRef]
66. Baumann, B.; Gotzinger, E.; Pircher, M.; Sattmann, H.; Schuutze, C.; Schlanitz, F.; Ahlers, C.; Schmidt-Erfurth, U.; Hitzenberger, C.K. Segmentation and quantification of retinal lesions in age-related macular degeneration using polarization-sensitive optical coherence tomography. *J. Biomed. Opt.* **2010**, *15*, 061704. [CrossRef]
67. Sharma, S.; Hartl, G.; Naveed, S.K.; Blessing, K.; Sharma, G.; Singh, K. Input polarization-independent polarization-sensitive optical coherence tomography using a depolarizer. *Rev. Sci. Instrum.* **2020**, *91*, 043706. [CrossRef]
68. Tang, P.; Wang, R. Stable fiber-based polarization-sensitive optical coherence tomography using polarization maintaining common-path interferometer. *J. Biomed. Opt.* **2020**, *25*, 116009. [CrossRef]
69. Abouraddy, A.F.; Nasr, M.B.; Saleh, B.E.A.; Sergienko, A.V.; Teich, M.C. *Quantum-Optical Coherence Tomography with Dispersion Cancellation*; American Physical Society: College Park, MD, USA, 2002.
70. Booth, M.C.; Di Giuseppe, G.; Saleh, B.E.A.; Sergienko, A.V.; Teich, M.C. Polarization-sensitive quantum-optical coherence tomography. *Phys. Rev. A* **2004**, *69*, 043815. [CrossRef]
71. Sukharenko, V.; Bikorimana, S.; Dorsinville, R. Birefringence and scattering characterization using polarization sensitive quantum optical coherence tomography. *Opt. Lett.* **2021**, *46*, 2799–2802. [CrossRef]
72. Schutze, C.; Teleky, K.; Baumann, B.; Pircher, M.; Gotzinger, E.; Hitzenberger, C.K.; Schmidt-Erfurth, U. Polarisation-sensitive OCT is useful for evaluating retinal pigment epithelial lesions in patients with neovascular AMD. *Br. J. Ophthalmol.* **2016**, *100*, 371–377. [CrossRef]
73. Schranz, M.; Roberts, P.K.; Motschi, A.R.; Hollaus, M.; Mylonas, G.; Sacu, S.; Pircher, M.; Hitzenberger, C.K.; Schmidt-Erfurth, U. Tracking of fibrosis growth in neovascular age related macular degeneration. *Investig. Ophthalmol. Vis. Sci.* **2022**, *63*, 1025–F0272.
74. Lejoyeux, R.; Benillouche, J.; Ong, J.; Errera, M.H.; Rossi, E.A.; Singh, S.R.; Dansingani, K.K.; da Silva, S.; Sinha, D.; Sahel, J.A.; et al. Choriocapillaris: Fundamentals and advancements. *Prog. Retin. Eye Res.* **2022**, *87*, 100997. [CrossRef]
75. Scholler, J.; Mazlin, V.; Thouvenin, O.; Groux, K.; Xiao, P.; Sahel, J.A.; Fink, M.; Boccara, C.; Grieve, K. Probing dynamic processes in the eye at multiple spatial and temporal scales with multimodal full field OCT. *Biomed. Opt. Express* **2019**, *10*, 731–746. [CrossRef]
76. Apelian, C.; Harms, F.; Thouvenin, O.; Boccara, A.C. Dynamic full field optical coherence tomography: Subcellular metabolic contrast revealed in tissues by interferometric signals temporal analysis. *Biomed. Opt. Express* **2016**, *7*, 1511–1524. [CrossRef]
77. Thouvenin, O.; Fink, M.; Boccara, C. Dynamic multimodal full-field optical coherence tomography and fluorescence structured illumination microscopy. *J. Biomed. Opt.* **2017**, *22*, 26004. [CrossRef]
78. Singh, R.; Cuzzani, O.; Binette, F.; Sternberg, H.; West, M.D.; Nasonkin, I.O. Pluripotent Stem Cells for Retinal Tissue Engineering: Current Status and Future Prospects. *Stem Cell Rev. Rep.* **2018**, *14*, 463–483. [CrossRef]
79. Ahmad, I.; Teotia, P.; Erickson, H.; Xia, X. Recapitulating developmental mechanisms for retinal regeneration. *Prog. Retin. Eye Res.* **2020**, *76*, 100824. [CrossRef]
80. Wright, L.S.; Pinilla, I.; Saha, J.; Clermont, J.M.; Lien, J.S.; Borys, K.D.; Capowski, E.E.; Phillips, M.J.; Gamm, D.M. VSX2 and ASCL1 Are Indicators of Neurogenic Competence in Human Retinal Progenitor Cultures. *PLoS ONE* **2015**, *10*, e0135830. [CrossRef] [PubMed]
81. Scholler, J.; Groux, K.; Goureau, O.; Sahel, J.A.; Fink, M.; Reichman, S.; Boccara, C.; Grieve, K. Dynamic full-field optical coherence tomography: 3D live-imaging of retinal organoids. *Light Sci. Appl.* **2020**, *9*, 140. [CrossRef] [PubMed]
82. Groux, K.; Verschueren, A.; Nanteau, C.; Clémençon, M.; Fink, M.; Sahel, J.A.; Boccara, C.; Paques, M.; Reichman, S.; Grieve, K. Dynamic full-field optical coherence tomography allows live imaging of retinal pigment epithelium stress model. *Commun. Biol.* **2022**, *5*, 575. [CrossRef] [PubMed]
83. Song, S.; Xu, J.; Wang, R.K. Long-range and wide field of view optical coherence tomography for in vivo 3D imaging of large volume object based on akinetic programmable swept source. *Biomed. Opt. Express* **2016**, *7*, 4734–4748. [CrossRef]
84. Pomerantzeff, O. Equator-plus camera. *Investig. Ophthalmol.* **1975**, *14*, 401–406.
85. Neubauer, A.S.; Yu, A.; Haritoglou, C.; Ulbig, M.W. Peripheral retinal changes in acute retinal necrosis imaged by ultra widefield scanning laser ophthalmoscopy. *Acta Ophthalmol. Scand.* **2005**, *83*, 758–760. [CrossRef]
86. Choudhry, N.; Golding, J.; Manry, M.W.; Rao, R.C. Ultra-Widefield Steering-Based Spectral-Domain Optical Coherence Tomography Imaging of the Retinal Periphery. *Ophthalmology* **2016**, *123*, 1368–1374. [CrossRef]
87. Everett, M.; Magazzeni, S.; Schmoll, T.; Kempe, M. Optical coherence tomography: From technology to applications in ophthalmology. *Transl. Biophotonics* **2021**, *3*, e202000012. [CrossRef]
88. Klein, T.; Wieser, W.; Eigenwillig, C.M.; Biedermann, B.R.; Huber, R. Megahertz OCT for ultrawide-field retinal imaging with a 1050 nm Fourier domain mode-locked laser. *Opt. Express* **2011**, *19*, 3044–3062. [CrossRef] [PubMed]
89. Gresores, N.J.; Singer, M.; Cairns, A.M.; Sinai, M.J.; Sadda, S.R. Evaluation of a Combined Ultra-wide Field SLO with SD OCT. *Investig. Ophthalmol.* **2018**, *59*, 664.

90. NIDEK Co., L. NIDEK Launches the Mirante SLO Model. Available online: https://www.nidek-intl.com/news-event/news/entry-4046.html (accessed on 1 August 2022).
91. NIDEK. *Scanning Laser Ophthalmoscope Mirante SLO/OCT Mirante SLO*; NIDEK: Gamagori, Japan, 2022.
92. SPECTRALIS Inc., H.E. Available online: https://business-lounge.heidelbergengineering.com/us/en/products/spectralis/spectralis/ (accessed on 1 August 2022).
93. Choudhry, N.; Sodhi, S. Peripheral OCT Imaging in Practice. *Retina Today*. 2021. Available online: https://retinatoday.com/articles/2021-apr/peripheral-oct-imaging-in-practice (accessed on 1 August 2022).
94. Optos. Silverstone. Optos Products. 2022. Available online: https://www.Opt.os.com/products/silverstone/ (accessed on 1 August 2022).
95. Optos. Monaco. Optos Products. 2022. Available online: https://www.Opt.os.com/products/Monaco/ (accessed on 1 August 2022).
96. Sodhi, S.K.; Golding, J.; Trimboli, C.; Choudhry, N. Feasibility of peripheral OCT imaging using a novel integrated SLO ultra-widefield imaging swept-source OCT device. *Int. Ophthalmol.* **2021**, *41*, 2805–2815. [CrossRef] [PubMed]
97. Uji, A.; Yoshimura, N. Application of extended field imaging to optical coherence tomography. *Ophthalmology* **2015**, *122*, 1272–1274. [CrossRef]
98. Mishra, D.K.; Shanmugam, M.P.; Ramanjulu, R.; Sagar, P. Comparison of standard and "innovative wide-field" optical coherence tomography images in assessment of vitreoretinal interface in proliferative diabetic retinopathy: A pilot study. *Indian J. Ophthalmol.* **2021**, *69*, 99–102. [CrossRef]
99. Mori, K.; Kanno, J.; Gehlbach, P.L. Retinochoroidal Morphology Described by Wide-Field Montage Imaging of Spectral Domain Optical Coherence Tomography. *Retina* **2016**, *36*, 375–384. [CrossRef]
100. De Pretto, L.R.; Moult, E.M.; Alibhai, A.Y.; Carrasco-Zevallos, O.M.; Chen, S.; Lee, B.; Witkin, A.J.; Baumal, C.R.; Reichel, E.; de Freitas, A.Z.; et al. Controlling for Artifacts in Widefield Optical Coherence Tomography Angiography Measurements of Non-Perfusion Area. *Sci. Rep.* **2019**, *9*, 9096. [CrossRef]
101. Ong, J.; Hariprasad, S.M.; Chhablani, J. A Guide to Accessible Artificial Intelligence and Machine Learning for the 21st Century Retina Specialist. *Ophthalmic Surg. Lasers Imaging Retin.* **2021**, *52*, 361–365. [CrossRef]
102. Rakocz, N.; Chiang, J.N.; Nittala, M.G.; Corradetti, G.; Tiosano, L.; Velaga, S.; Thompson, M.; Hill, B.L.; Sankararaman, S.; Haines, J.L.; et al. Automated identification of clinical features from sparsely annotated 3-dimensional medical imaging. *NPJ Digit. Med.* **2021**, *4*, 44. [CrossRef]
103. Zhang, G.; Fu, D.J.; Liefers, B.; Faes, L.; Glinton, S.; Wagner, S.; Struyven, R.; Pontikos, N.; Keane, P.A.; Balaskas, K. Clinically relevant deep learning for detection and quantification of geographic atrophy from optical coherence tomography: A model development and external validation study. *Lancet Digit. Health* **2021**, *3*, e665–e675. [CrossRef]
104. Kolb, J.P.; Klein, T.; Kufner, C.L.; Wieser, W.; Neubauer, A.S.; Huber, R. Ultra-widefield retinal MHz-OCT imaging with up to 100 degrees viewing angle. *Biomed. Opt. Express* **2015**, *6*, 1534–1552. [CrossRef] [PubMed]
105. Song, G.; Chu, K.K.; Kim, S.; Crose, M.; Cox, B.; Jelly, E.T.; Ulrich, J.N.; Wax, A. First Clinical Application of Low-Cost OCT. *Transl. Vis. Sci. Technol.* **2019**, *8*, 61. [CrossRef] [PubMed]
106. Jung, W.; Kim, J.; Jeon, M.; Chaney, E.J.; Stewart, C.N.; Boppart, S.A. Handheld optical coherence tomography scanner for primary care diagnostics. *IEEE Trans. Biomed. Eng.* **2011**, *58*, 741–744. [CrossRef]
107. Rufai, S.R. Handheld optical coherence tomography removes barriers to imaging the eyes of young children. *Eye* **2022**, *36*, 907–908. [CrossRef]
108. Nicholson, R.; Osborne, D.; Fairhead, L.; Beed, L.; Hill, C.M.; Lee, H. Segmentation of the foveal and parafoveal retinal architecture using handheld spectral-domain optical coherence tomography in children with Down syndrome. *Eye* **2022**, *36*, 963–968. [CrossRef]
109. Maldonado, R.S.; Izatt, J.A.; Sarin, N.; Wallace, D.K.; Freedman, S.; Cotten, C.M.; Toth, C.A. Optimizing hand-held spectral domain optical coherence tomography imaging for neonates, infants, and children. *Investig. Ophthalmol. Vis. Sci.* **2010**, *51*, 2678–2685. [CrossRef]
110. Malone, J.D.; El-Haddad, M.T.; Yerramreddy, S.S.; Oguz, I.; Tao, Y.K. Handheld spectrally encoded coherence tomography and reflectometry for motion-corrected ophthalmic optical coherence tomography and optical coherence tomography angiography. *Neurophotonics* **2019**, *6*, 041102. [CrossRef]
111. Chopra, R.; Wagner, S.K.; Keane, P.A. Optical coherence tomography in the 2020s-outside the eye clinic. *Eye* **2021**, *35*, 236–243. [CrossRef]
112. Wang, K.L.; Chen, X.; Stinnett, S.; Tai, V.; Winter, K.P.; Tran-Viet, D.; Toth, C.A. Understanding the variability of handheld spectral-domain optical coherence tomography measurements in supine infants. *PLoS ONE* **2019**, *14*, e0225960. [CrossRef]
113. Kanyo, E.; Knapp, A.; Ehlers, J.P. The Emerging Role of Intraoperative OCT for Retinal Surgery. *Retinal Phys.* 2021. Available online: https://www.retinalphysician.com/issues/2021/november-december-2021/the-emerging-role-of-intraoperative-oct-for-retina (accessed on 1 August 2022).
114. Dayani, P.N.; Maldonado, R.; Farsiu, S.; Toth, C.A. Intraoperative use of handheld spectral domain optical coherence tomography imaging in macular surgery. *Retina* **2009**, *29*, 1457–1468. [CrossRef] [PubMed]
115. Ehlers, J.P.; Dupps, W.J.; Kaiser, P.K.; Goshe, J.; Singh, R.P.; Petkovsek, D.; Srivastava, S.K. The Prospective Intraoperative and Perioperative Ophthalmic ImagiNg with Optical CoherEncE TomogRaphy (PIONEER) Study: 2-year results. *Am. J. Ophthalmol.* **2014**, *158*, 999–1007. [CrossRef] [PubMed]

116. Ehlers, J.P.; Modi, Y.S.; Pecen, P.E.; Goshe, J.; Dupps, W.J.; Rachitskaya, A.; Sharma, S.; Yuan, A.; Singh, R.; Kaiser, P.K.; et al. The DISCOVER Study 3-Year Results: Feasibility and Usefulness of Microscope-Integrated Intraoperative OCT during Ophthalmic Surgery. *Ophthalmology* **2018**, *125*, 1014–1027. [CrossRef]
117. Ehlers, J.P.; Uchida, A.; Srivastava, S.K. The Integrative Surgical Theater: Combining Intraoperative Optical Coherence Tomography and 3D Digital Visualization for Vitreoretinal Surgery in the DISCOVER Study. *Retina* **2018**, *38* (Suppl. 1), S88–S96. [CrossRef] [PubMed]
118. Ray, R.; Baranano, D.E.; Fortun, J.A.; Schwent, B.J.; Cribbs, B.E.; Bergstrom, C.S.; Hubbard, G.B., 3rd; Srivastava, S.K. Intraoperative microscope-mounted spectral domain optical coherence tomography for evaluation of retinal anatomy during macular surgery. *Ophthalmology* **2011**, *118*, 2212–2217. [CrossRef]
119. Ehlers, J.P.; Petkovsek, D.S.; Yuan, A.; Singh, R.P.; Srivastava, S.K. Intrasurgical assessment of subretinal tPA injection for submacular hemorrhage in the PIONEER study utilizing intraoperative OCT. *Ophthalmic Surg. Lasers Imaging Retin.* **2015**, *46*, 327–332. [CrossRef]
120. Grewal, D.S.; Carrasco-Zevallos, O.M.; Gunther, R.; Izatt, J.A.; Toth, C.A.; Hahn, P. Intra-operative microscope-integrated swept-source optical coherence tomography guided placement of Argus II retinal prosthesis. *Acta Ophthalmol.* **2017**, *95*, e431–e432. [CrossRef]
121. Liu, Y.; Holekamp, N.M.; Heier, J.S. Prospective, Longitudinal Study: Daily Self-Imaging with Home OCT for Neovascular Age-Related Macular Degeneration. *Ophthalmol. Retin.* **2022**. [CrossRef]
122. Chakravarthy, U.; Goldenberg, D.; Young, G.; Havilio, M.; Rafaeli, O.; Benyamini, G.; Loewenstein, A. Automated Identification of Lesion Activity in Neovascular Age-Related Macular Degeneration. *Ophthalmology* **2016**, *123*, 1731–1736. [CrossRef]

MDPI
St. Alban-Anlage 66
4052 Basel
Switzerland
www.mdpi.com

Journal of Clinical Medicine Editorial Office
E-mail: jcm@mdpi.com
www.mdpi.com/journal/jcm

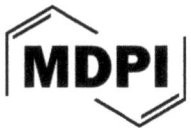

Disclaimer/Publisher's Note: The statements, opinions and data contained in all publications are solely those of the individual author(s) and contributor(s) and not of MDPI and/or the editor(s). MDPI and/or the editor(s) disclaim responsibility for any injury to people or property resulting from any ideas, methods, instructions or products referred to in the content.